AUTOIMMUNITY: ROLE, REGULATION AND DISORDERS

AUTOIMMUNITY: ROLE, REGULATION AND DISORDERS

FYNN L. VOGEL AND
LUCAS F. ZIMMERMAN
EDITORS

Nova Biomedical Books
New York

For permission to use material from this book please contact us:
Telephone 631-231-7269; Fax 631-231-8175
Web Site: http://www.novapublishers.com

Library of Congress Cataloging-in-Publication Data

Autoimmunity : role, regulation, and disorders / Fynn L. Vogel and Lucas F. Zimmermann (editors).
p. ; cm.
Includes bibliographical references and index.
ISBN 978-1-60456-833-2 (hardcover : alk. paper)
1. Autoimmunity. 2. Autoimmune diseases. I. Vogel, Fynn L. II. Zimmermann, Lucas F.
[DNLM: 1. Autoimmune Diseases. 2. Autoimmunity. WD 305 A93973 2008]
QR188.3A9845 2008
616.97'8--dc22

2008023151

Published by Nova Science Publishers, Inc. ✝ New York

Contents

Preface vii

Chapter 1 Benefits from Genome-Wide Association Studies: Identification of New Susceptibility Genes for Type 1 Diabetes **1**
Dimitry A. Chistiakov and Natalia V. Voronova

Chapter 2 Subclinical Atherosclerosis in Patients with Rheumatoid and Psoriatic Arthritis **57**
Elisabetta Profumo, Brigitta Buttari, Maria Elena Tosti, Rossana Scrivo, Antonio Spadaro, Chiara Tesori, Manuela Di Franco and Rachele Riganò

Chapter 3 Exogenous Nucleic Acids Contribute to Joint Inflammation in Rheumatoid Arthritis by Activating an Anti-Viral Interferon Response **69**
Mattias Magnusson and Andrej Tarkowski

Chapter 4 Antigenic Complementarity in the Induction of Autoimmunity: A Review **75**
Robert Root-Bernstein

Chapter 5 Autoimmune Initiation of Multiple Sclerosis: Molecular Aspects **113**
Fred C. Westall

Chapter 6 Potential Role of an Abnormal Proliferative, Reparative Response in Initiation and Maintenance of Sjögren's Syndrome, and the Beneficial Effects of Green Tea Polyphenols **149**
Douglas Dickinson, Kevin Gillespie, Isamu Kodani, Amy Camba and Stephen Hsu

Chapter 7	Coxsackievirus B3 Induced Autoimmune Heart Disease: Role of the Innate Immune Response in Controlling Autoimmunity *S. A. Huber and Jessica Schwartz*	**167**
Chapter 8	Innate Autoimmunity:Basic Mechanisms and Clinical Association *Maria Ramos and Ming Zhang*	**187**
Chapter 9	MHC-Anti MHC-Receptor Interactions Regulate Autoimmune Reactivity *Bent Rubin*	**199**
Chapter 10	Thyroid, Autoimmunity and Pregnancy *Roberto Negro*	**233**
Chapter 11	Autoantibody Profiles of an Asbestos-Exposed Population *Jean C. Pfau, David J. Blake and Marvin J. Fritzler*	**245**
Chapter 12	Shared Variable Domain Elements among Anti-Collagen Antibodies Reactive with Goodpasture Epitopes *Faustina N. Sackey, Kendra L. Congdon, Graham F. Brady, Helmut Hopfer, Ying Zhang, Katherine M. Mackin Amy G. Clark and Mary H. Foster*	**269**
Index		**283**

Preface

Autoimmunity is the failure of an organism to recognize its own constituent parts (down to the sub-molecular levels) as self, which results in an immune response against its own cells and tissues. Any disease that results from such an aberrant immune response is termed an autoimmune disease such as the disease multiple sclerosis or heart disease. This book provides new and important research on several autoimmune disorders and their processes.

Chapter 1 - With the relative failing of linkage and candidate gene association studies, there had been much sceptism about the ability of geneticists to identify genes for common, complex disorders. Vast amounts of resources were poured into these studies, with very limited success. In the field of genetics of type 1 diabetes (T1D), over more then twenty years of labor-intensive and cost-expensive efforts resulted in the identification only four causal loci predisposing to T1D as follows Human Leucocyte Antigens (HLA) class II, insulin gene region, cytotoxic T-lymphocyte associated 4 (CTLA-4), and protein tyrosine phosphatase, non-receptor member 22 (PTPN22). Recent technological advances, and a better understanding of the genetic architecture of complex diseases, has led to the development of the genome-wide association (GWA) study, which is a powerful new approach to identifying genes influencing predisposition to common, complex disease. For T1D, the implication of the GWA approach in 2005 resulted in rapid progress in discovery of new etiological variants. To date, the involvement to T1D pathogenesis is proven for several new genes such as interleukin 2 receptor alpha (IL2RA/CD25), interferon-induced helicase domain 1 (IFIH1), and small ubiquitin-related modifier 4 (SUMO4). An extended list of likely candidates for T1D susceptibility identified through the GWA approach includes protein-tyrosine phosphatase 2 (PTPN2), CD226 antigen, peroxisomal proliferator-activated receptor gamma (PPARG2), interleukin-2/interleukin-21 (IL2/IL21), disintegrin and metalloprotease 33 (ADAM33), and some other genes. For those, preliminary genetic findings should be supported by strong confirmations in other large-scale population GWA studies and functional analyses to find true causal variants. As a type of genetic research, GWA approach is still in its infancy. However, a great benefit to clinical medicine is expected in the years to come, and whilst prediction of disease and pharmacogenetics may eventually prove valuable, the greatest clinical benefit of GWA studies is likely to come from etiological insights into disease processes.

Chapter 2 - Accelerated development of atherosclerosis has been observed in patients with rheumatic diseases such as rheumatoid arthritis (RA) and psoriatic arthritis (PsA). It may be related to the inflammatory overload accompanied to the combination of an excessive production of reactive oxygen species with an impaired antioxidant defence capacity, leading to oxidative stress that may facilitate the development and progression of atherosclerosis. Compared with the general population, patients with RA die prematurely, mainly because of cardiovascular diseases but the mechanism by which premature atherosclerosis develops in RA is unknown. Recent data have demonstrated the prevalence of atherosclerosis also in patients with PsA, a chronic inflammatory autoimmune disease characterized by inflammatory arthritis and skin psoriasis. PsA shares some phenotypic characteristics with RA, even though the synovial inflammation of PsA is characterized by less macrophage infiltration and increased vascularity in comparison to RA inflammation. The increased cardiovascular risk in PsA and RA suggests the need to treat the inflammatory process and to monitor traditional atherosclerotic risk factors in these pathologies.

The aim of our study was to evaluate whether increased oxidative stress may be associated to the presence of subclinical atherosclerosis in patients with RA and in patients with PsA. For this purpose we determined the levels of oxidized low density lipoproteins (ox-LDL) and of nitric oxide (NO) in the sera obtained from 19 patients with RA, 20 with PsA and 20 sex- and age-matched healthy controls. Patients with RA fulfilled the American College of Rheumatology criteria, and patients with PsA fulfilled the CASPAR criteria. In all patients we evaluated the activity and duration of the disease and classical risk factors for atherosclerosis. Our results showed higher levels of ox-LDL and lower levels of NO in sera from patients with RA and PsA than in sera from healthy controls. Notably, higher serum levels of ox-LDL were observed in patients with an intima-media thickness (IMT) >1 than in those with an IMT ≤ 1, and higher serum levels of NO in patients with an IMT ≤ 1 than in those with an IMT >1, in patients with RA and PsA. Our data suggest that monitoring circulating levels of ox-LDL and NO in patients with RA and PsA could give information on the development of atherosclerotic disease and therefore could be useful to the clinical management of patients.

Chapter 3 - Viral infections may give rise to both transient arthralgias and chronic arthritides. In addition, flares in RA have been suggested to be precipitated during viral infection. Double-stranded RNA is expressed by most viruses and is one of the strongest activators of innate anti-viral immunity. In apparent absence of ongoing viral infection, such dsRNA is found at significantly higher levels in sera and synovial fluids of RA patients than in a control population of osteoarthritis patients. This dsRNA in the joint may well be pathogenic because intra-articular injection of viral dsRNA, but not eukaryotic-like ssRNA, is highly arthritogenic. The mechanisms by which dsRNA triggers inflammation potentially include the dsRNA receptors PKR, TLR3, RIG and/or MDA5, whose activation results in production of proinflammatory cytokines. The ability of dsRNA to induce experimental arthritis in mice is, however, not dependent on PKR or TLR3, because mice devoid of these receptors develop arthritis to the same extent as wt mice, indicating that other receptors including RIG and MDA-5 may be involved. Common for activation of all these signaling pathways is that they can culminate in production of type I IFN. Production of type I IFN is the immediate, anti-viral immune response upon viral infection that prevents and halts further viral replication. Mice unable to respond to type I IFN (IFNAR -/-) are completely protected against dsRNA-induced arthritis and injection of type I IFN intra-articularly into the knee of healthy mice results in a pronounced, but transient joint inflammation. Thus, if the immune response to a viral infection results in accumulation of type I IFN or deposition of dsRNA in the joint, then this defence may be directly harmful for the host by causing arthritis.

Chapter 4 - The causes of human autoimmune diseases remain a mystery. The reason may be that current theories based on molecular mimicry are overly simplistic, relying on single agent etiologies that do not explain how immune tolerance is broken. This essay presents a novel theory of autoimmunity based on evidence that autoimmune diseases result from concomitant exposure to multiple antigens that induce molecularly complementary immune responses. As in a normal immune response, each antigen induces a complementary antibody or T-cell response, but because the antigens are molecularly complementary, the resulting antibodies or T cells are also molecularly complementary. Antibodies or T cells against each antigen therefore mimic the structure of the other (complementary) antigen resulting in confusion as to what is "self" and "nonself", and thereby producing disregulation within the immune system. Significantly, complementary antibodies or T cells recognize each other as "nonself" and attach each other. The result is that autoimmunity is always characterized primarily by a "civil war" within the immune system itself. Diagnostic symptoms of this "civil war" are the circulating immune complexes and perivascular cuffing that occur in all autoimmune diseases. If, in addition, the antigens mimic other "self" proteins, then this "civil war" extends to other body systems. Epidemiological, clinical, and experimental evidence is presented for the presence of multiple concurrent infections preceding autoimmunity, for complementary antigens within these multiple infections, and for complementary immune responses to these antigens. Case studies include thrombocytopenia purpura, myocarditis, rheumatic fever, multiple sclerosis, and AIDS. Experimentally testable differences between the molecular mimicry, antiidiotype, and antigenic complementarity theory are presented. Mechanisms explaining prevention and suppression of animal models of autoimmunity are provided and their implications of the development of novel treatments for human autoimmune diseases discussed. The etiological implications discussed with regard to changes that the theory requires in applying Koch's postulates to autoimmune diseases. And the risks of initiating autoimmune diseases by delivering more and more vaccines concomitantly are discussed.

Chapter 5 - Multiple sclerosis (MS) is considered to be initiated by an autoimmune attack on myelin proteins by a mimic within a protein from some unidentified microorganism. Experimental allergic encephalomyelitis (EAE) is the model for MS. Different peptides from four myelin proteins are potent known EAE immunogens. The contribution of particular amino acids to encephalitogenicity within several immunogens and the minimum adjuvant requirements have been ascertained. Thus, the EAE initiation process at a molecular level is known. Using this EAE molecular information with known aspects of clinical MS, e.g. patient's age, variable histology, clinical immunological data, epidemiology, etc., the molecular initiation process of the autoimmune aspects of MS is defined. This definition includes: a.) type of organism providing the mimic, b.) estimation of single versus multiple immunogens, c.) location of the mimic, d.) involvement of adjuvant molecules and other inflammatory agents, e.) elucidation of magnetic resonance imaging (MRI) data, f.) dissection of confusing cellular immunology data, and g.) explanation of variable histological lesion locations. With this information various therapeutic options are discussed.

Chapter 6 - Sjogren's syndrome (SS), one of the major autoimmune disorders, causes destruction of the salivary and lacrimal glands, leading to dry mouth and dry eyes and subsequent clinical complications. SS is also associated with rheumatic disorders such as rheumatoid arthritis. Green tea polyphenols (GTPs), a complex mixture of substances, exerts anti-inflammatory and anti-apoptotic properties, which may protect tissues from--or at least delay--the onset of auto-immune disorders. We discovered that EGCG, the most potent of the GTPs, is able to suppress epithelial expression of autoantigens. The non-obese diabetic (NOD) mouse is a model for autoimmune insulin-dependent diabetes and SS-like disease. Previously, we showed that NOD mice fed with GTPs had lowered serum autoantibody levels and decreased submandibular gland lymphocyte infiltration. EGCG has the same effect. In NOD mice, cells in lymphocyte-infiltrated areas had an elevated apototic index in comparison to the epithelium in BALB/c control mice. In NOD mice fed with EGCG, apoptosis in infiltrated areas was reduced to BALB/c levels. However, in the non-infiltrated glandular epithelium of NOD mice, apoptosis was only modestly higher than in BALB/c, and the levels were not affected by EGCG. Remarkably, in the glandular epithelium of NOD mice fed with water, there was a significant increase in expression of the proliferation markers PCNA (an autoantigen) and Ki67. In contrast, expression in EGCG-fed animals was similar to BALB/c. Proteomic profiling of acinar cell proteins demonstrated alterations in NOD mice as compared to BALB/c that could in part be changed to the BALB/c expression pattern by dietary EGCG.

Our observations are consistent with a model for SS in which early lymphocyte – independent acinar cell abberations, detectable at the protein level, preceed and prime subsequent autoimmune reactions. The elevated proliferation observed in the glandular epithelium suggests an abnormal reparative response. A subsequent autoimmune attack on the acinar cells could amplify the priming signal by activation of apoptosis and autoantigen expression in infiltrates. One possible mechanism of induction is that acinar cells cannot integrate conflicting intrinsic pro-differentiation and abberant proliferation signals, leading to cell death as the default state. The beneficial effects of GTPs/EGCG likely result from their known pro-differentiation and anti-proliferation properties preventing otherwise undamaged cells from entering the default state. Complementary and alternative approaches such as green tea polyphenols could protect secretory glands from autoimmune-induced tissue destruction, and early detection of autoimmune risk for disease might be possible by examination of protein markers in saliva and serum.

Chapter 7 - Virus infections can initiate autoimmunity to self molecules, but not all infections have this effect. A deciding factor in whether infection induces autoimmunity is the nature of the innate immune response initiated by the pathogen. The innate immune system is the initial response to infection and not only helps control microbial growth but modulates the type and intensity of the developing adaptive (antigen-specific) immune response to the microbe. One type of cell affected by the innate immune system is the T regulatory cell. T regulatory cells are a special population of lymphocytes which can inhibit inflammation and autoimmunity. Control of T regulatory cell activation and/or function often determines whether autoimmunity will occur, and many factors, including the role of antigen-presenting cells, signaling through Toll-Like Receptors (TLRs), and innate effectors including natural killer cells and T cells expressing the gamma-delta (γδ) T cell receptor, affect T regulatory cell generation. This review discusses how virus infection, and the innate immune response it generates, determines whether T regulatory cells are activated.

Chapter 8 - Innate autoimmunity refers to that innate immune system recognizes self targets and initiate inflammatory response in a similar way as with pathogens. One novel example of this innate autoimmunity is ischemia-reperfusion (I/R) injury. Recent advance in this field reveals a general mechanism of I/R injury by which ischemic stress leads to expose a highly conserved self-antigen on the cell surface, and such antigen is recognized by the innate immune system resulting in acute inflammation. Studies of different I/R models showed that reperfusion of ischemic tissues elicits an acute inflammatory response involving serum complement system which is activated by natural IgM. A monoclonal natural IgM that initiates I/R injury has been identified. This led to the subsequent identification of nonmuscle myosin heavy chain type II A and C as the self-targets in two different tissues. In addition, studies of the downstream pathway of this innate response found that IgM binds initially to ischemic antigen providing a binding site for mannan binding lectin (MBL), which subsequently leads to activation of complement and results in tissue injury. The discovery of natural IgM mediated innate autoimmunity opens up a new area of biomedical research and may lead to the development of potential interventions for I/R injury.

Chapter 9 - Major histocompatibility complex class I or class II molecules (MHCI or MHCII) are cell surface proteins involved in cell-cell interactions in the immune system, and among other body-cells. Anti-MHC receptors may be germ line encoded like killer cell activating receptors (KAR) or killer cell inhibitory receptors (KIR) expressed in particular on NK and NKT cells but also on some T lymphocytes. Anti-MHC receptors on T lymphocytes are rearranged from V, D, J, and C gene segments encoding antigen T-cell receptors (TCR), which react with peptides associated with the MHCI or MHCII binding groves. Among the more than 10^{12} different possible TCR molecules, several bind self-peptide-MHC molecules with high avidity. Such T cells are deleted in the thymus by negative selection, and in principle only non-self reacting T cells emigrate from the thymus. However, thymus negative selections are not infallible, and self-reactive T cells do enter the periphery, and some aggressive, auto-reactive T cells induce autoimmune diseases. We will discuss four examples of auto-reactivity: 1) TCR anti-TCR reactivity in experimental autoimmune encephalomyelitis (EAE) and immunity against T-cell lymphomas, 2) auto-reactivity to self-proteins with modulated amino acids in rheumatoid arthritis, 3) the role of harmless autoimmune reactions in natural immunity, and 4) NKT cell – dendritic cell – NK cell interactions in autoimmune reactions against spontaneous tumors and in type I Diabetes. We will attempt to formulate a strong point for the important role of MHC anti-MHC reactions in the regulation of autoimmune reactivity.

Chapter 10 - Multiple and complex are the interactions involving the thyroid gland and the reproductive sphere, before and during pregnancy. The most common thyroid dysfunction in women of reproductive age is hypothyroidism due to thyroid autoimmunity (TAI), and widely identified are the complications due to hypothyroidism before and during pregnancy. Hypothyroidism increases the risk of menstrual irregularities, infertility and pregnancy morbidity. Furthermore, also isolated TAI is associated with infertility, and increased rate of miscarriage. But while the pathological mechanisms which link hypothyroidism and obstetrical complications are well known, the ones which link TAI and infertility, for example, remain largely speculative. In a condition where TAI and hypothyroidism are so strictly associated, these two entities can not be clear cut and represent the two sides of the same coin. Then, the hypothesized mechanisms which underlie obstetrical complications namely, autoimmunity *per se* and thyroid impairment, appear to be not mutually exclusive. Finally, among the complications due to TAI and hypothyroidism, of particular interest are the ones associated with the impaired neural development in the fetus and the following reduced intelligence quotient in the offspring.

Chapter 11 - Asbestos exposure is associated with autoimmune responses including increased serum immunoglobulins, positive autoantibody tests and immune complex deposition. Occupational and environmental asbestos exposures continue to occur world-wide, making this a current human health issue. The premise that asbestos exposure exacerbates autoimmunity is supported by recent studies from an asbestos exposed population in Libby, Montana, USA. Residents of Libby have experienced significant exposures to amphibole asbestos due to the mining of asbestos-contaminated vermiculite near the community over several decades. This community exhibits higher frequencies of positive anti-nuclear antibody (ANA) tests compared to an unexposed control population and what would be expected based on epidemiological data.

Systemic autoimmune diseases are characterized by autoantibody profiles that correspond to specific sets of intracellular components. These profiles can be used to help predict disease, establish a diagnosis as well as assess clinical progression. At this time, it is not known whether a discrete clinical or sub-clinical autoimmune entity is associated with amphibole asbestos exposure. However, asbestos exposure leads to clinical manifestations similar to systemic lupus erythematosus (SLE) in asbestos exposed mice. Therefore, we hypothesized that features of certain autoimmune diseases may be associated with asbestos exposure in humans. The purpose of this study was to determine whether a serological signature exists in this asbestos-exposed population, and to compare this profile with other known systemic autoimmune disease autoantibody profiles.

Our results indicate that autoantibodies from individuals exposed to amphibole asbestos primarily recognize chromatin, histone and Ro52, similar to patients with systemic lupus erythematosus (SLE). Anti-dsDNA and anti-Ro52 antibodies are also generated in a murine model of asbestos induced autoimmunity, which suggests that asbestos may drive similar immune phenomena in both humans and mice. In addition, we show that an unexpected number of subjects expressed the Scl-topoisomerase I (topo I: also referred to as Scl-70) antibody, typically seen in scleroderma. The subjects with anti-topo I tended to have higher levels of asbestos exposure and more severe lung disease compared to those without topo I, whereas there was no association with exposure or lung disease among people with anti-RNP (antibodies to ribonucleoprotein, common in SLE). Finally, we show that some Libby serum samples contained antibodies that bound fibroblasts, a phenomenon that is also seen in scleroderma. By comparison, neither rheumatoid factor (RF) nor anti-cyclic citrullinated peptide (CCP), markers for rheumatoid arthritis (RA), was substantially elevated in the Libby sample set. This information could be extremely valuable for improved screening of exposed populations. In addition, certain autoantibody profiles may serve as diagnostic or prognostic markers relative to asbestos exposure.

Chapter 12 - Patients and rodents with Goodpasture's syndrome develop severe glomerulonephritis and lung hemorrhage due to binding of pathogenic autoantibodies to the non-collagenous NC1 domain of the alpha3 chain of type IV collagen. To gain insight into origins of anti-collagen autoimmunity and to identify potential targets for therapeutic intervention, we analyzed the variable domains of five anti-alpha3(IV)NC1 monoclonal autoantibodies (mAb) obtained by fusion of splenocytes from C57BL/6 and SJL mice immunized with alpha3(IV)NC1collagen. Sequencing reveals that all mAb are minimally mutated and share use of IGHV1 (previously J558) and IGKV3 (formerly Vkappa21) subgroup genes, despite their origins from three different mice and two different strains. Use of a conserved combination of unmutated IG genes suggests that a restricted germline-encoded optimal binding site conformation dominates the antibody response to alpha3(IV)NC1 antigen. Preferential expression of the IGKV3 subgroup was also previously reported among pathogenic autoantibodies reactive with type II collagen in autoimmune arthritis, raising the possibility of structural similarities between seemingly disparate pathogenic collagen II and collagen IV epitopes. The C57BL/6- and SJL-derived anti-Goodpasture mAb differ in their use of D and J genes, using IGHD2-1 and IGHJ2 genes (IMGT® nomenclature, http://imgt.cines.fr) and IGHD1-1 and IGHJ4, respectively. However, both sets of mAb include four core amino acids with a conserved charge structure in the CDR3 of the heavy chain. The shared determinants present potential therapeutic targets on pathogenic anti-collagen B cells that escape central deletion *in vivo*.

In: Autoimmunity: Role, Regulation and Disorders
Editor: Fynn L. Vogel and L. F. Zimmermann

ISBN 978-1-60456-833-2

Chapter 1

Benefits from Genome-Wide Association Studies: Identification of New Susceptibility Genes for Type 1 Diabetes

Dimitry A. Chistiakov* and Natalia V. Voronova**

*Department of Molecular Diagnostics, National Research Center GosNIIgenetika, Moscow 113545, 1st Dorozhny Proezd 1, Russia

**Department of Diabetology, Endocrinology Research Center, Russian Academy of Medical Sciences, Moscow 117036, Dm. Ulyanov street 12

Abstract

With the relative failing of linkage and candidate gene association studies, there had been much sceptism about the ability of geneticists to identify genes for common, complex disorders. Vast amounts of resources were poured into these studies, with very limited success. In the field of genetics of type 1 diabetes (T1D), over more then twenty years of labor-intensive and cost-expensive efforts resulted in the identification only four causal loci predisposing to T1D as follows Human Leucocyte Antigens (HLA) class II, insulin gene region, cytotoxic T-lymphocyte associated 4 (CTLA-4), and protein tyrosine phosphatase, non-receptor member 22 (PTPN22). Recent technological advances, and a better understanding of the genetic architecture of complex diseases, has led to the development of the genome-wide association (GWA) study, which is a powerful new approach to identifying genes influencing predisposition to common, complex disease. For T1D, the implication of the GWA approach in 2005 resulted in rapid progress in discovery of new etiological variants. To date, the involvement to T1D pathogenesis is proven for several new genes such as interleukin 2 receptor alpha (IL2RA/CD25), interferon-induced helicase domain 1 (IFIH1), and small ubiquitin-related modifier 4 (SUMO4). An extended list of likely candidates for T1D susceptibility identified through the GWA approach includes protein-tyrosine phosphatase 2 (PTPN2), CD226 antigen,

* Tel : +7-495-315-0329; fax: +7-495-315-0501; E-mail: dimitry.chistiakov@eudoramail.com

peroxisomal proliferator-activated receptor gamma (PPARG2), interleukin-2/interleukin-21 (IL2/IL21), disintegrin and metalloprotease 33 (ADAM33), and some other genes. For those, preliminary genetic findings should be supported by strong confirmations in other large-scale population GWA studies and functional analyses to find true causal variants. As a type of genetic research, GWA approach is still in its infancy. However, a great benefit to clinical medicine is expected in the years to come, and whilst prediction of disease and pharmacogenetics may eventually prove valuable, the greatest clinical benefit of GWA studies is likely to come from etiological insights into disease processes.

Introduction

Type 1 diabetes (T1D) is the third most prevalent chronic disease of childhood, affecting up to 0.4% of children in some populations by age 30 years, with an overall lifetime risk of nearly 1% [1]. The disease is divided into two subtypes, autoimmune and idiopathic [2]. Etiology and pathogenesis of idiopathic T1D is yet to be identified. Most T1D is believed to be autoimmune in etiology, caused by autoimmune destruction of insulin-producing beta cells of the pancreas in genetically susceptible individuals. This results in complete dependence of affected subjects on exogenous insulin to regulate blood glucose levels.

The etiology of autoimmune T1D is only partially characterized, but it is recognized that both genetic and environmental factors are important in defining disease risk. T1D clusters in families but does not segregate with a known mode of inheritance [3]. The incidence and the age at onset of T1D in some populations have increased dramatically since 1950 [4]. These data, coupled with the incomplete concordance for the phenotype in monozygotic twins (30 – 70%), suggest that the penetrance of T1D predisposing alleles is strongly influenced by environmental factors [5].

T1D is strongly clustered in families with an overall genetic risk ratio (λ_S) of approximately 15 [6]. One locus has been shown to contribute strongly to this familial clustering and represent the primary determinant of IDDM1. There are the Human Leucocyte Antigen (HLA) class II genes residing within the Major Histocompatibility Complex (MHC) on chromosome 6p21. IDDM1 may account for nearly 40% of the observed familial clustering of type 1 diabetes, with a locus-specific λ_S of ~3 [7]. The frequency of HLA class II susceptibility alleles also correlates well with the population incidence of type 1 diabetes [8]. However, individuals carrying the high-risk haplotype DRB1*04-DQB1*0302/ DRB1*03-DQB1*0201 have only ~5% absolute risk of T1D in general population. In affected sibpair families, this haplotype provides increased but only ~20% risk [9]. Therefore, HLA alone could not explain the familial clustering of T1D.

It has been suggested that several or perhaps many non-HLA genes with minor effects should contribute to the genetic background of the disease. The suggestion has been supported by the evidence showing that in first- and second-degree relatives the observed risk of T1D declined in a pattern concordant with multiplicative effects of multiple loci.

In affected families, linkage analyses and association studies revealed around twenty non-HLA putative susceptibility loci. There are IDDM2 (chromosome 11p15), IDDM3 (15q26), IDDM4 (11q13), IDDM5 (6q25), IDDM6 (18q12-q21), IDDM7 (2q33), IDDM8 (6q27), IDDM9 (3q22-q25), IDDM10 (10p11-q11), IDDM11 (14q24-q31), IDDM12 (2q31-

q33), IDD13 (2q34-q35), IDDM15 (6q21), IDDM16 (14q32), IDDM17 (10q25), IDDM18 (5q33), GCK (7p15-p13), 1q42, 8q22-q24, 16q22-q24, and Xp11 [6, 10-12]. Even though statistical evidence supporting linkage for some of these regions was strong in the initial reports, most regions have not been clearly replicated in multiple populations [6, 13]. Of those loci, only three have been then defined by association and functional studies. There are the insulin gene region on chromosome 11p15 (locus IDDM2; [14]), the cytotoxic T lymphocyte antigen 4 (CTLA-4, IDDM12; [15]) on chromosome 2q33, and the PTPN22 gene encoding lymphoid protein tyrosine phosphatase (chromosome 1p13; [16]). We characterized these susceptibility genes earlier on [17].

A relatively low success of genetic association studies in finding T1D susceptibility genes could be explained by several reasons. A major barrier to T1D gene identification, given the likely weak locus-specific contribution (i.e. low λ_S) for non-HLA genes, is the employment of a rather small sample size in most case-control studies that is insufficient to detect genetic variants with modest effects (i.e. having Odds Ratio of less then 1.3 for association with T1D). Other reasons of inconsistent results in association studies included differences in research strategies and selection criteria of the cohorts studied, sample heterogeneity, etc. An absence of strong collaboration between groups and large, well-defined sample sets, often including both case-control and family datasets, also contributed negatively to the research progress in searching T1D susceptibility genes [18].

In 90th, several international consortia such as the Wellcome Trust Case-Control Consortium (WTCCC; http://www.wtccc.org.uk) and the National Institute of Diabetes and Digestive and Kidney Diseases (NIDDK)/Juvenile Diabetes Research Foundation (JDRF) Type 1 Diabetes Genetics Consortium (http://www.t1dgc.org) have been formed on the field of genetics of T1D. The consortia collected (and then shared) large-scale population datasets that have been recruited according to the well-defined selection standards, and released genetic data as soon as possible.

Application of a number of technical advances greatly accelerated research progress in T1D genetics. Possibility to amplify a whole-genome DNA with phi29 DNA polymerase resolved the problem associated with limiting DNA quantities. The high throughput analysis of thousands DNA samples became possible using robust chip technologies from Affimetrix and Illumina involved 100-500 thousands SNPs across a whole human genome. New developments in HapMap project resulted in dissecting complex architecture of the human genome, built from many and many thousands of extended blocks of the linkage disequilibrium (LD), and providing a comprehensive reference map (http://www.hapmap.org) [19].

Within last three years, the above achievements have been successfully employed in genome-wide association (GWA) studies to detect susceptibility genes in several common complex pathologies such as type 2 diabetes, hypertension, cancer as well as inflammatory and autoimmune disorders (autoimmune thyroid disease, rheumatoid arthritis (RA), T1D, systemic erythematosus (SLE), inflammatory bowel disease, asthma, etc.). For T1D, GWA scans resulted in the discovery and further confirmation of three new susceptibility genes in different large-scale population datasets. Thus, the number of T1D genes discovered within last two years is almost equal to that found in the duration of more then twenty years of extensively laborious but less conclusive efforts. In this review, we will consider these exciting findings that significantly improved our understanding of precise molecular mechanisms of T1D pathogenesis.

Genome-Wide Association Studies: Optimizing Strategies

Limitations of Whole-Genome Linkage Studies

Whole-genome linkage mapping was traditionally used to find disease-associated genes. This approach has been tremendously successful for the identification of genes conferring susceptibility to monogenic, or so-called 'Mendelian' disorders, whose etiology is genetically determined. For monogenic diseases, etiological variants cause monogenic disorders are often rare probably due to the negative selection against the disease alleles that associated with mortality and morbidity at early onset of the disease [20]. For linkage analysis, markers that flank the disease gene must segregate with the disease in families. Because Mendelian diseases are, by definition, caused by highly penetrant variants, markers within 10–20 centimorgans (cM) of the disease-causing alleles will cosegregate with the disease status.

In genome-wide linkage analysis, a whole-genome scan is performed using microsatellite markers distributed across a whole genome. However, in many common diseases, the aforementioned characteristics of Mendelian diseases might not apply. In some cases only, genome-wide linkage scans resolved genomic regions significantly linked to a disease, with the subsequent discovery of the causal variants. For T1D, mapping a susceptibility locus at the CTLA-4 gene region could serve as the example of the successful application of linkage analysis [21]. In most cases, linkage analysis has achieved only limited success, and the genes discovered usually explain only a small fraction of the overall heritability of the disease [22].

The lack of success can be addressed to various factors including the low heritability of most complex traits, inadequately powered study designs and imprecise definition of phenotypes. Exploiting larger sample sizes and denser marker maps could improve the results of linkage analysis [23, 24]. However, even if statistically significant evidence of linkage is obtained, extensive candidate gene studies are still required to identify a disease gene within the region of linkage usually exceeding 10 cM (~10 megabases).

Linkage analysis is usually has a limited success to find common genetic variants that have modest effects on disease [25]. The typical frequencies of variants that underlie common disease are largely unknown, but common variants (with frequencies of >1%) have been proposed to influence disease susceptibility [26]. The common variants might contribute to common diseases, whose susceptibility alleles might not be under intense negative selection [27]. There are enough examples of common variants contributing to a common disease, most of which increase the risk of disease by two-fold or less when examined in large population datasets. Some of these well-established disease-susceptibility alleles could never be detected by linkage analysis. For example, the Arg620Trp variant of PTPN22 that affects the risk to T1D would only be detected using linkage studies of over one million affected sib pairs [28]. Consistent with this calculation, the numerous genome-wide linkage studies of T1D were unable to identify the PTPN22 locus as a region of significant linkage [23, 29, 30]. Because it is reasonable to suppose that common alleles as well as rare alleles will contribute to common disease and because linkage analysis has poor power for finding common alleles that have low penetrance, a strategic complement to linkage analysis is desirable.

Candidate-Gene Approaches

Candidate gene studies are frequently used as a practical alternative to linkage analysis. The selection of putative genes (so-called functional candidates) is based on their functional significance and potential involvement in the pathogenesis of a disease. If these genes are located within the susceptibility locus, significantly linked to the disease, and their function could be related to the pathogenic mechanism, they might be considered as positional candidates [31].

The most comprehensive analysis of candidate genes is obtained by resequencing the entire gene in cases and controls and searching for a variant (or set of variants), which is enriched or depleted in disease cases. However, since such studies are still laborious and expensive, they have been usually limited to the coding regions of one or a few candidate genes [32].

Association studies using common allelic variants are cheaper and simpler than the complete resequencing of candidate genes [33]. Breafly, association studies compare the frequency of alleles (genotypes) of a particular variant between disease cases and controls. Alternative approaches include using family-based controls to avoid the potential problem of population stratification. Candidate-gene association studies have identified many of the genes that are known to contribute to susceptibility to common disease [34, 35]. However, these studies rely on having predicted the identity of the correct gene or genes, usually on the basis of biological hypotheses or the location of the candidate within a previously determined region of linkage. Even if these hypotheses are broad (for example, involving the testing of all genes in the insulin-signaling pathway), they will, at best, identify only a fraction of genetic risk factors, even for diseases whose pathophysiology is relatively well understood. When the fundamental physiological defects of a disease are unknown, the candidate-gene approach will clearly be inadequate to fully explain the genetic basis of the disease.

Prerequisites for Genome-Wide Association Studies

In GWA approach, most of the genome is involved for searching polymorphic markers (and then causal genetic variants) significantly associated with a disease. Because no assumptions are made about the genomic location of the causal variants, this approach could exploit the strengths of association studies without having to guess the identity of the causal genes. The GWA approach therefore represents an unbiased and comprehensive option that can be attempted even in the absence of convincing evidence regarding the function or location of the causal genes. Since thousands and thousands markers have to be evaluated in

GWA study, this approach is expected to be enormously expensive and laborious. However, recent technical advances have moved GWA studies from the futuristic to the realistic.

To date, powerful technologies are developed by Affimetrix and Perlegen for throughput genotyping of large population datasets comprising thousands individual DNA samples. These technologies are based on commercially available platforms, which contain high dense panels of single nucleotide polymorphisms (SNPs) distributed across a whole genome. For example, Affimetrix have developed several mapping sets consisted of the oligonucleotide microarrays of 100K, 500K and 1.2M SNPs. These sets cover a significant portion of the genome. The higher density of SNPs in the platform makes cheaper the cost of genotyping [36]. Currently, the lowest prices are estimated to be around $0.50 per genotype [37]. However, the HapMap project plans to include information on ~300 million genotypes, and the United States National Institutes of Health recently approved proposals to determine an additional 600 million genotypes at $0.01 per genotype. This cost is approaching that required to make genome-wide association studies feasible; once this falls to 0.001 US$ per genotype, such studies could become routine (for example, 500,000 genotypes could be typed for only $500 per individual).

Another crucial advance towards enabling efficient GWA studies is the availability of the dbSNP database (http://www.ncbi.nlm.nih.gov/dbSNP). The database now contains nearly 10 million SNPs, including most of the ~11 million SNPs with minor allele frequencies (MAF) of 1% or greater that are estimated to exist in the human genome [37]. The determination of LD patterns on a genome-wide scale through the HapMap project also greatly increases the efficiency of GWA approaches, particularly those that use markers selected on the basis of LD.

Choosing Markers for Genome-Wide Association Studies

LD-Based Markers

To be useful, markers tested for association must either be the causal allele or be in LD with the causal allele [38]. Most of the genome falls into segments of strong LD, within which variants are strongly correlated with each other, and most chromosomes carry one of only a few common haplotypes [39].

Resequencing of several large genomic regions (of ~500 kb) performed as a part of the Encyclopedia of DNA Elements (ENCODE; http://www.genome.gov/10005107) project showed that most of the roughly 11 million common SNPs in the genome have groups of neighbours that are all nearly perfectly correlated with each other - the genotype of one SNP perfectly predicts those of correlated neighbouring SNPs. Thus, one SNP can thereby serve as a proxy for many others in an association screen. Once the patterns of LD are known for a given region, a few SNPs can be chosen such that, individually or in haplotypes, they capture most of the common variation within the region [40].

The precise number of tag SNPs needed is yet to be determined, and will depend on the methods used to select SNPs, the degree of long-range LD between blocks and the efficiency with which SNPs in regions of low LD can be tagged [41].Various algorithms have been proposed for selecting tag SNPs [42, 43]; the optimal method will depend partly on which of the many methods for searching for associations is employed (using haplotypes, single markers, multiple markers and so on).

Missense SNPs

The missense approach was proposed by Botstein and Risch [44] who suggested that association studies should be focused on missense SNPs. Because a typical gene contains one or two missense SNPs [45], this strategy would require the genotyping of only 30,000–60,000 SNPs. However, in contrast to Mendelian disorders, in which causal missense SNPs are highly penetrant and often lead to severe phenotypes, in complex traits, causal missense variants have a rather modest effect.

To support the missense variant approach, Botstein and Risch [44] have pointed out that the small list of common variants that have been reliably associated with common disease include a large proportion of missense variants. However, this argument is undermined by a significant ascertainment bias. It is difficult to estimate a true proportion of causal variants that involve missense changes. Moreover, SNPs in coding regions are implicitly accepted as 'the answer' when an association with a missense variant is detected, often without the functional scrutiny that is required for a SNP in a non-coding region, and often despite the presence of many nearby variants that might be equally or more strongly associated with disease. Therefore, for example, the missense variant of the CTLA-4 gene, i.e. the Thr17Ala substitution, showed a reliable association with T1D and other autoimmune diseases only because it is in strong LD with a regulatory polymorphism in a non-coding region, which is more strongly associated with disease and is therefore more likely to be causal [15].

When compared, the human and mouse genomes showed that a significant amount of non-coding DNA is highly conserved [46]. The functional role of the conserved non-coding regions has been supported experimentally [47, 48]. Polymorphisms in the non-coding regions could also have an important role in the genetics of biomedical traits. Indeed, a modification of the missense approach to include SNPs in these conserved regions has also been proposed Botstein and Risch [44]. However, a large number of additional SNPs required would sacrifice the efficiency of the missense approach and would result in studies that are similar in scale to the indirect LD approach.

Rare Alleles

Current SNP platforms comprising more then million randomly selected SNPs (or a few hundred thousand that have been optimally selected on the basis of LD) seem to provide more or less complete coverage of the genome. However, it is important to note that none of the existing marker sets will be optimal for detecting the effects of rare variants with frequencies of 1% or less. Even if rare alleles have strong effects, they might be difficult to detect by association methods because they are less well represented in SNP databases and because tag SNP approaches are currently designed to tag common SNPs (usually with frequencies >5%).

Population-genetic considerations indicate that most rare alleles with frequencies <5% are likely to have arisen relatively recently (because old alleles tend to either disappear or become common), so there will have been less time for recombination and mutation to disrupt the haplotype on which they arose. Indeed, rare variants are expected to be on single, long haplotypes, as has been observed [49]. Recently, Lin et al. [50] have proposed an exhaustive search of all haplotypes that could greatly increase power to detect rare variants with strong effects. Using similar approach (i.e., through the detection of all haplotypes composed of common variants), Verrneire and coauthors [51] have identified rare alleles of the CARD15 gene with frequencies of <5% strongly associated with inflammatory bowel disease.

How to Increase Efficiency of the Genome-Wide Association Approach?

Sample Size: Enlarge or Minimize?

The most serious limitation of genome-wide studies is the high cost and significant effort required to genotype hundreds of thousands of SNPs per individual. Because of this high cost, there is pressure to limit the sample size, with a consequent reduction in power. To override these problems, a multi-stage approach will be helpful [52]. This approach can reduce the amount of genotyping required, without sacrificing power. In stage 1, the full set of SNPs is genotyped in a fraction of samples, and a liberal p-value threshold is used to identify a subset of SNPs with putative associations. In the second and possibly third stages, the SNPs identified from the first stage are retested at more stringent p-values in populations that are larger or of a similar size. The results of this can then be used to distinguish the few true-positive associations identified in stage 1 from the many false-positive results that occur by chance.

How should the thresholds used in these analyses be defined? Using the standard Bonferroni correction (for example, as suggested by Risch and Merikangas [53] to use for genome-wide studies a conservative p-value threshold of 5×10^{-8} equivalent to a p-value of 0.05 after a Bonferroni correction for 1 million independent tests) leads to the requirement of inappropriately low p-values (and therefore inappropriately large sample sizes).

Many alternative strategies for defining significance thresholds have been proposed including a permutation testing to empirically assess the probability of having observed a particular result by chance, frequentist approaches for estimating experiment-wide significance, and Bayesian approaches for assessing the likelihood that an association is genuine [54, 55]. It should be stressed that genuine associations can achieve thresholds that survive correction for multiple testing if enough samples are genotyped (either as a single study or as a combined analysis of several studies). For example, the association of the variable number of tandem repeats mutation in the insulin gene with T1D has overall p-value that survives even conservative genome-wide corrections for multiple testing [56].

Pooling of the samples, in which equal amounts of DNA from multiple individuals are mixed into a single well before genotyping, greatly decreases the number of samples required for genotyping in GWA [57]. However, this requires the extremely accurate determination of small differences in allele frequency to detect alleles with modest effects, while still using high-throughput, low-cost genotyping platforms. Since pooled genotyping only measures allele frequencies, it would be more difficult to identify variants with pure recessive effects using this strategy: under a recessive model, the difference in genotype frequencies between cases and controls will be more pronounced than the difference in allele frequencies. Another limitation of pooling strategy in study of complex disease is the need to made a different pool for each phenotype, thereby reducing the cost savings. Nevertheless, because of the potentially dramatic cost savings, large-scale empirical trials of several different pooled genotyping technologies might be valuable, including direct comparisons with individual genotyping data on the same samples to assess sensitivity and specificity.

Avoiding False-Positive Associations

The most widely occurred source of systematic bias is the population stratification due to the ethnic admixture. Population stratification is the presence of multiple subgroups within a population that differ in disease prevalence This can lead to the overrepresentation of one or more subgroups among the individuals selected as disease cases in association studies. If a genetic marker has different frequencies in the different subgroups, false-positive associations can ensue.

Several approaches have been suggested to detect or correct for population stratification by typing dozens of unlinked markers [58, 59]. Typing unlinked markers in well-matched case-control studies showed that the large-scale stratification is unlikely in well-matched populations [59, 60]. However, mild stratification is difficult to rule out, and can be shown to exist in well-matched studies of historically admixed populations if enough markers are typed or if the right phenotype is chosen [61]. Fortunately, the large number of markers typed in a GWA study will permit the extremely precise assessment of stratification, allowing for either the appropriate upward correction of p-values (with a concurrent loss of power) or the rematching of cases and controls on the basis of genotypes at a large number of random loci [62].

Another way of avoiding stratification is to use family-based samples. This approach has several theoretical advantages: as well as being immune to stratification [63], these samples can be used to determine whether an allele has different effects on disease when it is inherited maternally or paternally [64], and discordant sib designs [65] can control for the effects of shared environment. However, the most commonly used family-based design, the transmission disequilibrium test (TDT; [63]) is susceptible to technical artefacts.

The potential contribution of genotyping errors to false-positive TDT associations has been characterized [66]. The techniques to minimize random genotyping error rates in TDT analyses have been also described, including tests that take errors into account, with some accompanying loss of power [67]. Missing data could be an important cause of false-positive associations in TDT, even when reasonable quality control measures are used. The impact of missing heterozygotes is most important with alleles that are rare enough to avoid violation of Hardy-Weinberg equilibrium, but are still common enough to achieve low p-values. False-positives are also observed under other scenarios, especially missing homozygotes of the rare allele. Therefore, data completeness is important for TDTs, especially for rarer alleles. Nevertheless, despite the above potential artefacts and other associated difficulties, family-based approaches might still be of significant value because they avoid stratification and might allow the use of more powerful statistical methods.

Towards a Complete SNP Map

Obtaining a complete SNP map plays a crucial role in increasing resolution of GWA studies. By exploiting the LD between nearby loci, which is an important and widespread feature of the genome, it is now possible to survey in an association study a significant proportion of the common variation of a large number of genes that occur in regions of high LD [68]. Cost efficiency can be gained, as it is not necessary to genotype SNPs that are in strong LD with other SNPs; this can be done by choosing a subset set of SNPs known as tag SNPs that capture most of the allelic variation in a region [40].

The degree of LD between alleles at two loci can be described in terms of the metric r^2. An r^2 is informative in association analyses because it is inversely proportional to the sample size that is required for detecting disease association given a fixed genetic risk [69]. An r^2 of 1 indicates perfect LD, and there is no loss of power when using a marker tag SNP instead of directly genotyping the disease causal variant. Therefore, the general consensus is that an r^2 of 0.8 or greater is sufficient for tag SNP mapping to obtain a good coverage of untyped SNPs, allowing genotyping of a lower number of marker SNPs with relatively small losses in power. So, if we knew the identity of all the common SNPs in a region and there was LD between them, then by iterative pair-wise comparisons, the optimal set of tags could be chosen.

The coverage provided by the HapMap have reached at least 1 SNP per 4-5 kb by the end of 2006, and that about 300,000 tag SNPs will need to be genotyped to cover 50% of the genome at an r^2 of 0.8 or greater. However, even with an average density of 1 SNP every 2.5 kb, ~25% of SNPs will still not be captured adequately by LD and tag SNPs [70]. To tag most variants with MAFs of >0.1, as many as 500,000 more SNPs might be required to cover in a comprehensive fashion the remaining 25% of the genome that shows lower LD. Nevertheless, as few as 75,000 tag SNPs might well cover 25% of the genome (in regions of high LD), a vast increase in efficiency over a candidate gene-by-gene approach. Further cost-efficiency and power could be gained by choosing not only the regions of highest LD, but also those regions that contain the highest density of genes.

For a complete SNP map with contiguous coverage (with every SNP or other polymorphism having an r^2 of at least 0.8 with a SNP that can be genotyped robustly), it is not necessary to obtain near complete genome sequences from a large number of unrelated individuals. The tag SNP selection is estimated to require resequencing for only a relatively small number of individuals: 32 individuals, or 64 chromosomes, might be sufficient to provide $r^2 \geq 0.8$ for more than 98% of cases, and this is consistent with previous studies for different tag SNP methods [70, 71].With current sequencing technology, this is a massive task, but emphasis could be placed on resequencing regions of lower LD (perhaps 20% of the genome).

Future Prospects

Despite the caveats outlined above, GWA studies of the role of common variants in complex disease will be carried out in the near future. Initial studies will define more accurately the principal factors, which have been summarized above, that can reduce the power of such studies. To make GWA studies a true practical, large sample sizes should be used, biases taken into account, multiple-testing issues addressed and replication studies carried out, therefore optimizing experimental design, statistical power and cost efficiency. A set of SNPs must be chosen that comprehensively captures the common variation across the genome. Accumulating the data necessary to choose such SNPs is one of the main goals of the human HapMap project, which is due to be completed by the end of 2008. Methods for selecting such SNPs, and for using them efficiently for tests of association, are being developed and refined. Other proposed large sets of markers should be similarly assessed to determine how completely they survey variation across the genome. Complete genome resequencing in a larger population of cases and controls is required to cover the complete spectrum of coding and non-coding variants and, indeed, provide opportunity to test both rare and common variants for roles in disease.

Advances in Genome-Wide Association Studies: The Identification of New Genes Underlying Susceptibility to Type 1 Diabetes

Within last three years, due to the employment of GWA approaches in genetics of T1D, cur understanding of molecular and genetic roots of the pathogenesis of T1D have been significantly enriched by the identification of three new genes conferring susceptibility to the disease. There are interleukin 2 receptor alpha (IL2RA/CD25), interferon-induced helicase domain 1 (IFIH1), and small ubiquitin-related modifier 4 (SUMO4). Additionally, preliminary data on association with T1D have been obtained for a disintegrin and metalloprotease 33 (ADAM33), peroxisomal proliferator-activated receptor gamma (PPARG2), protein-tyrosine phosphatase 2 (PTPN2), CD226 antigen and some other genes. These loci are shown to have a modest genetic effect in the etiology of T1D, which could be detected only with the involvement of well-powered, large-scale population datasets exploited in current GWA studies.

Interleukin 2 Receptor Alpha

Genetic Analyses

The region of linkage to T1D involving the IL2RA/CD25 gene was recently mapped on chromosome 10p14-q11 linkage in the largest family-based study to date (1,435 families), with the second highest logarithm of odds score (LOD=3.21, nominal $p=1.2\times10^{-4}$, $\lambda_S=1.12$) outside the HLA region [30]. Actually, linkage of T1D to 10p14-q13 (IDDM10 locus) was supported again by this and past whole-genome scans [23, 72]. However, analyses of the strong positional and functional candidate gene GAD2 failed to show that this gene is a T1D susceptibility locus [73, 74].

In 2005, Vella et al. [75], using a tag SNP approach, mapped the IL2RA/CD25 gene as a susceptibility locus for T1D on chromosome 10p15.1. The investigators tested 20 tag SNPs with MAF>0.05 encompassing a 48-kb region of the IL2RA/CD25 gene and observed a highly significant association with T1D, with multilocus test p-value of $6.5x10^{-8}$, in a large population dataset (3,521 cases and 3,930 controls) from UK. The association was independently replicated in the family-based study envolved 740 affected Caucasian families from UK and US, providing a multilocus test p-value of $7.3x10^{-3}$ [75].

The association between IL2RA and T1D was then confirmed in the Canadian family collection (949 nuclear family trios) [76]. Two of the 12 IL2RA SNPs genotyped [rs706778 (A/G) and rs3118470 (C/T)] showed statistically significant association with T1D (OR=1.27 and 1.28, p=$6.96x10^{-4}$ and $8.63x10^{-4}$, respectively). Both SNPs are located in the 5' end of the long intron 1 within 3 kb of each other, are in high LD (r^2=0.613), and confer similar ORs. They map to the second LD block, which encompasses the 5' flanking region, the first exon, and the 5' end of intron 1 of IL2RA The A-C haplotype was associated with an increased T1D risk. (OR=1.26, p= 3.02×10^{-4}) [76].

Although the initial association was found using tag SNPs for the IL2RA region, the causal variant could be outside and unrelated to the functional candidate gene, IL2RA, possibly in the flanking gene IL15RA, which is also a strong functional candidate [77] or in the other neighboring gene that encodes RNA binding motif protein 17 (RBM17). IL-2RA and IL-15RA are structurally related molecules involved in the regulation of T cells, although often with opposing roles. For instance, IL-15RA inhibits IL-2–mediated activation-induced cell death (AICD), whereas IL-2RA promotes AICD [78].

To clarify this, Lowe et al. [79] analyzed LD structure within a 190-kb region containing the IL2RA, IL15RA and RBM17 genes. The IL15RA gene was found to lie in an LD block separate from that containing IL2RA. This excluded IL15RA from the further analysis. However, there was no clear breakdown in LD in the 21-kb region between IL2RA and RBM17 (Figure 1). The GWA study of the IL2RA gene region revealed 18 nonsynonymous SNPs strongly associated with T1D ($p<10^{-6}$) in 2,965 affected individuals and 2,548 control samples from UK, with one marker (ss52580109) the most highly associated with the disease (p=$7.83x10^{-11}$; OR for minor allele A = 0.63).

Assuming that ss52580109 was either the causal variant or in strong LD with the causal variant, Lowe et al. [79] analyzed polymorphisms in a 500-kb extended IL15RA-IL2RA-RMB17 region and found four SNPs in perfect LD (r^2=1) with ss52580109.These markers have been genotyped in an additional large case-control collection, and for one of those, ss52580101, the highest association was observed (p=$3.37x10^{-20}$; OR for minor allele A = 0.65). However, the marker rs11597367 added significantly to ss52580101, indicating that ss52580101 alone could not explain the association of the region with T1D. The two causal variants are found to act multiplicatively, and consequently, and the haplotype ORs can be represented as products of the effects of the two SNPs (OR for the major-major alleles (C from ss52580101 and T from ss11597367) is 2.04). The association of ss52580101 and rs11594656 with T1D was replicated in a large independent family collection. Again, there was no support for a haplotype-specific effect [79]. Thus, it is impossible to distinguish between these two SNPs, therefore suggesting that there are two ancestrally distinct causal alleles that are marked by these SNPs.

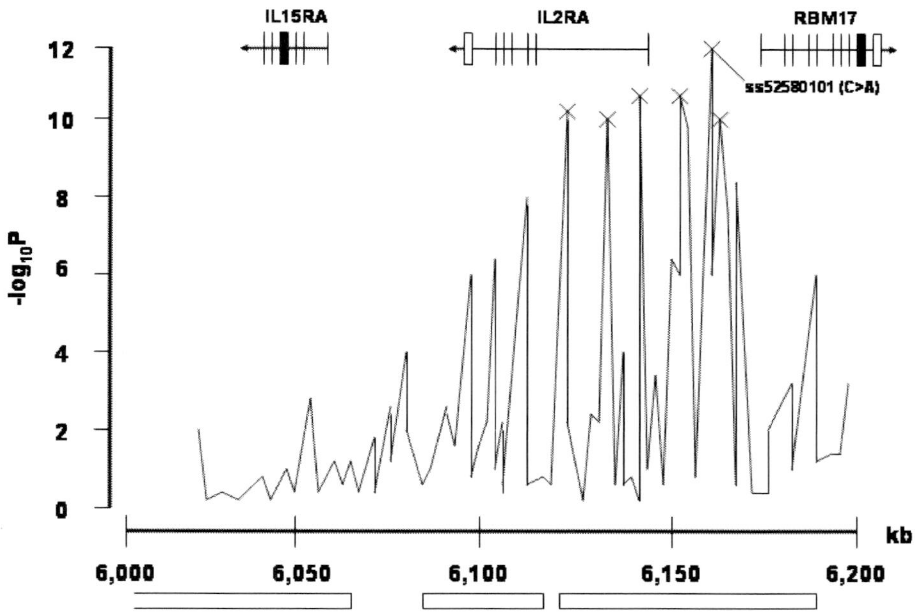

Figure 1. Results of the association analysis of tag SNPs within the 190-kb extended region, contained the IL15RA, IL2RA, and RBM17 genes, in the large population collection of UK diabetic patients and controls. The vertical scale defines the strength of association (-log$_{10}$ of a P-value for every tag SNP tested). The horizontal scale represents a physical distance in kilobases (kb) from a p-terminus of chromosome 10. Crosses (X) denote SNPs in perfect linkage disequilibrium (LD; r^2=1) with the most significant SNP, ss52580101(C>A). From left to right, crosses represent rs12722522(C>T), rs12722508 (T >A), rs12722495 (A>G), ss52580073(G>A), ss52580101(C>A), and ss52580109 (G>A). Open boxes on the bottom show extended LD blocks.

Importantly, the set of 20 IL2RA SNPs used in the initial study [75] was recently evaluated for association with Graves' disease (GD) in 1896 GD UK patients and 1822 geographically matched controls [80]. A significant association was observed, with a multilocus test p-value of 4.5 x 10^{-4}. This indeed could suggest the functional significance of the IL2RA/CD25 locus as a general autoimminity gene, contributing to the pathogenesis of at least two organ-specific autoimmune diseases such as GD and T1D. However, this evidence should be further supported by additional well-powered studies, involving large population and family collections.

Functional Studies

The two most associated markers of IL2RA, ss52580101 and rs11594656 have been evaluated for functional significance [79]. The ss52580101 showed association with serum concentration of soluble IL-2RA (sIL2-RA), a product of the proteolytic cleavage of membrane-bound IL-2RA after the induction of T cell proliferation [81]. Individuals with two copies of the ss52580101 major disease susceptibility allele (G/G) have lowered concentrations of log sIL-2RA then carriers of one or more copies of the protective allele (G/A and A/A). Similarly, patients carrying two copies of the major susceptible allele (T/T) of the rs11594656 were associated with lower concentrations of sIL-2RA compared with those having the protective allele (T/A and A/A). This therefore suggests both SNPs are functional. The SNPs are independently associated with serum concentration of sIL2-RA, accounting for 8.2% of the total variance in $\log_{10}$-transformed sIL-2RA concentrations; rs11594656 alone accounted for 6.6% and ss52580101 alone accounted for 2.3% of the total variance [79].

The functional significance provide a strong support that the ss52580101 and rs11594656 to be etiological variants for T1D susceptibility on chromosome 10p15. Both are located in the 5' regulatory region of the IL2RA/CD25 gene but do not affect none of eight putative regulatory elements implicated in the regulation of IL2-RA expression in response to stimuli such as IL-2-, tumor necrosis beta (TNFa)- and T-cell receptor (TcR)-mediated costimulation [82]. However, these polymorphisms could disrupt putative CpG dinucleotides. The methylation of CpG is important in the transcriptional regulation of genes either by physically disrupting the binding of transcriptional proteins to a gene or by allowing the binding of methyl-CpG–binding domain proteins, which recruit chromatin remodeling proteins such as histone deacetylases, inactivating chromatin and thus silencing gene expression [83]. The 5' region of the IL2RA gene is shown to be highly acetylated in both resting and activated T cells [84]. Therefore, it is possible that the SNPs may be involved in either enhancing or disrupting histone remodeling and, consequently, may indirectly disrupt IL2RA transcription.

Putative Role of IL-2RA in the Etiology of T1D

A role of IL2RA as the susceptibility gene in the pathogenesis of T1D could be related to the reduced levels of sIL-2RA in the susceptible allele carriers. Stimulated in vitro monocytes from peripheral blood of T1D patients are shown produced less sIL-2RA than those from control subjects [85]. The decreased concentrations of sIL-2RA could be associated with reduced proliferation of a variety of lymphocytes, including CD4+CD25+ regulatory T cells whose depletion and altered function directly contribute to T1D pathogenesis [86].

Regulatory T cells are crucial in maintaining self-tolerance. CD25 is upregulated upon engagement of the TcR, but a small subset of CD4+ T-cells express it constitutively upon their maturation in the thymus. They constitute the population of CD4+CD25+ regulatory T cells that are anergic to TcR signals and potently suppress activated T-cells in a contact-dependent and cytokine-independent fashion [87]. As direct evidence of the importance of CD4+CD25+T cells in type 1 diabetes, the transfer of CD4+CD25+ T cells prevented autoimmune diabetes in recipient non-obese diabetic (NOD) mice [88]. CD4+CD25+ T cells depend on IL-2 for their growth and survival, and the IL-2 signaling effect is mainly mediated by IL-2RA (Figure 2) [89, 90]. Furthermore, an IL-2RA-dependent proliferation of CD4+CD25+ regulatory T cells could be strongly linked to their efficiency in the immune suppression and indeed explain a suggested role of this immune receptor in general autoimmunity.

Alteration of the IL-2/IL-2RA Pathway Is a Common Mechanism of Susceptibility to Autoimmune Diabetes in Humans and NOD Mice

Recent findings discovered IL-2RA as a new susceptibility gene for T1D extended a number of loci that underline shared genetic background for autoimmune diabetes in humans and NOD mice. Earlier studies showed that shared susceptibility to T1D in the human and mouse could be attributed to the MHC class II antigens, representing human IDDM1 and murine Idd1 loci [91]. A second common locus includes CTLA-4 (human IDDM7) and ctla4 (mouse idd5.1). Recently, a significant role of PTPN22 was described in human diabetes. The mouse has a PTPN22 ortholog, ptpn8 encoding PEST-domain enriched tyrosine phosphatase. Genetic alterations in ptpn8 have been shown to contribute to diabetes susceptibility in the NOD mouse [92].

Human and mouse also share the IL-2/IL-2RA pathway of controlling autoimmunity. The il2 represents a causal gene in the susceptibility locus idd3 on murine chromosome 3 [93-96]. Mouse strains carrying either Idd3 susceptibility (NOD or 129 strains) or protective (B6 strain) alleles exhibited no difference in the steady state level of Il2 RNA [97]. Therefore, the reduction in diabetes conferred by Idd3-protective alleles is not due to differences in the level of transcription of the Il2 gene.

Mouse strains carrying an Idd3 susceptibility allele have a proline at position 6 of the mature interleukin-2, whereas strains carrying an Idd3-protective allele have a serine [94, 97]. Different IL2 allotypes have different glycosylation profiles, and this also correlates with the presence or absence of proline at position 6 [97]. Although these glycosylation differences have no effect on the ability of IL2 to stimulate proliferation of IL2-dependent cell lines, they may affect the half-life of the molecule leading to a functional deficiency in circulating IL2. IL2 was shown to bind to heparan sulfate in vivo, and this bound IL2 is functional in both promoting T-cell activation and stimulating activation-induced cell death [98]. The binding to heparan sulfate may well be altered by differences in glycosylation, thereby influencing in vivo availability of IL2.

NOD mice are genetically resistant to the induction of the islet allograft tolerance, and this tolerance is substantially determined by the Idd3 region gene. The resistance to the islet allograft tolerance induction overlaps in the mechanism, by which the Idd3 resistance locus improves self-tolerance and the induction of allotolerance [99]. Mice that are deficient in the action of IL2, either through the targeted disruption of the Il2 structural gene itself or the genes encoding the α or β chains of its receptor, developed a variety of autoimmune diseases [100]. Studies in IL2 and IL2 receptor knockout mice have shown that the cytokine plays a nonredundant role during Fas-mediated apoptosis of activated T cells, one of the central processes in immune homeostasis [101]. Finally, the engineered haplodeficiency of Il2 gene expression in NOD mice was found to not only reduce T cell IL-2 production by two-fold but also mimic the autoimmune dysregulatory effects of the naturally occurring susceptibility alleles of Il2. Reduced IL-2 production correlated with the reduced function of CD4+ CD25+ regulatory T cells, which are critical for maintaining immune tolerance [102]. These studies suggest on a crucial role of the IL2/IL2RA regulatory pathway in immune homeostasis, whose disturbances (likely, through the impaired function CD4+ CD25+ regulatory T cells) could induce islet autoimmunity and T1D. Dysregulation of the IL2/IL2RA-mediated pathway therefore might represent one of the general ways of inducing autoimmunity since the IL2RA gene is found to predispose to T1D and GD in humans [79, 80], while the murine idd3 locus is associated not only with diabetes but also defines susceptibility to experimental autoimmune encephalomyelitis and autoimmune ovarian dysgenesis induced by neonatal thymectomy, a disease dependent on regulatory T cell function [103-105].

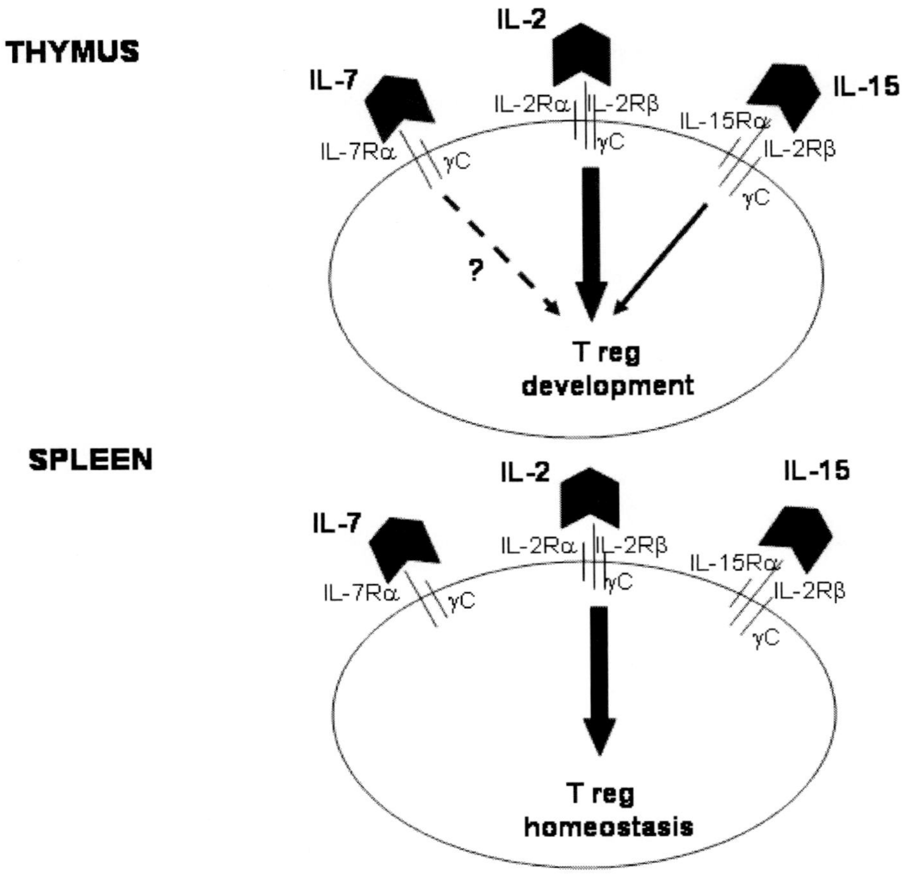

Figure 2. Cytokine-dependent regulation of CD4+CD25+ regulatory T (Treg) cells. In the thymus, IL-2 plays a predominant role in the regulation of Treg development. In the absence of IL-2, IL-15 is sufficient for proliferation of the Treg. Other γC-dependent cytokine, IL-7 may also play a minor role in the control of Treg development. In the spleen, IL-2-dependent signaling leads to the suppression of both Il-7Rα and IL-15Rα chains. Therefore, the mature Tregs becomes primarily dependent on IL-2 for their survival and expansion.

Interferon-Induced Helicase C Domain 1

Genetic Analyses

A GWA scan of a large UK case-control collection (nearly 3800 samples) using over 6,500 nonsynonymous SNPs reveal several SNPs located in non-HLA genomic regions and highly associated with T1D [106]. The third most associated SNP was rs1990760 (Ala946Thr) from the gene interferon induced with helicase C domain 1 (IFIH1) on chromosome 2q24.3 (OR for the minor allele G = 0.82, $P=4.73x10^{-5}$). Regenotyping of a panel of SNPs in the 236-kb region containing the entire IFIH1 gene and 5' part of the neighboring KCNH7 gene found no SNPs significantly added to the association between the rs1990760 and T1D, hence suggesting that this marker could be a true causal variant for T1D [107]. The association of the missence Ala946Thr variant of IFIH1 with T1D was then confirmed in the independent cohort of affected patients of European ancestry (1799 diabetic families), providing OR for the G allele of 0.88 (P=4.63x10^{-3}).

Furthermore, the Ala946Thr polymorphism showed strong association with GD in a large dataset of UK Whites (1204 cases and 892 controls). The Ala allele was highly associated with a higher risk of GD (OR=1.47; P=1.9x10^{-6}) [108]. Analysis of the causal marker of IFIH1 for possible relationship to systemic autoimmune disease such as RA in a large cohort of UK Caucasians (965 RA patients and 988 healthy controls) showed no significant association [109]. These results provide evidence for the putative involvement of IFIH1 in the pathogenesis of GD suggesting for a role of this gene in organ-specific autoimmunity related to the development of T1D and GD. However, more studies are required to support this suggestion.

Potential Role of IFIH1 in T1D

The codon 946 SNPs resides in exon 15 of the IFIH1 gene, outside of the functional portions of the enzyme such as the helicase or CARD domains, and therefore the biological effects of this variant are unknown (Figure 3) [110]. Although the variant does lie in a region that is highly conserved between mammals, suggesting functional importance. Indeed, the functional significance of the etiological variation in IFIH1 explaining its contribution to the pathology remains to be elucidated.

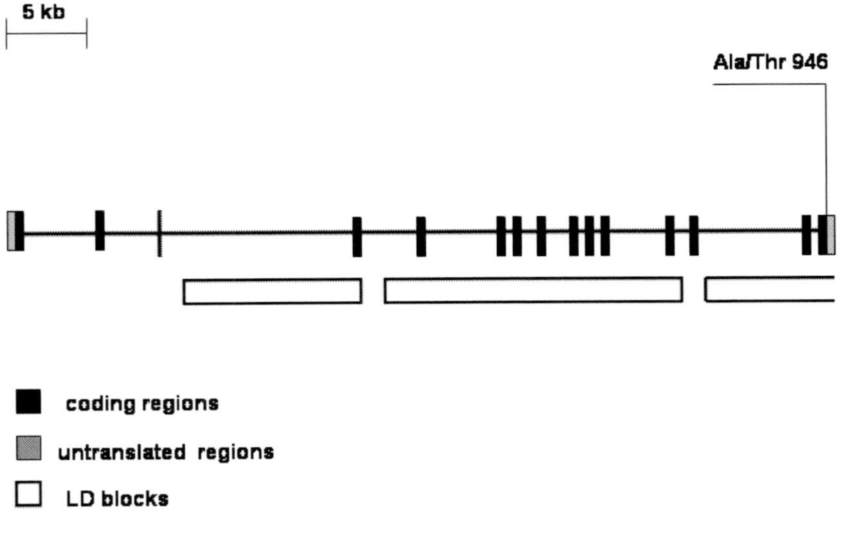

Figure 3. Structure of the interferon induced with helicase domain 1 (IFIH1) gene. The IFIH1 gene spans 51.5 kb on chromosome 2q24.3. The causal missense SNP (Ala/Thr 946) associated with both type 1 diabetes and Graves' disease situated in exon 15.

Despite no association between this genetic variant and RA was detected, IFIH1 mRNA levels were greater in RA patients compared with healthy controls [109]. However, there are no functional studies that could explained the association of the helicase gene with T1D or GD. Genetic analysis did not ruled out the possibility of the location of the etiological marker within other genes situated in the disease-associated region on 2q24.3, including functional candidates, such as fibroblast activation protein (FAP), grancalcin (GCA), and a potassium voltage-gated channel and subfamily H member 7 (KCNH7) [107].

IFIH1, also referred to as mda-5 or Helicard, is an early type I interferon (IFN) β–responsive gene, which may contribute to the apoptosis of virally infected cells in antiviral immune responses, thus making it a sensor or pathogen recognition receptor for viral infection [111]. Double-strand viral RNA is sensed via a helicase domain resulting in the activation of an N-terminal caspase recruitment domain (CARD), which activates several key downstream pathways including NF-κB and IRF3 [112]. The genetic association of IFIH1 with T1D may be explained by the reported link with preceding viral infections and islet cell autoimmunity [113].

To date, 13 different viruses including enteroviruses, rubella, mumps, rotavirus, parvovirus, and cytomegalovirus are known to induce the autoimmune response against beta-cells in humans and animals. However, clinical evidences for viral-induced diabetes in humans are controversial and far to be conclusive [114]. Viruses can promote islet autoimmunity through the direct lysis of beta-cells, bystander activation of self-reactive T cells, loss of regulatory T cells, and molecular mimicry. In animals, the src kinases, particularly hck, play the important role in the activation of macrophages and subsequent production TNFα, IL-1β, and nitric oxide, leading to the destruction of insulin-producing cells, which results in the development of viral-induced diabetes. In DR-BB rats infected with Kilham rat virus, the finely tuned balance of CD45RC+CD4+ T cells is disrupted, leading to the selective activation of beta-cell-cytotoxic effector T lymphocytes (Th1-like CD45RC+CD4+ T cells and CD8+ T cells) and downregulation of regulatory Th2-like CD45RC-CD4+ T cells [115].

Thus, discovery of the IFIH1 gene involved to the antiviral immunity and associated with T1D should promote a new wave of studies focused on the detailed explanation of the pathogenic mechanism of the induction of T1D in genetically predisposed individuals with viral infection.

Small Ubiquitin-Like Modifier 4

Genetic Studies Revealed the Ethnic-Specific Association of SUMO4 with Type 1 Diabetes

The association between the causal variant encoding the methionine-to-valine substitution at codon 55 (M55V) of the small ubiquitin-like modifier 4 (SUMO4) gene was reported as the causal variant of IDDM5 on chromosome 6q25 [116, 117]. Further studies consistently replicated the association in multiple Asian populations (Japanese, Korean and Chinese), providing an overall OR=1.29 ($p=7.0 \times 10^{-6}$; reviewed by Ikegami et al. [118, 119], Noso et al. [120], and Wang et al. [121]). In Caucasians, the analyses of SUMO4 association with T1D produced negative results [122-125] except the dataset from the North-Central Florida, US [116, 126]. Only in Swedish patients, the M55 variant was not associated with diabetes by itself but increased the risk in the subset positive for the high-risk HLA-DR3/DR4 [127]. Hence, the SUMO4 M55V polymorphism seems to be specifically associated with T1D in Asians.

The association of the etiological R620W variant of PTPN22 could represent another example of the ethnic-specific association with T1D. In contrast to SUMO4, the PTPN22 R620W was found to show association with the disease in Caucasians but not in Asians because this marker is absent in Asians [128]. However, the M55V SNP of SUMO4 is a common polymorphism in Caucasians, with MAF of approximately 0.4-0.5.

The inconsistence of the results in Caucasians probably could be explained by the heterogeneity in family datasets used in the association studies. The cause for the heterogeneity remains to be determined. One possible explanation for the heterogeneity is that the IDDM5 interval may contain multiple T1DM susceptibility genes, which may contain both susceptible and protective alleles that are in different linkage disequilibrium patterns in different populations.

In Japanese, in addition to T1D, the M55V marker of SUMO4 showed association with other autoimmune diseases: autoimmune thyroid disease (OR=1.52; P=0.0041) and RA (OR=1.53; P=0.027) [129], suggesting for the general role of SUMO4 in autoimmunity. However, studies in Caucasians involved larger population cohorts failed to show association with neither RA [130-132] nor SLE [133]. Although further well-powered studies are definitely required to replicate the association of SUMO4 with autoimmunity in Japanese, the loss of association in Caucasians may be explained with epistasis between SUMO4 and other loci, influencing the direction of the association. Complex gene–environment interactions may exist that could render an allele predisposing in one population yet protective in another. The IDDM5 locus is a large region, containing several other candidates for the role of a general autoimmunity gene. Those include the estrogen receptor 1 gene (ESR1), vasoactive intestinal peptide (VIP) and the three UL16-binding protein genes (ULBP1–3).

Functional Studies Supporting a Role of SUMO4 in Autoimmunity

The M55V SNP was shown to alter the sequence of the PKC phosphorylation site (at position 54–56), which appears to be important for the molecular conformation and functional activity of SUMO4 [116]. In carriers of the predisposing M55 allele of SUMO4, the ability of SUMO4 to conjugate to IkBα is reduced resulting in less effective downregulation of the transcriptional activity of NFκB, a factor that is crucial for expression of many genes including immunomodulatory and heat shock genes [121]. As result, the in vivo expression of IL12-p40 and heat shock transcription factors, representing NF-kB-dependent genes, was 2-3-fold higher in the presense of the Met55 allele [116, 134].

SUMO4 is a member of a highly conserved protein family [134]. In contrast to a broad expression of other members of the SUMO family, the expression of SUMO4 is restricted to several tissues including pancreas and pancreatic beta-cells that makes this protein an attractive candidate for putative contribution in the etiology of diabetes [135]. SUMO binding to a target protein mediates posttranslational modification, that is, sumoylation. The sumoylation is a remarkably versatile regulatory mechanism of protein function involved in the regulation of immune response and cellular apoptosis with implication in signal transduction, protein targeting, DNA repair, and RNA processing [136]. The negative feedback network for SUMO4 in the NF-κB signaling pathway leads to the suppression of NF-κB-dependent expression of a variety of genes including inflammatory cytokines and immune costimulators and inhibitors (Figure 4) [137]. Therefore, in individuals carrying the

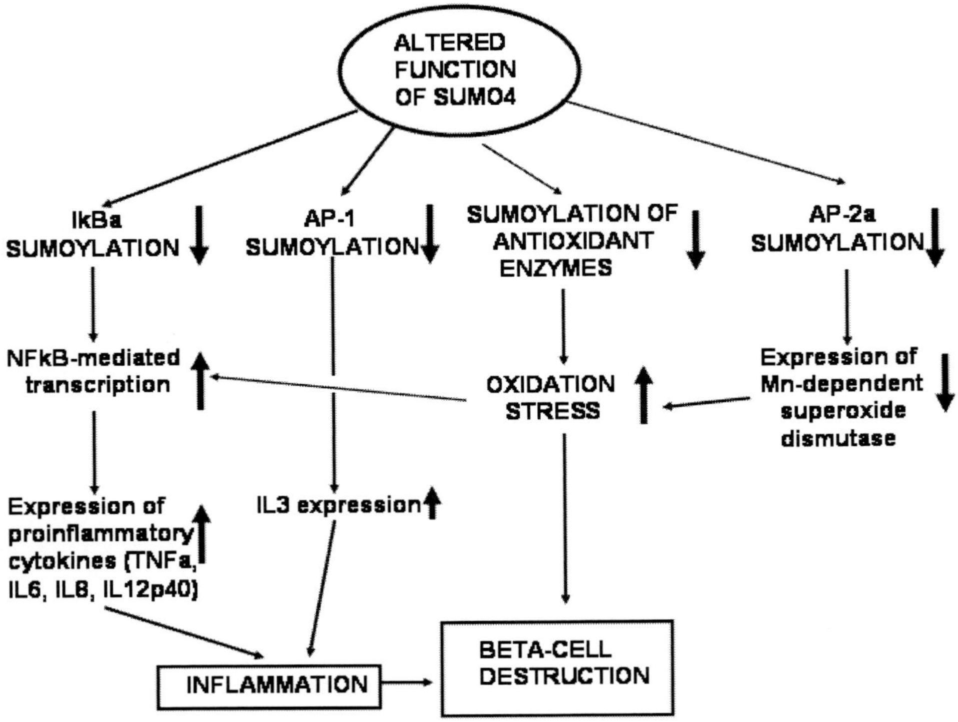

Figure 4. Possible mechanisms of the involvement of SUMO4 in the development of type 1 diabetes. Impaired function of SUMO4 could result in reduced sumoylation of IkBα and AP-1 that leads to the overexpression of NFκB- and AP-1-dependent proinflammatory cytokines and then to the activation of inflammatory response directed against beta-cells. Additionally, reduced activity of SUMO4 could affect symoylation of (and probably expression) of antioxidant enzymes and hence enhance oxidative stress. Oxidative stress directly or indirectly (through the induction of NFκB) causes beta-cell disruption and death. However, the effects of SUMO4 sumoylation on antioxidant enzymes are yet to be established. Additional mechanisms by which SUMO4 might contribute to the pathogenesis of T1D are needed to be elucidated.

higher risk Met55 variant of SUMO4, the expression of inflammatory cytokines is increased, a pathway is known to be implicated in autoimmune diseases.

The development of T1D is characterized with autoimmune-induced cellular stress that leads to the beta-cell destruction [138]. Many anti-stress proteins (Cu/Zn-dependent superoxide dismutase, catalase, peroxidoferrins, chaperons, valosin-containing protein, etc.) are the substrate for SUMO4-mediated sumoylation (Figure 4) [116], and therefore SUMO4 sumoylation of these anti-stress proteins could be a protective mechanism against intracellular stress by competing with ubiquitylation and thus stabilizing key anti-stress proteins by protecting them against degradation. Nevertheless, the molecular mechanisms by which SUMO4 contributes to T1D pathogenesis are still elusive and need further clarification.

Peroxisomal Proliferator-Activated Receptor-Gamma2 – A Link between Type 1 and Type 2 Diabetes?

The peroxisomal proliferator-activated receptor γ isoform 2 (PPARG2) is an established susceptibility marker for T2D. The PPARG2 gene encodes a member of the nuclear receptor superfamily that has regulatory functions in adipocyte differentiation and glucose homeostasis [139]. PPARγ is a target for a large family of antidiabetic drugs, the thiazolidinediones, that act as PPARγ agonists and increase hepatic and peripheral insulin action in T2D [140]. In isoform 2 of the receptor, the causal variant for T2D is a proline-to-alanine substitution in codon 12. An OR of 1.27 was estimated for the Pro allele of isoform 2 (p-value $=2.0\times10^{-8}$) in T2D [141]. This association is supported by functional data, as in vitro studies have shown that the protective Ala allele decreases the DNA-binding affinity of the PPARγ2, thus reducing its transcriptional activity [142].

However, Eftychi et al. [143] found a significantly preferable transfer of the risk allele Pro from parents to probands in a large family dataset (2,355 T1D families) of the European descent providing OR of 1.15 (p=0.018). In Danish family collection (490 families), the Ala allele was significantly overtransmitted to non-affected siblings suggesting for association with reduced risk of T1D (p=0.024) [144]. In addition, the Ala allele of PPARγ2 has been shown to be associated with greater exercise-induced improvement of insulin sensitivity measures in Finnish T1D patients [145].

The genetic data suggest that the Pro12Ala PPARG2 could represent an etiological variant not only for T2D but also for T1D, with the Pro12 allele as a common risk marker for both types of diabetes. Another locus responsible for shared susceptibility to both diseases was found in the insulin gene but with predisposition determined by opposite alleles of the 5' variable number tandem repeat locus [146].

Studies in NOD mice support the evidence for a role of PPARγ in autoimmune diabetes. Thiazolidinediones possess anti-inflammatory properties and decrease diabetes incidence in NOD mice [147]. The expression of PPARγ2 is increased in NOD mice, contributing to the bone loss through changes in marrow composition that results in decreased mature osteoblasts and increased adipose accumulation [148].

The Ala12 variant of PPARγ2 showed in vitro reduced binding to the PPAR-responsive element of several genes [142, 149]. Several studies have reported increased insulin sensitivity in carriers of the Ala12variant [142, 150, 151]. It would be interesting to test whether this marker is associated with the reduced beta-cell function that could explain the impact of PPARγ2 in diabetes. It might be hypothesized that increased insulin sensitivity decreases the secretory demand on the beta-cell modifying the phenotype, e.g. the age at clinical diabetes onset or the progression to clinical diabetes. This phenotype might be modulated by the Pro12Ala variant of PPARγ2.

PPARs can also repress gene expression in a DNA-binding–independent manner, by antagonizing the activities of other signal-dependent transcription factors such as NF-κB and activator protein-1 (AP-1) [152]. Therefore, altered activity of PPARγ may correlate with decreased PPAR-mediated signaling and hence increase transcriptional activity of NF-κB and AP-1 that enhances expression of proinflammatory cytokines, a prerequisite of beta-cell destruction. This could explain anti-inflammatory and anti-diabetic properties of PPARγ agonists in NOD mice. It is also shown that the agonists of PPARγ can reduce diabetic incidence in NOD mice through the suppression of intercellular adhesion molecule 1 expression (ICAM-1) and alteration of Th1/Th2 cytokine balance [153].

Intercellular Adhesion Molecule 1

Genetic Analyses

The ICAM1 gene coding for intercellular adhesion molecule 1, or CD54 antigen, is a strong functional candidate for T1D in the susceptibility locus on chromosome 19p13 mapped in UK affected sibpair families [154]. For a common polymorphism Lys469Glu (K469E) of ICAM1, case-control and family-based studies provided highly inconsistent results for association with T1D (see Tables 1 and 2).

We performed a simple meta-analysis that showed in pooled Scandinavian case-control samples, the patients homozygous for the E469 allele of the K469E marker have increased risk of T1D (p=0.0027; Table 1). Similarly, a meta-analysis in the combined family dataset (Romanian+Finnish+Dannish) also revealed a significantly more preferential transfer of the E469 allele to affected offsprings compared to non-diabetic siblings (p=0.00045; Table 2).

Nejencev et al. [160] found no association of the K469E with T1D in TDT analysis of a large multiethnic collection of 3695 families of European descent. However, the authors reported the association for another marker of ICAM1, Gly241Arg (R241G), with the R241 allele associated with lower risk of diabetes (relative risk (RR) = 0.91, p=0.03) [160]. In Swedish population, the association of a new common polymorphism (rs281432, C/G) found in intron 2 of the ICAM1 gene was recently showed (Figure 5) [158]. The C allele of this new marker was related to higher risk of disease (OR=1.644; p=0.026).

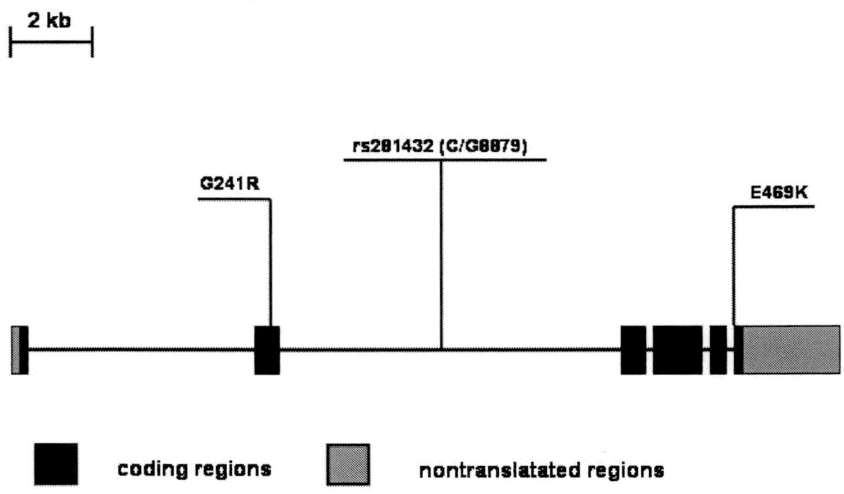

Figure 5. Structure of the intercellular adhesion molecule 1 (ICAM1) gene. The ICAM1 gene spans 15.5kb on chromosome 19p13. The location of three polymorphisms (G241R, rs281432, and E469K) that showed association with T1D is shown.

Table 1. Case-control studies of the ICAM1 K469 variant for association with type 1 diabetes

Population	n	Genotype, n (%)			p	Allele, n (%)		p	Ref.
K469E polymorphism		E/E	E/K	K/K		E469	K469		
Japanese									
Controls	171	21 (12.3)	87 (50.8)	63 (36.8)	-----	129 (37.7)	213 (62.3)	-----	[155]
Cases	164	30 (18.2)	77 (46.9)	57 (34.8)	NS	137 (41.8)	191 (58.2)	NS	
Young-onset T1D cases	90	10 (11.1)	40 (44.4)	40 (44.4)	NS	60 (33.3)	120 (66.7)	NS	
Young-onset T1D cases	74	20 (27.0)	37 (50.0)	17 (23.0)	0.0076	77 (52.0)	71 (48.0)	0.038	
Danish									
Controls	461	146 (31.7)	228 (49.4)	87 (18.9)	----	520 (56.4)	402 (43.6)	----	[156]
Cases	252	69 (27.4)	143 (56.7)	40 (15.9)	NS	281 (55.8)	223 (44.2)	NS	
Finnish									
Controls	212	55 (25.9)	106 (50.0)	51 (24.1)	----	216 (50.9)	208 (49.1)	----	[157]
Cases	218	57 (26.1)	103 (47.2)	58 (26.6)	NS	217 (49.7)	219 (50.2)	NS	
Swedish									
Controls	187	52 (27.8)	87 (46.5)	48 (25.7)	----	191 (51.1)	183 (48.9)	----	[158]
Cases	430	104 (24.3)	273 (63.4)	53 (12.3)	< 0.0001	481 (55.9)	379 (44.1)	NS	
All Scandinavians									
Controls	860	253 (29.4)	421 (48.9)	186 (21.7)	----	927 (53.9)	793 (46.1)	----	
Cases	900	230 (25.6)	519 (57.7)	151 (16.7)	0.0027	979 (54.4)	821 (45.6)	NS	

NS, nonsignificant.

Table 2. Family-based studies for association of ICAM-1 with type 1 diabetes

Population	n	Transmission to offspring		p	Reference
K469E polymorphism		K469 allele, n (%)	E469 allele, n (%)		
Romanian					
Unaffected	136	61 (47.3)	68 (52.7)	NS	[159]
Affected	212	70 (36.4)	122 (63.6)	0.0001	
Finnish					
Unaffected	60	46 (56.1)	36 (43.9)	NS	[157]
Affected	102	53 (50.0)	53 (50.0)	NS	
Danish					
Unaffected	252	104 (53.3)	91 (46.7)	NS	[156]
Affected	414	148 (48.5)	157 (51.5)	NS	
All Caucasians					
Unaffected	448	211 (52.0)	195 (48.0)	NS	
Affected	728	271 (44.9)	332 (55.1)	0.00045	
R241G polymorphism		R241 allele, n (%)	G241 allele, n (%)		
Finnish (affected)	1622	418	477	0.046	
British (affected)*	1467	235	295	0.014	
US Caucasians (affected)	573	102	198	NS	
Norwegian (affected)	366	70	65	NS	[160]
Romanian (affected)	307	55	39	NS	
Nothern Irish (affected)	268	58	62	NS	
All affected	4603	938	1036	0.003	

NS, nonsignificant.

Due to the significant inconsistence of the case-control and family studies, it is difficult to conclude whether the ICAM1 gene plays a role in the pathogenesis of T1D. The ICAM1 gene region needs to be further evaluated by GWA study in a large case-control sample using a high density of SNP markers. In a recent GWA scan, Todd et al. [161] found a suggestive association with T1D for SNP marker rs1051738 (OR=0.84; $p=1.51x10^{-4}$), representing an amino acid substitution (A479E) in the PDE4A gene (encodes cAMP-dependent phosphodiesterase 4A) on chromosome 19p13, in a large case-control dataset from UK (3,400 affected subjects and 3,300 controls). However, the association of this marker has not been replicated in the independent population collection (2,700 cases and 3,500 controls) [161].

Functional Studies and Possible Role of ICAM-1 in T1D

The E469K SNP is located in exon 6 encoding for Ig-like domain 5 [162]. Although the 5th Ig-like domain is not known to be involved in ligand binding, it has been shown to play a role for adhesion of B cells and dendritic cells [163]. The domain has also been demonstrated to be the ICAM-1-immunodominant epitope [164]. A recent study showed that the codon 469 SNP affects ICAM-1 mRNA splicing pattern and TPA-induced apoptosis [165]. The polymorphism is located at the three-base position upstream of the splice donor site that produces an alternatively spliced short isoform (ICAM-1S). The E469 variant correlates with lower amount of ICAM-1S mRNA [165]. Since the short isoform of ICAM-1 has no transmembrane and intracellular domain, ICAM-1 signal transduction and cell-cell contact including Fas-FasL interaction may be influenced. Iwao et al. [165] observed an increased apoptosis in peripheral blood mononuclear cells of an individual with the E/E genotype. These findings could highlight a role of the allele E469 as a risk factor in various inflammatory diseases and, probably, in diabetes. In addition, if the amino acid position 469 plays a role in the interaction between domain 1 and domain 5, this variation may affect dimerization of ICAM-1 molecule [166]. This may lead to the functional changes of heterozygous, though further studies will be needed.

The G241R marker resides in exon 4 that encodes the functionally important Ig-like domain 3 [162]. This domain is recognized by the integrin Mac-1. G241 is conserved across mammalian species and is also seen in immunoglobulin-like domains of other molecules (for example, in the μ chain of IgM). Thus, a non-conservative amino acid change from glycine to arginine might have a functional effect, which should be established in direct functional studies. Yang et al. [167] have reported a significant difference between anti-neutrophil cytoplasmic antibodies (ANCA)-positive and ANCA-negative patients with inflammatory bowel diseases in the frequency of the G241R polymorphism of ICAM-1. However, no interaction was detected between the presence/absence of self-antibodies against GAD65, a major antigen in T1D, and the codon 241 ICAM-1 gene polymorphism in Japanese patients [155].

The precise role of ICAM-1 in diabetes is not well established. ICAM-1 is a 90-kDa cell surface glycoprotein belonging to the immunoglobulin superfamily and it is involved in the firm attachment of leucocytes to endothelium [168]. It is likely that this adhesion molecule contributes to lymphocyte-endothelial cell interactions and accumulation of inflammatory monocytes into the pancreas [169]. ICAM-1 is shown to participate in the extravasation of lymphocytes from the circulation into the inflamed pancreas [170]. The expression of ICAM-1 on pancreatic β-cells was detected by electron microscopy, suggesting that ICAM-1 could be involved in the killer lymphocyte-mediated cytolysis of pancreatic beta-cells in T1D [171]. Treatment with monoclonal antibodies against ICAM-1 (or against soluble form of ICAM-1) and leukocyte function-associated antigen-1 (LFA-1) inhibited ICAM-1/LFA-1 interaction and prevented the development of insulitis in murine autoimmune diabetes [172, 173]. The latter finding is of potential human relevance since elevated circulating ICAM-1 levels have been found in human subjects prior or at onset of T1D [174]. A role of the soluble form of ICAM-1 in T1D needs to be further elucidated because this might provide an important functional link to the E469K variant of the molecule as a putative etiological marker for diabetes on chromosome 19p13.

Protein Tyrosine Phosphatase, Non-Receptor 2

The PTPN2 gene encoding T-cell protein tyrosine phosphatase (TC-PTP) is located on chromosome 18p11, a genomic region that provides a highly significant evidence for association with T1D in recent GWA scans [161, 175]. There are three common disease-associated SNPs located either within the PTPN2 gene (e.g., rs1893217 (C/T) and rs478582 (C/T) in intron 2 and 6, respectively) or near this gene (rs2542151, G/T) (Figure 6). Both SNPs of PTPN2 associated with diabetes are located within a 114 kb-long LD block that includes the entire PTPN2 gene [176].

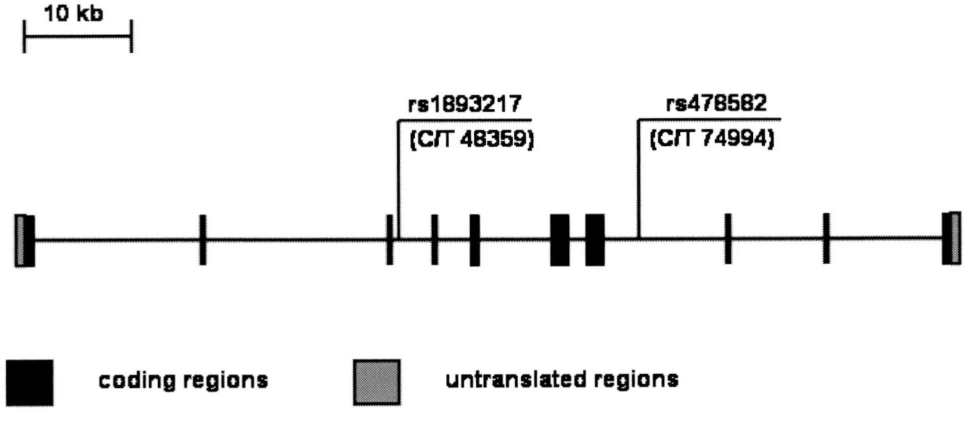

Figure 6. Structure of the protein tyrosine phosphatase, non-receptor 2 (PTPN2) gene encoding T-cell protein tyrosine phosphatase. The PTPN2 gene encompasses nearly 100 kb on chromosome 18p11 and includes 10 exons. The location of two SNPs associated with type 1 diabetes is shown.

Furthermore, the PTPN2 gene might represent a general autoimmunity locus. The T1D-associated rs2542151 marker also showed strong association with Grohn's disease (OR=1.15; $p=3.16x10^{-8}$) in a GWA-based search analysis of 1,182 affected and 2,024 control individuals from UK [177]. In addition, both markers within PTPN2 (rs1893217 and rs478582) that showed association with T1D were found to be associated with Graves' disease (OR=1.13

(p=0.0251) for rs1893217 and OR=0.91 (p=0.0239) for rs478582) [161]. These findings provide a strong evidence for the presence of a common susceptibility locus for T1D, GD and Grohn's disease on chromosome 18p11, with PTPN2 as a causal gene. However, additional studies are necessary to confirm this. All three disease-associated polymorphisms require functional evaluations to find an etiological marker(s) responsible for autoimmunity in the 18p11 genomic region.

The PTPN2 gene represents an attractive functional candidate for autoimmunity since it encodes T-cell protein phosphatase, a key negative regulator of inflammation [178]. TC-PTP and protein tyrosine phosphatase 1B (PTP1B), both are closely related to each other, negatively regulate insulin receptor (IR) signaling in peripheral tissues [179]. PTP1B and TC-PTP function in a coordinated and temporally distinct manner to achieve an overall regulation of IR phosphorylation and signaling [180]. The level and the extent of dephosphorylation of the IR and its downstream substrates reflect the balance between insulin-induced-IR self-phosphorylation, which stimulates the receptor kinase activity, and the PTPs that dephosporylate the IR and downstream substrates. Impaired IR signaling is linked to insulin resistance in T2D. It has been postulated that inhibition of such PTPs will result in prolonged insulin signaling, potentially counteracting T2D-associated insulin resistance [181]. The PTP1B locus have mapped to chromosome 20q13.1-q13.2, a region identified as a quantitative trait linked to insulin resistance and obesity [182, 183]. PTP1B, a collaborator of TC-PTP in regulating IR-mediated signaling, is an established therapeutic target for T2D [181].

TC-PTP is also involved in immune cell signaling [184]. Mice deficient for TC-PTP develop an inflammatory disorder characterized by chronic myocarditis, gastritis, and nephritis due to widespread tissue mononuclear cell infiltration. The pleiotropic defects observed in TC-PTP$^{-/-}$ mice indicate that TC-PTP targets a substrate or class of substrates involved in numerous signaling pathways in the immune response. In the TC-PTP-deficient mouse, the mononuclear cell infiltration results in dramatic increase of inflammatory cytokines (IFN-γ, TNF-α, and IL-2) and NO production that lead to massive myocyte and hepatic necrosis [185]. These findings suggest that TC-PTP downregulates IL-2 and IFN-γ-mediated signaling (that leads to the activation of macrophages and induction of the inflammatory response) through dephoshorylaton of JAK1 and JAK3 tyrosine kinases, participating in activation of the receptors for these cytokines (Figure 7) [186].

The systemic inflammation in the TC-PTP$^{-/-}$ mice is accomplished by higher levels of TNF-α in the serum that recruits and attracts monocytes and macrophages to sites of inflammation. TC-PTP is able to suppress TNF-α-mediated activation immune cells via binding to TRAF2, a component of TNF-α-signaling pathway, which targets TC-PTP to Src kinase (and hence to the subsequent inhibition of Erk-dependent signaling) (Figure 7) [187].

In addition, TC-PTP implies in the dephosphorylation of the downstream JAK effectors, the STATs that regulate transcription of many genes in the nuclear. STAT1, STAT5a and STAT5b are shown to be substrates for TC-PTP [188, 189]. Dephosphorylation of STAT5a/b by TC-PTP is associated with blocking the prolactin signaling [188]. These data suggest for a key role of TC-PTP in the regulation of inflammatory response and provide an essential background for putative involvement of certain TC-PTP variants in inflammatory and autoimmune diseases that need to be elucidated.

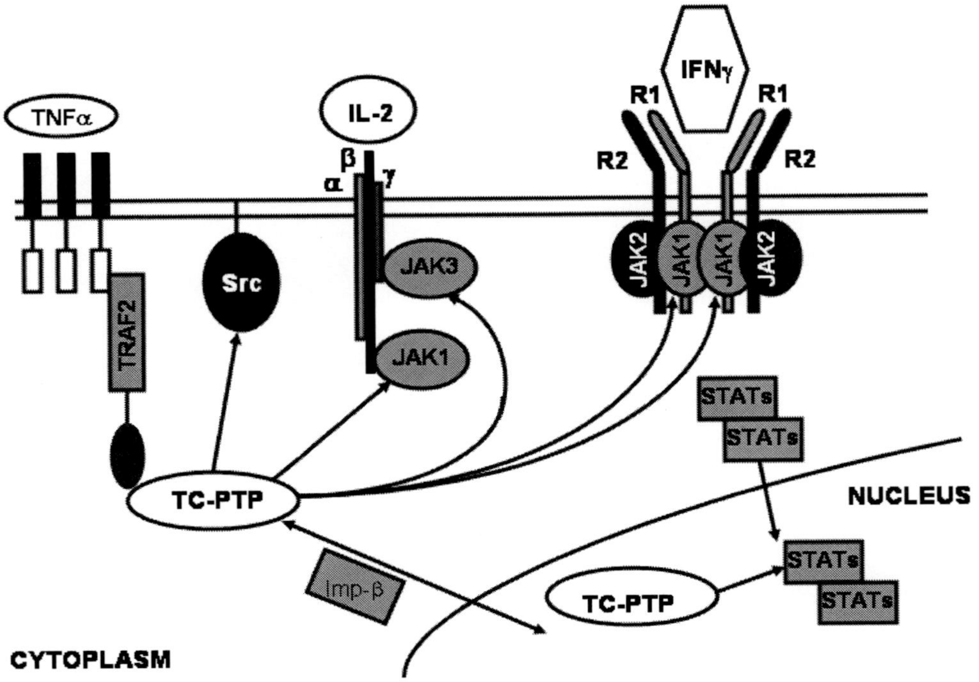

Figure 7. Substrates targeted by T-cell protein tyrosine phosphatase (TC-PTP). TC-PTP negatively regulates JAK/STAT signaling that leads to the induction of the inflammatory reaction. TC-PTP downregulates signaling mediated by proinflammatory cytokines (IFN-γ, TNF-α, IL-2) through the dephosphorylation of JAK1, JAK3 and Src kinases, which activate downstream signaling pathways induced by binding of the cytokines to their receptors. As a part of the complex with Importin-β (Imp-β), TC-PTP is able to shuttle from the cytoplasm to the nucleus, where the enzyme can dephosphorylate STATs, the molecules involved in signal transduction and activation of the transcription of a number of genes.

Other Genes

A Disintegrin and Metalloprotease Domain 33

Recently, an association with T1D was observed for rs2787094 (G/C) SNP in two independent family-based studies from UK, providing OR of 0.78 ($p=0.0004$) and 0.77 ($p=4.4\times10^{-6}$) in the 1st and 2nd datasets, respectively [190]. However, the association has not been supported by case-control analysis in 4,326 cases and 4,610 controls ($p=0.57$) [190]. The rs2787094 is located at position of +2900 or +2978 of the 3'UTR (exon 22) of the long and short isoform of a disintegrin and metalloprotease domain 33 (ADAM33), respectively.

The ADAM33 gene is located on chromosome 20p13, a region contained a proven susceptibility locus for asthma, bronchial hyperresponsiveness, and proriasis [191-194]. However, disease-associated SNPs for asthma and psoriasis lie in opposite ends of the gene: asthma markers reside the transcriptional regulatory region of intron 2 [195], while psoriasis markers are situated at 3'end of ADAM33 [194], where the diabetes-associated rs2787094 marker is located. The function of this SNPs is unclear, but some 3'UTR SNPs have been suggested to be involved in alternative splicing, splicing efficiency or mRNA turnover [196].

An alternative splicing could play an important role in the pathogenic role of ADAM33 since a variety of splice variants have been described [197].

ADAM33 belongs to the family of type 1 Zn^{2+}-dependent metalloproteases. Members of this family are membrane-anchored proteins structurally related to snake venom disintegrins, and have been implicated in a variety of biological processes involving cell-cell and cell-matrix interactions, including fertilization, muscle development, and neurogenesis. A major function of active ADAMs having a protease catalytic domain is proteolytic release of cell surface membrane proteins such as cytokines, growth factors, and receptors [198]. A physiological function of ADAM33 remains to be evaluated. Cleavage studies with synthetic peptides showed that the protease is able to in vitro digest insulin B chain and TNF-related activation-induced cytokine that makes a potential link between the ADAM33 function and diabetes [199].

CD226 Antigen

The region 18q22 showed consistent association with T1D in two large GWA studies [161, 175]. In the last GWA scan, a marker rs763361 (G/A) in the T lymphocyte costimulation gene CD226 was found to be strongly associated with disease (RR=1.18 for the minor allele A; $p_{overall}=1.38x10^{-8}$) in both case-control and family-based studies [161]. The rs763361 SNP also showed association with GD in a large case-control collection of UK patients (a total of 5,800 affected and healthy individuals), providing RR of 1.10 (p=0.0182) [161]. Hence, for CD226, preliminary results suggest for its role in conferring susceptibility to two organ-specific autoimmune diseases (T1D and GD).

CD226 is an excellent functional candidate for autoimmunity on chromosome 18q22. This gene encodes an intercellular adhesion molecule, a 65 kDa transmembrane glycoprotein that constitutively expressed on the surface of a variety of immune cells including natural killer (NK) cells, platelets, monocytes, peripheral blood T lymphocytes, and in a small subset of B cells [200]. CD226 is a member of Ig-superfamily and contains two Ig-like domains in its extracellular domain (Figure 8). The codon 307 polymorphism resides in the functionally important cytoplasmic domain that is responsible for signal transduction. However, it is unknown yet (and therefore, needs to be tested) whether this amino acid substitution influences the function of the CD226 cytosolic tail. CD226 antigen is involved in the lymphocyte function–associated antigen 1 (LFA-1)-mediated costimulatory signaling for triggering naive T cell differentiation and proliferation [201].

In CD4+ T lymphocytes, both LFA-1 and CD226 are recruited upon antigen recognition by the TCR. Phosphorylation of CD226 with TCR/CD3-induced serine protein kinase C (PKC) leads to physical association between CD226 and LFA-1 that takes CD226 into the lipid raft compartment [202]. Fyn protein tyrosine kinase phosphorylates the CD226 molecule thereby playing a role in the transduction of LFA-induced costimulatory signal for T cell proliferation and differentiation (Figure 9) [203].

In NK cells, CD226 cooperates with other triggering NK receptors in the induction of NK-mediated cytotoxicity [204]. The expression of CD226 in NK T cells from SLE patients is strongly suppressed likely due to the defective expression of the TCR ζ chain and increased intracellular free calcium concentration [205]. Consequently, the NK cells in SLE are highly vulnerable to anti-CD95-induced apoptosis, which is therefore triggered by CD226

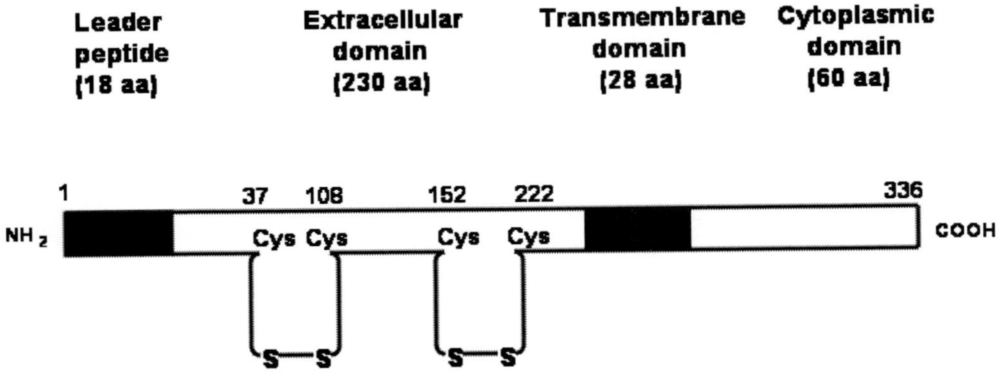

Figure 8. Schematic structure of the molecule of CD226 antigen. A CD226 precursor consists of 336 amino acid (a.a.) redidues. Proteolytic cleavage of the 18 a.a. signal sequence results in the formation of the 318 a.a. mature receptor molecule that comprises the extracellular, transmembrane, and cytoplasmic domains. The extracellular domain consists of two immunoglobulin-like subdomains and contains four cysteins linked with disulfide bridges.

antigen [206]. These findings highlight possible involvement of CD226 in autoimmunity. However, more studies are required to understand a role of this antigen in T1D and other autoimmune disorders.

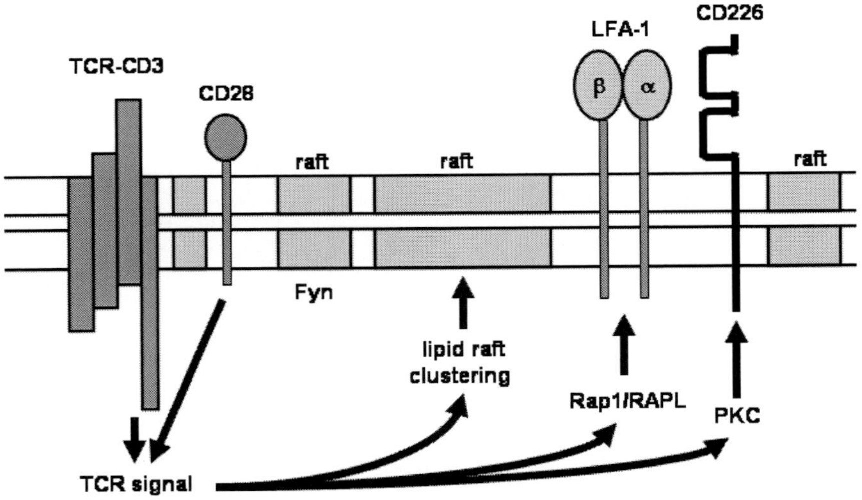

Figure 9. T-cell receptor (TCR) -induced recruitment of LFA-1 and CD226 in CD4+ T cell. Antigen presentation to TCR and costimulatory signal from CD28 activate the T cell. TCR-mediated signaling induces the formation of compartmentalized clusters with lipid rafts and association between small GTPase RAP with its activator RAPL. The RAP/RAPL complex associates with LFA-1. The TCR-mediated signal also induces the serine phosphorylation of CD226 by protein kinase C (PKC). The complex with RAP/RAPL/LFA-1 then accumulates in the lipid raft compartment, into which CD226 associates with LFA-1. Once activated LFA-1 binds its ligand ICAM expressed on the antigen-presenting cells, the LFA-1-mediated signal induces tyrosine phosphorylation of Fyn present in lipid raft compartment, by which DNAM-1 is then tyrosine phosphorylated, and mediates co-stimulatory signal for CD4+ Tcell proliferation and differentiation.

The 763361 marker of CD226 is predicted to be functional. This SNP resides in the final 3' exon 7 and alters the exon splicing silencer (ESS) sequence [161]. The disease-susceptible minor allele A (encodes Ser307) maintains the wild-type ESS sequence. This nucleotide position is crucial in splicing exon 7 of CD226 and is highly conserved in vertebrates. Therefore, compared to the resistant Gly307 allele, the predisposing Ser307 allele would have higher silencer function that reduces the productive splicing of exons 6 and 7. Indeed, the less mature CD226 mRNA production is expected to lead to less expression of CD226 antigen on the surface and less T cell activation [161]. However, this hypothesis needs to be supported by functional analyses in the future.

C-Type Lectin Domain Family 16, Member A

The SLEC16A (KIAA0350) gene encoding C-type lectin domain family 16, member A represents a causal gene conferring susceptibility to T1D on chromosome 16p13. The rs12708716 (A/G) SNP located in intron 19 of KIAA0350 showed a strong evidence for association with T1D in a large GWA scan for susceptibility markers to seven common diseases (trend p-value of 9.24×10^{-8}; OR for homozygous AA = 1.55) [175]. The association of this marker was then replicated in the second GWA screen of 4,000 affected individuals and 5,000 control subjects for T1D-predisposing loci (OR=0.83 for the minor allele G; $p=7.07\times10^{-9}$) [161].

Further analysis of the LD structure in the KIAA0350 gene region showed that this gene lies alone within the 233 kb-long LD block on chromosome 16p13.13, which is flanked but distinct from the neighboring strong functional candidates, CIITA (activator of the MHC class II gene) and SOCS1 (suppressor of cytokine signaling) (Figure 10) [207]. A GWA analysis of the extended KIAA0350 region in the Canadian dataset revealed a highly significant association with T1D (OR for a minor allele of 0.65-0.67; nominal p-value of less then 10^{-8}) for three SNPs, rs2903692 (A/G), rs725613 (C/A) and rs17673553 (G/A), located within the KIAA0350 [207]. All three markers were in strong LD to each other.

Studies are underway to characterize the functional role of KIAA0350. The predicted protein product of KIAA0350 exhibits similarities to a subset of adhesion and immune function signaling molecules. This gene encodes a protein with a calcium-dependent, or C-type, lectin-binding domain structure. Proteins of this type are known to be involved with calcium current flux, and the predicted function of the protein encoded by KIAA0350 includes sugar binding. The C-type lectins are known for their recognition of various carbohydrates and are crucial for processes that range from cell adhesion to pathogen recognition [208]. The C-type lectin domain family 16, member A, encoding by the KIAA0350 gene is a 'non-classical' C-type lectin that lacks the residues involved in calcium binding. It shown that SLEC16A is highly expressed in different NK cell lines and dendritic cells, hence, suggesting for a putative role of this surface receptor in innate immunity and recognition of the MHC class I and related molecules [209, 210].

The etiological variant of SLEC16 remains to be found and then functionally characterized. Hakonarson and coauthors [207] have attempted to evaluate functional relevance of a synonymous SNP in exon 19 (rs2286973, A/G) that is in strong LD with rs725613 and rs2903692, but found no influence of this polymorphism to a steady-state mRNA. However, they observed the highest levels of SLEC16A mRNA in the NKL cell line that is only one of four NK lines tested homozygous for the risk allele A of rs2903692. This could suggest on a potential functional significance of this T1D-aasosiated marker.

V-erb-b2 Erythroblastic Leukemia Viral Oncogene Homolog 3 (Avian)

A marker rs2292239 (C/A) located in intron 7 at nucleotide 8288 of the ERBB3 gene showed consistently association with T1D in two GWA screens, with an overall p-value of 6.46×10^{-19} (OR=1.28) [161, 175]. The ERBB3 gene resides on chromosome 12q13 and codes for a homolog of avian V-erb-b2 erythroblastic leukemia viral oncogene 3. The association of ERBB3 with T1D needs further confirmation in additional studies involving large datasets.

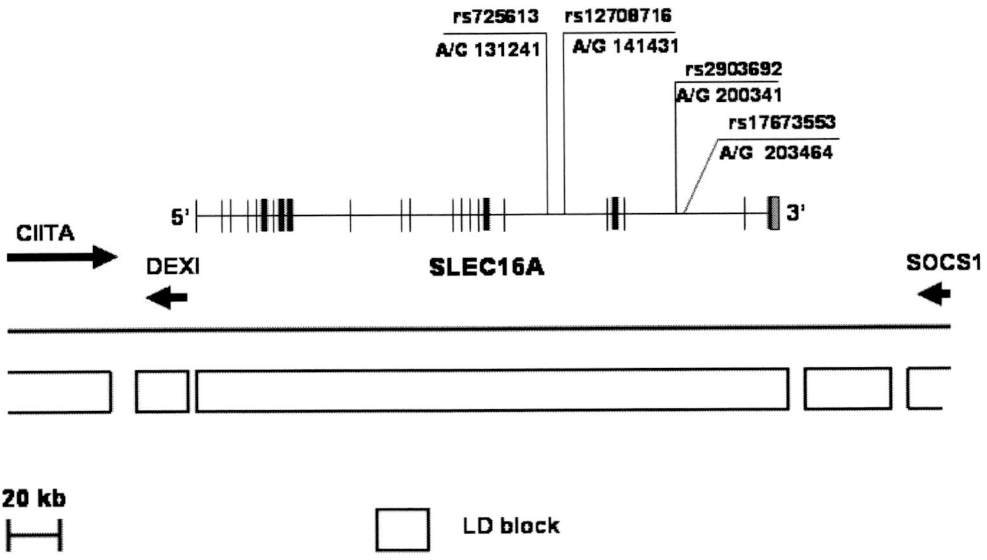

Figure 10. A 380-kb chromosome 16p13.13 region containing the SLEC16A (C-type lectin domain family 16, member A), CIITA (class II, major histocompatibility complex, transcactivator), DEXI (dexamethasone-induced transcript), and SOCSI (suppressor of cytokine signaling 1) genes. The entire SLE16A (KIAA0350) gene lies within the 233-kb LD block. The exon-intron structure of SLE16A is shown. The positions of SNPs the most highly associated with T1D are presented.

This gene encodes a member of the epidermal growth factor receptor (EGFR) family of receptor tyrosine kinases. This membrane-bound protein has a neuregulin-binding domain but not an active kinase domain. It therefore can bind this ligand but not convey the signal into the cell through protein phosphorylation. However, it forms heterodimers with other EGF receptor family members, which do have kinase activity. Heterodimerization leads to the activation of pathways, which lead to proliferation or differentiation of a variety of cell types [211]. Amplification of this gene and/or overexpression of its protein have been reported in numerous cancers, including prostate, bladder, and breast tumors. Alternate transcriptional splice variants encoding different isoforms have been characterized. Interestingly, one ERBB3 isoform lacks the intermembrane region and is secreted outside the cell. This form acts to modulate the activity of the membrane-bound form [212].

In cultured hepatocytes, a suppression of ERBB3 expression by insulin through the downregulation of PI3 kinase was observed [213]. In diabetic rats, with altered insulin-dependent metabolism, the ERBB3 expression is reduced and associated with erectile dysfunction that is a consequence of neurovascular abnormalities and hypertension [214]. Due to the pivotal function of ERBB3 in the development of the nervous system [215], this evidence could suggest for a potential role of this receptor in neuronal complications of diabetes.

The TENR-IL2-IL21 Region

The TENR-IL2-IL21 genomic region on human chromosome 4q27 corresponds to the susceptibility locus for autoimmune diabetes idd3 on murine chromosome 3 [216]. Two recent GWA studies found that two SNP (rs17388568 and rs3136534) located within this region are significantly associated with T1D [161, 175]. The most associated marker rs17388568 (G/A) showed association with disease in case-control dataset and affected families, providing OR of 1.11 (for allele A; $p_{overall}$=5.57x10^{-5}) [161]. Both disease-associated markers are situated 5' the IL2 gene; the 17388568 SNP is located in intron 8 of ADAD1 (TENR) encoding adenosine deaminase containing domain 1 (testis specific) (Figure 11). The product of the ADAD1 gene is expressed exclusively in testis, has ability to bind to a variety of RNAs and contributes to testis-specific heterogeneous nuclear RNA packaging, alternative splicing and probably to nuclear/cytoplasmic transport of mRNAs [217].

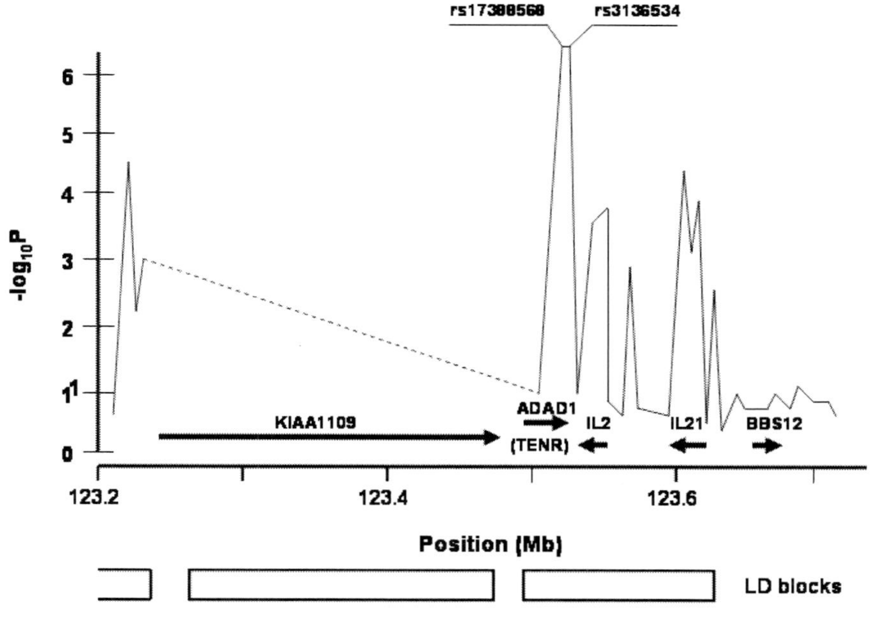

Figure 11. A plot reflecting the strength of association with T1D of SNPs on chromosome 4q27. The vertical scale defines the strength of association (-log_{10} of a P-value for every tag SNP tested). The horizontal scale represents a physical distance in megabases (Mb) from a p-terminus of chromosome 4. Positions of the most associated markers (rs17388568 and rs3136534) are shown. Since the IL2 gene shares the same LD block with the ADAD1 gene, the etiological variant that needs to be found is likely to lie within the IL2 gene. However, association with IL21 could not be ruled out because this gene remains to be a strong functional candidate for susceptibility to T1D on chromosome 4q27.

It is unlikely that ADAD1 could play a role in T1D pathogenesis due to its function and testis-specific expression. However, the chromosome region 4q27 has two strong positional and functional candidates, IL-2 and IL-21, both involved in immune regulation. We have discussed above the role of the causal gene Il2 in the etiology of diabetes in NOD mice. Similarly, either IL2 or IL21 is likely to confer susceptibility to T1D in humans. The IL-2 and IL21 genes both share the same LD block with ADAD1 (Figure 11), and hence rs17388568 and rs3136534 could be in LD with etiological marker(s) located in the IL2 gene.

Furthermore, the TENR-IL2-IL21 region is shown to be involved in susceptibility to multiple autoimmune and inflammatory diseases such as T1D, GD [161], RA [218], celiac disease [219], and probably systemic sclerosis [220]. Thus, this locus harbors a susceptibility gene involved in general autoimmunity. An etiological variant(s) controlling susceptibility to T1D and general autoimmunity on chromosome 4q27 has to be identified. Besides IL-2, IL-21 also represents a strong functional candidate due to its important role in maintaining T cell homeostasis [221]. In NOD mice, lymphopenia and its compensatory homeostatic expansion are observed to drive autoimmunity against pancreatic beta-cells trough their enhanced responses to IL-21 [222]. Asano et al. [223, 224] studied association of IL-21 with T1D in Japanese but obtained inconsistent results.

The Rregion 5p13

A significant association with T1D on chromosome 5p13 was observed in the last GWA [161]. Of the most-associated 14 SNPs, three were in strong LD with each other. There are rs3194051, rs6897932 (both in the IL7 receptor (IL7R) gene), and rs 1445898 in the CAPSL gene (Figure 12). All three disease-associated markers cause amino acid substitutions. The rs1445898 (A/G) is situated in exon 3 and causes a glutamine-to-arginine change in codon 75 (Q75R) of CAPSL. The CAPSL gene encodes calcyphosine-like protein with unknown function that has two Ca^{2+}-binding motifs. The Q75R dimorphism resides in one of these motifs and indeed could be potentially functional. Calcyphosine is a Ca2+-binding protein, which functions in Ca2+-dependent signaling in the central nervous system and peripheral neurons [225].

The rs3194051 (G/A) SNP resides in exon 8 of the IL7R gene and leads to a valine-to-isoleucine change in codon 356 (V356I). The marker rs6897932 (T/C) is located in exon 6 of IL7R and changes isoleucine to threonine in position 244 (I244T). The rs6897932 is shown to be functional since it alters the sequence of putative ESS and hence influences the amount of soluble and membrane-bound isoforms of the IL-7R [226]. Furthermore, the I244T polymorphism showed a strong association with multiple sclerosis (MS) that makes this marker a likely etiological variant explaining susceptibility to autoimmune diseases (T1D and MS) on chromosome 5p37 [226-229].

In the 5p13 susceptibility locus, IL-7R represents the strongest functional candidate for a causal gene due to emerging role of its ligand, interleukin-7, in maintaining naïve and memory T cell homeostasis in peripheral immune system and preventing apoptosis of T lymphocytes [230]. The IL7R gene encodes the alpha-chain of the interleukin-7 receptor, which associates with the interleukin 2 receptor gamma-chain (IL2RG) to form the functional receptor molecule [231]. The IL2RG is a common gamma chain shared by the receptors of various cytokines, including interleukin 2, 4, 7, 9, and 15 [232]. The IL-7R plays a critical role in the V(D)J recombination during lymphocyte development. A mouse, fully or even partially deficient for Il7r, develops severe combined immunodeficiency syndrome accompanied with markedly reduced circulating T cells [233].

A role of IL-7/IL-7R-mediated pathway in T1D needs to be clarified. The IL-7/IL-7R-dependent regulation of immune tolerance is associated with CD4+CD25+ regulatory T cell function, a subset of T cells, that express considerably higher levels of the IL-7 receptor

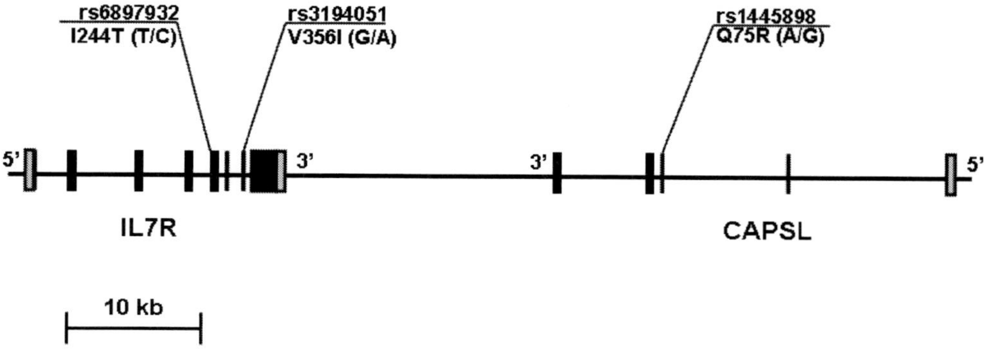

Figure 12. Structure of the interleukin-7 receptor (ILR7) and calcyphosine-like (CAPSL) genes containing SNPs (rs6897932, rs3194051, and rs1445898) highly associated with T1D. All three SNPs are in strong linkage disequilibrium.

alpha-chain than CD4+CD25- T lymphocytes [234] \. IL-7 plays a critical role in survival of this subset of Tregs and, together with other cytokines, IL-2, IL-4, and IL-15, maintains an optimal suppressive potency of CD4+CD25+ Tregs [234, 235]. In MS patients, an altered expression of both IL-7 and its receptor is shown [229]. Disturbances in IL-7/IL-7R expression could influence both survival and suppressive function of the CD4+CD25+ Tregs and break the peripheral tolerance thereby causing autoimmunity.

Conclusion

With the relative failing of linkage and candidate gene association studies, there had been much sceptism about the ability of geneticists to identify genes for common, complex disorders. Vast amounts of resources were poured into these studies, with very limited success. Recent technological advances, and a better understanding of the genetic architecture of complex diseases, has led to the development of the GWA study, which is a powerful new approach to identifying genes influencing predisposition to common, complex disease. Genome-wide studies are 'hypothesis-free' and allow the identification of previously unsuspected genes and pathways in disease aetiology. The initial success of many GWA studies has certainly brought much excitement to the genetics community, and we finally have the ability to systematically identify the genetic variants underlying a range of common disorders.

For T1D, a majority of loci discovered in GWA studies need independent confirmation by other GWA scans, with exploiting well-characterized, large-scale population and family cohorts. In some cases, it is difficult to distinguish between two or several highly associated SNPs due to the strong LD. Implication of denser SNP microarray platforms should help in genetic dissection of these LD blocks to identify a true etiological marker. Genetic findings should be supported by comprehensive functional analyses to characterize a role of a putative causal variant in etiology of diabetes. This provides the opportunity to discover new targets to develop new effective antidiabetic drugs and therapeutic approaches.

Is should be stressed that many of the new loci associated with T1D also predispose to other autoimmune diseases. This could be attributed to IL2RA/CD25, PTPN2, IL2/IL21, CD226, IL7R and likely SUMO-4, the genes with proven or putative susceptibility for T1D. These genes are involved in the immune regulation, particularly in controlling T-cell homeostasis, and hence alterations in these genes could underline T-cell mediated autoimmunity. The discovery of causal genetic markers for general autoimmunity greatly benefits understanding general pathophysiological mechanisms of autoimmune pathology and design of common strategies in the treatment of autoimmune diseases with shared etiology and shared genetic background.

As a type of genetic research, GWA approach is still in its infancy, and as we have only just acquired the ability, through GWA studies, to identify a large number of common disease genes, it is unsurprising that there has been no major impact of this research on clinical practice as yet. We expect there will be a great benefit to clinical medicine in the years to come, and whilst prediction of disease and pharmacogenetics may eventually prove valuable, the greatest clinical benefit of GWA studies is likely to come from etiological insights into disease processes.

References

[1] Rewers, M.J. (1991). The changing face of the epidemiology of insulin-dependent diabetes mellitus (IDDM): research designs and models of disease causation. *Annals of Medicine, 23*, 419–426.

[2] Knowler, W.C., Lebovitz, H., Lernmark, A., Nathan, D., Palmer, J., Rizza, R., Saudek, C., Salomon, B., Lenschow, D.J., Rhee, L., Ashourian, N., Singh, B., Sharpe, A. and Bluestone, J.A. (2000). B7/CD28 costimulation is essential for the homeostasis of the CD4+CD25+ immunoregulatory T cells that control autoimmune diabetes. *Immunity, 12,* 431– 440.

[3] Noble, J.A., Valdes, A.M., Cook, M., Klitz, W., Thomson, G. and Erlich, H.A. (1996). The role of HLA class II genes in insulin-dependent diabetes mellitus: molecular analysis of 180 Caucasian, multiplex families. *American Journal of Human Genetics, 59*, 1134–1148.

[4] Onkamo, P., Vaananen, S., Karvonen, M. and Tuomilehto, J. (1999). Worldwide increase in incidence of type 1 diabetes: the analysis of the data on published incidence trends. *Diabetologia, 42*, 1395–1403.

[5] Hirshhorn, J.N. (2003). Genetic epidemiology of type 1 diabetes. *Pediatric Diabetes, 4,* 87–100.

[6] Pociot, F. and McDermott, M.F. (2002). Genetics of type 1 diabetes mellitus. *Genes and Immunity,* 3, 235–249.

[7] Rich, S.S. (1990). Mapping genes in diabetes: a genetic epidemiological perspective. *Diabetes, 39,* 1315–1319.

[8] Ronningen, K.S., Keiding, N. and Green, A. (2001). EURODIAB ACE Study Group: Europe and diabetes: correlations between the incidence of childhood-onset type I diabetes in Europe and HLA genotypes. *Diabetologia, 44, Suppl. 3,* B51–B59.

[9] Valdes, A.M., Noble, J.A., Genin, E., Clerget-Darpoux, F., Erlich, H.A. and Thomson, G. (2001). Modeling of HLA class II susceptibility to type 1 diabetes reveals an effect associated with DPB1. *Genetic Epidemiology, 21,* 212–223.

[10] Bell, G.I., Horita, S. and Karam, J.H. (1984). A polymorphic locus near the human insulin gene is associated with insulin-dependent diabetes mellitus. *Diabetes, 33,* 176 – 183.

[11] Davies, J.L., Kawaguchi, Y., Bennett, S.T., Copeman, J.B., Cordell, H.J., Pritchard, L.E., Reed, P.W., Gough, S.C.L., Jenkins, S.C., Palmer, S.M., Balfour, K.M., Row, B., Farrall, M., Barnett, A.H., Bain, S.C. and Todd, J.A. (1994). A genome-wide search for human type 1 diabetes susceptibility genes. *Nature, 371,* 130 –136.

[12] Hashimoto, L., Habita, C., Beressi, J., Delepine, M., Besse, C., Cambon-Thomsen, A., Deschamps, I., Rotter, J., Djoulah, S., James, M., Froguel, P., Weissenbach, J., Lathrop, G.M. and Julier, C. (1994). Genetic mapping of a susceptibility locus for insulin-dependent diabetes mellitus on chromosome 11q. *Nature, 371,*161–164.

[13] Melanitou, E., Fain, P. and Eisenbarth, G.S. (2003). Genetics of type 1A (immune mediated) diabetes. *Journal of Autoimmunity, 21,* 93–98.

[14] Julier, C., Lucassen, A., Villedieu, P., Delepine, M., Levy-Marchal, C., Danze, P.M., Bianchi, F., Boitard, C., Froguel, P. and Bell, J. (1994). Multiple DNA variant association analysis: application to the insulin gene region in type I diabetes. *American Journal of Human Genetics, 55,* 1247–1254.

[15] Ueda, H., Howson, J.M., Esposito, L., Heward, J., Snook, H., Chamberlain, G., Rainbow, D.B., Hunter, K.M., Smith, A.N., Di Genova, G., Herr, M.H., Dahlman, I., Payne, F., Smyth, D., Lowe, C., Twells, R.C., Howlett, S., Healy, B., Nutland, S., Rance, H.E., Everett, V., Smink, L.J., Lam, A.C., Cordell, H.J., Walker, N.M. Bordin, C., Hulme, J., Motzo, C., Cucca, F., Hess, J.F., Metzker, M.L., Rogers, J., Gregory, S., Allahabadia, A., Nithiyananthan, R., Tuomilehto-Wolf, E., Tuomilehto, J., Bingley, P., Gillespie, K.M., Undlien, D.E., Ronningen, K.S., Guja, C., Ionescu-Tirgoviste, C., Savage, D.A., Maxwell, A.P., Carson, D.J., Patterson, C.C., Franklyn, J.A., Clayton, D.G., Peterson, L.B., Wicker, L.S., Todd, J.A and Gough, S.C. (2003). Association of the T-cell regulatory gene CTLA4 with susceptibility to autoimmune disease. *Nature, 423,* 506 –511.

[16] Bottini, N., Musumeci, L., Alonso, A., Rahmouni, S., Nika, K., Rostamkhani, M., MacMurray, J., Meloni, G.F., Lucarelli, P., Pellecchia, M., Eisenbarth, G.S., Comings, D. and Mustelin, T. (2004). A functional variant of lymphoid tyrosine phosphatase is associated with type I diabetes. *Nature Genetics, 36,* 337–338.

[17] Chistiakov, D.A. (2007). New advances in the genetics and treatment of type 1 diabetes mellitus and late diabetic complications. New York, USA: Nova Publishers, Inc.

[18] Todd, J.A. (2006). Statistical false positive or true disease pathway? *Nature Genetics, 38,* 731-733.

[19] The International HapMap Consortium (2003). The international HapMap project. *Nature, 426,* 789–796.

[20] Pritchard, J.K. (2001). Are rare variants responsible for susceptibility to complex diseases? *American Journal of Human Genetics, 69,* 124–137.

[21] Nistico, L., Buzzetti, R., Pritchard, E., Van der Auwera, B., Giovanni, C., Bosi, E., Larrad, M.T., Rios, M.G., Chow, C.C., Cockram, C.S., Jakobs, K., Mijovic, C., Bain, S.C., Barnett, A.H., Vandewalle, C.L., Shuit, F., Gorus, F.K., Tosi, R., Pozzilli, P. and Todd, J.A. (1996). The CTLA-4 gene region of chromosome 2q33 is linked to, and associated with, type 1 diabetes. *Human Molecular Genetics, 5,* 1075–1080.

[22] Altmuller, J., Palmer, L.J., Fischer, G., Scherb, H. and Wjst, M. (2001). Genome-wide scans of complex human diseases: true linkage is hard to find. *American Journal of Human Genetics, 69,* 936–950.

[23] Cox, N. J., Walephorst, B., Morrison, V.A., Johnson, L., Pinchuk, L., Spielman, R.S., Todd, J.A. and Concannon, P. (2001). Seven regions of the genome show evidence of linkage to type 1 diabetes in a consensus analysis of 767 multiplex families. *American Journal of Human Genetics, 69,* 820–830.

[24] Sawcer, S.J., Maranian, M., Sunglehurst, S., Yeo, T., Compston, A., Daly, M.J., De Jager, M.J., Gabriel, S., Hafler, D.A., Ivinson, A.J., Lander, E.S., Rioux, J.D., Walsh, E., Gregory, S.G., Schmidt, S., Pericak-Vance, M.A., Barcellos L., Hauser, S.L., Oksenberg, J.R., Kenealy, S.J. and Haines, J.L. (2004). Enhancing linkage analysis of complex disorders: an evaluation of high-density genotyping. *Human Molecular Genetics, 13,* 1943–1949.

[25] Risch, N.J. (2000). Searching for genetic determinants in the new millennium. *Nature, 405,* 847–856.

[26] Chakravarti, A. (1999). Population genetics — making sense out of sequence. *Nature Genetics, 21,* 56–60.

[27] Reich, D.E. and Lander, E.S. (2001). On the allelic spectrum of human disease. *Trends in Genetics, 17,* 502–510.

[28] Gregersen, P.K. (2005). Gaining insight into PTPN22 and autoimmunity. *Nature Genetics, 37*, 1300-1301.

[29] European Consortium for IDDM Genome Studies. (2001). A genome wide scan for type 1-diabetes susceptibility in Scandinavian families: identification of new loci with evidence of interactions. *American Journal of Human Genetics, 69,* 1301-1313.

[30] Concannon, P., Erlich, H.A., Julier, C., Morahan, G., Nerup, J., Pociot, F., Todd, J.A. and Rich, S.S.; Type 1 Diabetes Genetics Consortium. (2005). Type 1 diabetes: evidence for susceptibility loci from four genome-wide linkage scans in 1,435 multiplex families. *Diabetes, 54,* 2995-3001.

[31] Tabor, H.K., Risch, N.J. and Myers, R.M. (2002). Candidate-gene approaches for studying complex genetic traits: practical considerations. *Nature Reviews Genetics, 3,* 391–397.

[32] Hirschhorn, J.N. and Altshuler, D. (2002). Once and again — issues surrounding replication in genetic association studies. *Journal of Clinical Endocrinology Metabolism, 87,* 4438–4441.

[33] Cardon, L.R. and Bell, J.I. (2001). Association study designs for complex diseases. *Nature Reviews Genetics, 2,* 91–99.

[34] Hirschhorn, J.N., Lohmueller, K., Byrne, E. and Hirschhorn, K. (2002). A comprehensive review of genetic association studies. *Genetic Medicine, 4,* 45–61.

[35] Lohmueller, K.E., Pearce, C.L., Pike, M., Lander, E.S. and Hirschhorn, J.N. (2003). Meta-analysis of genetic association studies supports a contribution of common variants to susceptibility to common disease. *Nature Genetics, 33,* 177–182.

[36] Matsuzaki, H., Loi, H., Donq, S., Tsai, Y.Y., Fang, J., Low, J., Di, X., Li, W.M., Yang, G., Liu, G., Huang, J., Kennedy, G.C., Ryder, T.B., Mercus, G.A., Walsh, P.S., Shriver, M.D., Puck, J.M., Jones, K.W. and Mei, R. (2004). Parallel genotyping of over 10,000 SNPs using a one-primer assay on a high-density oligonucleotide array. *Genome Research, 14,* 414–425.

[37] Kruglyak, L. and Nickerson, D.A. (2001).Variation is the spice of life. *Nature Genetics, 27,* 234–236.

[38] Jorde, L.B. (2000). Linkage disequilibrium and the search for complex disease genes. *Genome Research, 10,* 1435–1444.

[39] Daly, M.J., Rioux, J.D., Schaffner, S.F., Hudson, T.J. and Lander, E.S. (2001). High-resolution haplotype structure in the human genome. *Nature Geneics, 29,* 229–232.

[40] Johnson, G. C., Esposito, L., Barratt, B.J., Smith, A.N., Heward, J., Di Genova, G., Ueda, H., Cordell, H.J., Eaves, I.A., Dudbridge, F., Twells, R.C., Payne, F., Hughes, W., Nutland, S., Stevens, H., Carr, P., Tuomilehto-Wolf, E., Tuomilehto, J., Gough, S.C., Clayton, D.G. and Todd, J.A. (2001). Haplotype tagging for the identification of common disease genes. *Nature Genetics, 29,* 233–237.

[41] Carlson, C.S., Eberle, M.A., Kruglyak, L. and Nickerson, D.A. (2004). Mapping complex disease loci in whole-genome association studies. *Nature, 429,* 446–452.

[42] Ke, X. and Cardon, L.R. (2003). Efficient selective screening of haplotype tag SNPs. *Bioinformatics, 19,* 287–288.

[43] Stram, D.O., Honman, C.A., Hirschholm, J.N., Altshuler, D., Kolonel, L.N., Henderson, B.E. and Pike, M.C. (2003). Choosing haplotype-tagging SNPs based on unphased genotype data using a preliminary sample of unrelated subjects with an example from the Multiethnic Cohort Study. *Human Heredity, 55,* 27–36.

[44] Botstein, D. and Risch, N. (2003). Discovering genotypes underlying human phenotypes: past successes for mendelian disease, future approaches to complex disease. *Nature Genetics, 33 (Suppl.),* 228-237.

[45] Cargill, M., Altshuller, D., Ireland, J., Sklar, P., Ardlie, K., Patil, N., Shaw, N., Lane, C.R., Lim, E.P., Kalyanaraman, N., Nemesh, J., Ziaugra, L., Friedland, L., Roffe, A., Warrington, J., Lipshutz, R., Daley, G.Q. and Lander, E.S. (1999). Characterization of single-nucleotide polymorphisms in coding regions of human genes. *Nature Genetics, 22,* 231–238 (1999).

[46] Waterston, R.H., Lindlad-Toh, K., Birney, E., Rogers, J., Abril, A.F., Agarwal, P., Agarwala, R., Ainscough, R., Alexandersson, M., An, P., Antonarakis, S.E., Attwood,

J., Baertsch, R., Bailey, J., Barlow, K., Beck, S., Berry, E., Birren, B., Bloom, T., Bork, P., Botcherby, M., Bray, N., Brent, M.R., Brown, B.G., Brown, S.D., Bult, C., Burton, J., Butler, J., Campbell, R.D., Carcinci, P., Cawley, S., Chiaromonte, F., Chinwalla, A.T., Church, D.M., Clamp, M., Clee, C., Collins, F.S., Cook, L.L., Copley, R.R., Coulson, A., Couronne, O., Cuff, J., Curwen, V., Cutts, T., Daly, M., David, R., Davies, J., Delehaunty, K.D., Deri, J., Dermitzakis, E.T., Dewey, C., Dickens, N.J., Diekhans, M., Dodge, S., Dudchak, I., Dunn, D.M., Eddu, S.R., Elnitski, L., Emes, R.D., Eswara, P., Eyras, E., Felsenfeld, A., Fewell, G.A., Flicek, P., Foley, K., Frankel, W.N., Fulton, L.A., Fulton, R.S., Furey, T.S., Gage, D., Gibbs, R.A., Glusman, G., Gnerre, S., Goldman, N., Goodstadt, L., Grafham, D., Graves, T.A., Green, E.D., Gregory, S., Guigo, R., Guyer, M., Hardison, R.C., Haussler, D., Hayashizaki, Y., Hillier, L.W., Hinrichs, A., Hlavina, W., Holzer, T., Hsu, F., Hua, A., Hubbard, T., Hunt, A., Jackson, I., Jaffe, D.B., Johnson, L.S., Jones, M., Jones, T.A., Joy, A., Kamal, M., Karlsson, E.K., Karolchik, D., Kasprzyk, A., Kawai, J., Keibler, E., Kells, C., Kent, M.J., Kirby, A., Kolbe, D.L., Korf, I., Kucherlapati, R.S., Kulbokas, E.J., Kulp, D., Landers, T., Leger, J.P., Leonard, S., Letunic, I., Levine, R., Li, J., Li, M., Lloyd, C., Lucas, S., Ma, B., Maglott, D.R., Mardis, E.R., Matthews, L., Mauceli, E., Mayer, J.H., McCarthy, M., McCombie, W.R., McLaren, S., McLay, K., McPherson, J.D., Meldrim, J., Meredith, B., Mesirov, J.P., Miller, W., Miner, T.L., Mongin, E., Montgomery, K.T., Morgan, M., Mott, R., Mullikin, J.C., Muzny, D.M., Nash, W.E., Nelson, J.O., Nhan, M.N., Nicol, P., Ning, Z., Nusbaum, O., O'Connor, M.J., Okazaki, Y., Oliver, K., Overton-Larty, E., Pachter, I., Parra, G., Pepin, K.H., Peterson, J., Revzner, P., Plumb, R., Pohl, C.S., Poliakov, A., Ponce, T.C., Ponting, P.C., Potter, S., Quail, M., Reymond, A., Roe, B.A., Roskin, K.M., Rubin, E.M., Rust, A.G., Santos, S., Sapojnikov, V., Schultz, J., Schwartz, M.S., Schwartz, S., Scott, C., Seaman, S., Searle, S., Sharpe, T., Sheridan, A., Shownkeen, R., Sims, S., Singer, J.B., Slater, G., Smit, A., Smith, D.R., Spencer, B., Stabenau, A., Stange-Thomann, N., Sugnet, C., Suyama, M., Tesler, G., Rhompson, J., Torrents, D., Trevaskis, E., Tromp, J., Ucla, C., Ureta-Vidal, A., Vinson, J.P., Von Niederhausern, A.C., Wade, C.M., Wall, M., Weber, R.J., Weiss, R.B., Wendl, M.C., West, A.P., Wetterstrand, K., Wheeler, R., Whelan, S., Wierzbowski, J., Willey, D., Williams, S., Wilson, R.K., Winter, E., Worley, K.C., Wyman, D., Yang, S., Yang, S.P. Zdobnov, E.P., Zody, M.C. and Lander, E.S. (2002). Initial sequencing and comparative analysis of the mouse genome. *Nature, 420,* 520–562.

[47] Pennacchio, L.A. and Rubin, E.M. (2001). Genomic strategies to identify mammalian regulatory sequences. *Nature Reviews Genetics, 2,* 100–109.

[48] Thomas, J.W., Touchman, J.W., Blakesley, R.W., Bouffard, G.G., Beckstrom-Sternberg, S.M., Margulies, E.H., Blanchette, M., Siepel, A.C., Thomas, P.J., McDowell, J.C., Maskeri, B., Hansen, N.F., Schwartz, M.S., Weber, R.J., Kent, W.J., Karolchik, D., Bruen, T.C., Bevan, R., Cutler, D.J., Schwartz, S., Elnistski, L., Idol, J.R., Prasad, A.B., Lee-Lin, S.Q., maduro, V.V., Summers, T.J., Portnoy, M.E., Dietrich, N.L., Akhter, N., Ayele, K., Benjamin, B., Cariaga, K., Brinkley, C.P., Brooks, S.Y., Granite, S., Guan, X., Gupta, J., Haghighi, P., Ho, S.L., Huang, M.C., Karlins, E., Laric, P.L., Legaspi, R., Lim, M.J., Maduro, Q.L., Masiello, C.A.,

Mastrian, S.D., McCloskey, J.C., Pearson, R., Stantripop, S., Tiongson, E.E., Tran, J.T., Tsurgeon, C., Vogt, J.L., Walker, M.A., Wetherby, K.D., Wiggins, L.S., Young, A.C., Zhang, L.H., Osoegawa, K., Zhu, B., Zhao, B., Shu, C.L., De Jong, P.J., Lawrence, C.E., Smit, A.F., Chakravarti, A., Haussler, D., Green, P., Miller, W. and Green, E.D. (2003). Comparative analyses of multispecies sequences from targeted genomic regions. *Nature, 424,* 788–793.

[49] Kamatani, N., Sekine, A., Kitamoto, T., Iida, A., Saito, S., Kogame, A., Inoue, E., Kawamoto, M., Harigai, M. and Nakamura, Y. (2004). Large-scale single-nucleotide polymorphism (SNP) and haplotype analyses, using dense SNP maps, of 199 drug-related genes in 752 subjects: the analysis of the association between uncommon SNPs within haplotype blocks and the haplotypes constructed with haplotype-tagging SNPs. *American Journal of Human Genetics, 75,* 190–203.

[50] Lin, S., Chakravarti, A. and Cutler, D.J. (2004). Exhaustive allelic transmission disequilibrium tests as a new approach to genome-wide association studies. *Nature Genetics, 36,* 1181–1188.

[51] Vermeire, S., Wild, G., Kocher, K., Cousineau, J., Dufresne, L., Bitton, A., Langelier, D., Pare, P., Lapointe, G., Cohen, A., Daly, M.J. and Rioux, J.D. (2002). CARD15 genetic variation in a Quebec population: prevalence, genotype-phenotype relationship, and haplotype structure. *American Journal of Human Genetics, 71,* 74–83.

[52] Lowe, C.E., Cooper, J.D., Chapman, J.M., Barratt, B.J., Twells, R.C., Green, E.A., Savage, D.A., Guja, C., Ionescu-Tirgoviste, C., Tuomilehto-Wolf, E., Tuomilehto, J., Todd, J.A. and Clayton, D.G. (2004). Cost-effective analysis of candidate genes using htSNPs: a staged approach. *Genes in Immunity, 5,* 301–305.

[53] Risch, N.J. and Merikangas, K. (1996). The future of genetic studies of complex human diseases. *Science, 273,* 1516–1517.

[54] Storey, J.D. and Tibshirani, R. (2003). Statistical significance for genomewide studies. *Proceedings of the National Academy of Sciences of USA, 100,* 9440–9445.

[55] Wacholder, S., Chanock, S., Garcia-Closas, M., El Ghormli, L. and Rothman, N. (2004). Assessing the probability that a positive report is false: an approach for molecular epidemiology studies. *Journal of the National Cancer Institute, 96,* 434–442.

[56] Barratt, B. J., Payne, F., Lowe, C.E., Hermann, R., Healy, B.C., Harold, D., Concannon, P., Gharani, N., McCarthy, M.I., Olavesen, M.G., McCormack, R., Guja, C., Ionescu-Tirgoviste, C., Undlien, D.E., Ronningen, K.S., Gillespie, K.M., Tuomilehto-Wolf, E., Tuomilehto, J., Bennett, S.T., Clayton, D.G., Cordell, H.J. and Todd, J.A. (2004). Remapping the insulin gene/IDDM2 locus in type 1 diabetes. *Diabetes, 53,* 1884–1889.

[57] Sham, P., Bader, J.S., Craig, I., O'Donovan, M. and Owen, M. (2002). DNA pooling: a tool for large-scale association studies. *Nature Reviews Genetics, 3,* 862–871.

[58] Devlin, B. and Roeder, K. (1999). Genomic control for association studies. *Biometrics, 55,* 997–1004.

[59] Freedman, M.L., Reich, D., Penney, K.L., McDonald, G.J., Mignault, A.A., Patterson, N., Gabriel, S.B., Topol, E.J., Smoller, J.W., Pato, C.N., Pato, M.T., Petrushen, T.L., Kolonel, L.N., Lander, E.S., Sklar, P., Henderson, B., Hirschorn, J.N. and Altshuler, D.

(2004). Assessing the impact of population stratification on genetic association studies. *Nature Genetics, 36,* 388–393.

[60] Ardlie, K.G., Lunetta, K.L. and Seielstad, M. (2002). Testing for population subdivision and association in four case-control studies. *American Journal of Human Genetics, 71,* 304–311.

[61] Marchini, J., Cardon, L.R., Phillips, M.S. and Donnelly, P. (2004). The effects of human population structure on large genetic association studies. *Nature Genetics, 36,* 512–517.

[62] Pritchard, J.K., Stephens, M., Rosenberg, N.A. and Donnelly, P. (2000). Association mapping in structured populations. *American Journal of Human Genetics,* 67,170–181.

[63] Spielman, R.S. and Ewens, W.J. (1996). The TDT and other family based tests for linkage disequilibrium and association. *American Journal of Human Genetics, 59,* 983–989.

[64] Frayling, T.M., Walker, M., McCarthy, M.I., Evans, J.C., Allen, L.I., Lynn, S., Ayres, S., Millauer, B., Turner, C., Turner, R.C., Sampson, M.J., Hitman, G.A., Ellard, S. and Hattersley, A.T. (1999). Parent-offspring trios: a resource to facilitate the identification of type 2 diabetes genes. *Diabetes, 48,* 2475–2479.

[65] Horvath, S. and Laird, N.M. (1998). A discordant-sibship test for disequilibrium and linkage: no need for parental data. *American Journal of Human Genetics, 63,* 1886–1897.

[66] Mitchell, A.A., Cutler, D.J. and Chakravarti, A. (2003). Undetected genotyping errors cause apparent overtransmission of common alleles in the transmission/ disequilibrium test. *American Journal of Human Genetics, 72,* 598–610.

[67] Gordon, D., Haynes, C., Ioannidis, C., Patel, S.B., Bowcock, A.M. and Ott, J. (2004). A transmission disequilibrium test for general pedigrees that is robust to the presence of random genotyping errors and any number of untyped parents. *European Journal of Human Genetics, 12,* 752–761.

[68] Gabriel, S.B., Schaffner, S.F., Nguyen, H., Moore, J.M., Roy, J., Blumenstiel, B., Higgins, J., DeFelice, M., Lochner, A., Faggart, M., Liu-Cordero, S.N., Rotimi, C.N., Adeyemo, A., Cooper, R., Ward, R., Lander, E.S., Daly, M.J. and Altshuler, D. (2002). The structure of haplotype blocks in the human genome. *Science, 296,* 2225–2229.

[69] Pritchard, J.K. and Przeworski, M. (2001) Linkage disequilibrium in humans: models and data. *American Journal of Human Genetics, 69,* 1–14.

[70] Wang, W.Y. and Todd, J.A. (2003). The usefulness of different density SNP maps for disease association studies of common variants. *Human Molecular Genetics, 12,* 3145–3149.

[71] Carlson, C.S., Eberle, M.A., Rieder, M.J., Smith, J.D., Kruglyak, L. and Nickerson, D.A. (2003). Additional SNPs and linkage disequilibrium analyses are necessary for whole-genome association studies in humans. *Nature Genetics, 33,* 518–521.

[72] Concannon, P., Gogolin-Ewens, K.J., Hinds, D., Wapelhorst, B., Morrison, V.A., Stirling, B., Mitra, M., Farmer, J., Williams, S.R., Cox, N.J., Bell, G.I., Risch, N. and Spielman, R.S. (1998). A second-generation screen of the human genome for susceptibility to insulin-dependent diabetes mellitus (IDDM). *Nature Genetics, 19,* 292–296.

[73] Wapelhorst, B., Bell, G.I., Risch, N., Spielman, R.S. and Concannon, P. (1995). Linkage and association studies in insulin-dependent diabetes with a new dinucleotide repeat polymorphism at the GAD65 locus. *Autoimmunity, 21,* 127–130.

[74] Johnson, G.C., Payne, F., Nutland, S., Stevens, H., Tuomilehto-Wolf, E., Tuomilehto, J. and Todd, J.A. (2002). A comprehensive, statistically powered analysis of GAD2 in type 1 diabetes. *Diabetes, 51,* 2866 –2870.

[75] Vella, A., Cooper, J.D., Lowe, C.E., Walker, N., Nutland, S., Widmer, B., Jones, R., Ring, S.M., McArdle, W., Pembrey, M.E., Strachan, D.P., Dunger, D.B., Twells, R.C., Clayton, D.G. and Todd, J.A. (2005). Localization of a type 1 diabetes locus in the IL2RA/CD25 region by use of tag single-nucleotide polymorphisms. *American Journal of Human Genetics, 76,* 773-779.

[76] Qu, H.Q., Montpetit, A., Ge, B., Hudson, T.J. and Polychronakos, C. (2007). Toward further mapping of the association between the IL2RA locus and type 1 diabetes. *Diabetes, 56,* 1174–1176.

[77] Fehniger, T.A. and Caligiuri, M.A. (2001). Interleukin 15: biology and relevance to human disease. *Blood, 97,* 14–32.

[78] Waldmann, T.A. (2006). Biology of interleukin-2 and interleukin-15: implications for cancer therapy and vaccine design. *Nature Reviews Immunology, 6,* 595–601.

[79] Lowe, C.E., Cooper, J.D., Brusko, T., Walker, N.M., Smyth, D.J., Bailey, R., Bourget, K., Plagnol, V., Field, S., Atkinson, M., Clayton, D.G., Wicker, L.S. and Todd, J.A. (2007). *Nature Genetics, 39,* 1074-1082.

[80] Brand, O.J., Heward, J.M., Franklyn, J.A., Cooper, J.D., Todd, J.A. and Gough, S.C.L. (2007). Association of the interleukin-2 receptor alpha (IL-2Ralpha)/CD25 gene region with Graves' disease using a multilocus test and tag SNPs. *Clinical Endocrinology, 66,* 508–512.

[81] Robb, R.J. and Kutny, R.M. (1987). Structure-function relationships for the IL 2-receptor system. IV. Analysis of the sequence and ligand-binding properties of soluble Tac protein. *Journal of Immunology, 139,* 855–862.

[82] Kim, H.P., Imbert, J. and Leonard, W.J. (2006). Both integrated and differential regulation of components of the IL-2/IL-2 receptor system. *Cytokine and Growth Factors Reviews, 17,* 349–366.

[83] Klose, R.J. and Bird, A.P. (2006). Genomic DNA methylation: the mark and its mediators. *Trends in Biochemical Science, 31,* 89–97.

[84] Roh, T.Y., Cuddapah, S., Cui, K. and Zhao, K. (2006). The genomic landscape of histone modifications in human T cells. *Proceedings of the National Academy of Sciences of USA, 103,* 15782–15787.

[85] Giordano, C., Panto, F., Caruso, C., Modica, M.A., Zambito, A.M., Sapienza, N., Amato, M.P. and Galluzzo, A. (1989). Interleukin 2 and soluble interleukin 2-receptor secretion defect in vitro in newly diagnosed type I diabetic patients. *Diabetes, 38,* 310–315.

[86] Tree, T.I., Roep, B.O. and Peakman, M. (2006). A mini meta-analysis of studies on CD4+CD25+ T cells in human type 1 diabetes: report of the Immunology of Diabetes Society T Cell Workshop. *Annals of the New York Academy of Sciences, 1079,* 9–18.

[87] Shevach, E.M. (2001).Certified professionals: CD4+CD25+ suppressor T cells. *Journal of Experimental Medicine, 193,* F41–F46.

[88] Salomon, B., Lenschow, D.J., Rhee, L., Ashourian, N., Singh, B., Sharpe, A. and Bluestone, J.A. (2000). B7/CD28 costimulation is essential for the homeostasis of the CD4+CD25+ immunoregulatory T cells that control autoimmune diabetes. *Immunity, 12,* 431– 440.

[89] Randolph, D.A. and Fathman, C.G. (2006). CD4+CD25+ regulatory T cells and their therapeutic potential. *Annual Reviews in Medicine, 57,* 381– 402.

[90] Burchill, M.A., Yang, J., Vang, K.B. and Farrar, M.A. (2007). Interleukin-2 receptor signaling in regulatory T cell development and homeostasis. *Immunology Letters, 114,* 1-8.

[91] Ikegami, H., Fujisawa, T., Makino, S. and Ogihara, T. (2003). Congenic mapping and candidate sequencing for type 1 diabetes in the NOD mouse. *Annals of the New York Academy of Sciences, 1005,* 196-204.

[92] Wicker, L.S., Clark, J., Fraser, H.J., Garner, V.E., Gonzales-Munoz, A., Healy, B., Howlett, S., Hunter, K., Rainbow, D., Rosa, R.L., Smink, L.J., Todd, J.A. and Peterson, L.B. (2005). Type 1 diabetes genes and pathways shared by humans and NOD mice. *Journal of Autoimmunity, 25 (Suppl.),* 29-33.

[93] Lord, C.J., Bohlander, S.K., Hopes, E.A., Montague, C.T., Hill, N.J., Prins J.-B., Peterson L.B., Wicker, L.S., Todd, J.A. and Denny, P. (1995) Mapping of the diabetes polygene Idd3 on mouse chromosome 3 using novel congenic strains. *Mammalian Genome, 6,* 563–570.

[94] Denny, P., Lord, C.J., Hill, N.J., Goy, J.V., Levy, E.R., Podolin, P.L., Peterson, L.B., Wicker, L.S., Todd, J.A. and Lyons, P.A. (1997). Mapping of the IDDM locus Idd3 to a 0.35 cM interval containing the Interleukin-*2* gene. *Diabetes, 46,* 695–700.

[95] Lyons, P.A., Armitage, N., Argentina, F., Denny, P., Hill, N.J., Lord, C.J., Wilusz, M.B., Peterson, L.B., Wicker, L.S. and Todd, J.A. (2000). Congenic mapping of the type 1 diabetes locus, region of mouse chromosome 3: identification of a candidate, to a 780-kb Idd3 segment of ancestral DNA by haplotype mapping. *Genome Research, 10,* 446-453.

[96] Ikegami, H., Fujisawa, T., Makino, S. and Ogihara, T. (2002). Genetic dissection of type 1 diabetes susceptibility gene, Idd3, by ancestral haplotype congenic mapping. *Annals of the New York Academy of Sciences, 958,* 325–328.

[97] Podolin, P.L., Wilusz, M.B., Cubbon, R.M., Pajvani, U., Lord, C.J., Todd, J.A., Peterson, L.B., Wicker, L.S. and Lyons, P.A. (2000). Differential glycosylation of interleukin-2, the molecular basis for the NOD Idd3 type 1 diabetes gene? *Cytokine, 12,* 477–482.

[98] Wrenshall, L.E. and Platt, J.L. (1999). Regulation of T cell homeostasis by heparan sulfate-bound IL-2. *Journal of Immunology, 163,* 3793–3800.

[99] Pearson, T., Weiser, P., Markees, T.G., Serreze, D.V., Wicker, L.S., Peterson, L.B., Cumisky, A.-M., Shultz, L.D., Mordes, J.P., Rossini, A.A. and Greiner D.L. (2004). Islet allograft survival induced by costimulation blockade in NOD mice is controlled by allelic variants of Idd3. *Diabetes, 53,* 1972–1978.

[100] Hunig, T. and Schimpl, A. (1998). The IL-2 deficiency syndrome. A lethal disease caused by abnormal lymphocyte survival. In: *Cytokine knockouts* (ed. S.K. Durum and K. Muregge), pp. 1–19, Totowa, New Jersey, USA: Humana Press, Inc.

[101] Refaeli, Y., Van Parijs, L., London, C.A., Tschopp, J. and Abbas, A.K. (1998). Biochemical mechanisms of IL2-regulated Fas-mediated T cell apoptosis. *Immunity, 8,* 615–623.

[102] Yamanouchi, J., Rainbow, D., Serra, P., Howlett, S., Hunter, S., Garner, V.E.S., Gonzalez-Munoz, A., Clark, J., Veijola, R., Cubbon, R., Chen, S.-L., Rosa, R., Cumiskey, A.M., Serreze, D.V., Gregory, G., Rogers, J., Lyons, P.A., Healy, B., Smink, L.J., Todd, J.A., Peterson, L.B., Wicker, L.C. and Santamaria, P. (2007). Interleukin-2 gene variation impairs regulatory T cell function and causes autoimmunity. *Nature Genetics, 39,* 329-337.

[103] Teuscher, C., Wardell, B., Lunceford, J., Michael, S. and Tung, K. (1996). Aod2, the locus controlling development of atrophy in neonatal thymectomy-induced autoimmune ovarian dysgenesis, co-localizes with Il2, Fgfb and Idd3. *Journal of Experimental Medicine, 183,* 631–637.

[104] Encinas, J., Wicker, L.S., Peterson, L.B., Mukasa, A., Teuscher, C., Sobel, R., Weiner, H.L., Seidman, C.E., Seidman, J.G. and Kuchroo, V.K. (1999). QTL influencing autoimmune diabetes and encephalomyelitis map to a 0.15-cM region containing Il2. *Nature Genetics, 21,* 158–160.

[105] Samy, E., Parker, L., Sharp, C. and Tung, K. (2005). Continuous control of autoimmune disease by antigen-dependent polyclonal CD4+CD25+ regulatory T-cells in the regional lymph node. *Journal of Experimental Medicine, 202*, 771–781.

[106] Clayton, D.G., Walker, N.M., Smyth, D.J., Rask, R., Cooper, J.D., Maier, L.M., Smink, L.J., Lam, A.C., Ovington, N.R., Stevens, H.E., Nutland, S., Howson, J.M., Faham, M., Moorhead, M., Jones, H.B., Falkowski, M., Handenbol, P., Willis, T.D. and Todd, J.A. (2005). Population structure, differential bias and genomic control in a large-scale, case-control association study. *Nature Genetics, 37,* 1243–1246.

[107] Smyth, D.J., Cooper, J.D., Bailey, R., Field, S., Burren, O., Smink, L.J., Guja, C., Ionescu-Tirgoviste, C., Widmer, B., Dunger, D.B., Savage, D.A., Walker, N.M., Clayton, D.G. and Todd, J.A. (2006). A genome-wide association study of nonsynonymous SNPs identifies a type 1 diabetes locus in the interferon-induced helicase (IFIH1) region. *Nature Genetics, 38,* 617-619.

[108] Sutherland, A., Davies, J., Owen, C.J., Vaikkakara, S., Walker, C., Cheetham, T.D., James, R.A., Perros, P., Donaldson, P.T., Cordell, H.J., Quinton, R. and Pearce S.H.S. (2007). Genomic polymorphism at the interferon-induced helicase (IFIH1) locus contributes to Graves' disease susceptibility. *Journal of Clinical Endocrinology and Metabolism, 92,* 3338–3341.

[109] Marinou, I., Montgomery, D.S., Dickson, M.C., Binks, M.H., Moore, D.J., Bax, D.E. and Wilson, A.G. (2007). The interferon induced with helicase domain 1 A946T polymorphism is not associated with rheumatoid arthritis. *Arthritis Research and Therapy, 9:* R40.

[110] Kang, D.-C., Gopalkrishnan, R.V., Lin, L., Randolph, A., Valerie, K., Pestka, S., Fisher, P.B. (2004). Expression analysis and genomic characterization of human

melanoma differentiation associated gene-5, mda-5: a novel type I interferon-responsive apoptosis-inducing gene. *Oncogene, 23,* 1789–1800.

[111] Andrejeva, J., Childs, K.S., Young, D.F., Carlos, T.S., Stock, N., Goodbourn, S. and Randall, R.E. (2004). The V proteins of paramyxoviruses bind the inducible RNA helicase, mda-5, and inhibit its activation of the IFN-beta promoter. *Proceedings of the National Academy of Sciences of USA, 101,* 17264–17269.

[112] Yoneyama, M., Kikuchi, M., Matsumoto, K., Imaizumi, T., Miyagishi, M., Taira, K., Foy, E., Loo, Y.-M., Gale, M., Jr., Akira, S., Yonehara, S., Kato, A. and Fujita, T. (2005). Shared and unique functions of the DExD/H-box helicases RIG-I, MDA5, and LGP2 in antiviral innate immunity. *Journal of Immunology, 175,* 2851–2858.

[113] Van der Werf, N., Kloese, F.G., Rozing, J., Hillebrandt, J.L. (2007). Viral infections as potential triggers of type 1 diabetes. *Diabetes Metabolism Research and Reviews, 23,* 169-183.

[114] Jun, H.S. and Yoon, J.W. (2001). The role of viruses in type 1 diabetes: two distinct cellular and molecular pathogenic mechanisms of virus-induced diabetes in animals. *Diabetologia, 44,* 271-285.

[115] Yoon, J.W. and Jun, H.S. (2006). Viruses induce type 1 diabetes in animals. *Annals of the New York Academy of Sciences, 1079,* 138-146.

[116] Guo, D., Li, M., Zhang, Y., Yang, P., Eckenrode, S., Hopkins, D., Zheng, W., Purohit, S., Podolsky, R.H., Muir, A., Wang, J., Dong, Z., Brusko, T., Atkinson, M., Pozzilli, P., Zeider, A., Raffel, L.J., Jacob, C.O., Park, J., Serrano-Rios, M., Larrad, M.T., Zhang, Z., Garchon, H.J., Bach, J.F., Rotter, J.I., She, J.X. and Wang, C.Y. (2004). A functional variant of SUMO4, a new I kappa B alpha modifier, is associated with type 1 diabetes. *Nature Genetics, 36,* 837–841.

[117] Owerbach, D., Pina, L. and Gabbay, K.H. (2004). A 212-kb region on chromosome 6q25 containing the TAB2 gene is associated with susceptibility to type 1diabetes. *Diabetes, 53,* 1890–1893.

[118] Ikegami, H., Fujisawa, T., Kawabata, Y., Noso, S. and Ogihara, T. (2006). Genetics of type 1 diabetes: similarities and differences between Asian and Caucasian populations. *Annals of the New York Academy of Sciences, 1079,* 51-59.

[119] Ikegami, H., Kawabata, Y., Noso, S., Kawabata, Y. and Ogihara, T. (2007). Genetics of type 1 diabetes in Asian and Caucasian populations. *Diabetes Research and Clinical Practice, 77 (Suppl.),* S116–S121.

[120] Noso, S., Ikegami, H., Fujisawa, T., Kawabata, Y., Asano, K., Hiromine, T., Sugihara, S., Lee, I., Kawasaki, E., Awata, T. and Ogihara, T. (2006). Association of SUMO4, as a candidate gene for IDDM5, with susceptibility to type 1 diabetes in Asian populations. *Annals of the New York of Academy of Sciences, 1079,* 41-46.

[121] Wang, C.-Y., Podolsky, R. and She, J.-X. (2006). Genetic and functional evidence supporting SUMO4 as a type 1 diabetes susceptibility gene. *Annals of the New York Academy of Sciences, 1079,* 257-267.

[122] Kosoy, R. and Concannon, P. (2005). Functional variants in SUMO4, TAB2, and NFkB and the risk of type 1 diabetes. *Genes and Immunity, 6,* 231–235.

[123] Smyth, D.J., Howson, J.M.M., Lowe, C.E., Walker, N.M., Lam, A.C., Nutland, S., Hutchings, J., Tuomilehto-Wolf, E., Tuomilehto, J., Guja, C., Ionescu-Tirgoviste, C.,

Undlien, D.E., Ronningen, K.S., Savage, D., Dunger, D.B., Twells, R.C., McArdle, W.L., Strachan, D.P. and Todd, J.A. (2005). Assessing the validity of the association between the SUMO4 M55V variant and risk of type 1 diabetes. *Nature Genetics, 37,* 110-111.

[124] Sedimbi, S.K., Shastry, A., Park, Y., Rumba, I. and Sanjeevi, C.B. (2006). Association of SUMO4 M55V polymorphism with autoimmune diabetes in Latvian patients. *Annals of the New York Academy of Sciences, 1079,* 273-277.

[125] Caputo, M., Cerrone, G.E., Mazza, C., Cedola, N., Targovnik, H.M. and Gustavo, D.F. (2007). No evidence of association of CTLA-4 -318 C/T, 159 C/T, 3' STR and SUMO4 163 A/G polymorphism with autoimmune diabetes. *Immunological Investigations, 36,* 259–270.

[126] Wang, C.Y., Yang, P. and She, J.X. (2005). Assessing the validity of the association between the SUMO4 M55V variant and risk of type 1 diabetes. *Nature Genetics, 37,* 112–113.

[127] Sedimbi, S.K., Luo, X.R., Sanjeevi, C.B., Lernmark, A., Landin-Olsson, M., Arnqvist, H., Bjorck, E., Nystrom, L., Ohlson, L.O., Schersten B, Ostman, J., Aili, M., Baath, L.E., Carlsson, E., Edenwall, H., Forsander, G., Granstrom, B.W., Gustavsson, I., Hanas, R., Hellenberg, L., Hellgren, H., Holmberg, E., Hornell, H., Ivarsson, S.A., Johansson, C., Jonsell, G., Kockum, K., Lindblad, B., Lindh, A., Ludvigsson, J., Myrdal, U., Neiderud, J., Segnestam, K., Sjoblad, S., Skogsberg, L., Stromberg, L., Stahle, U., Thalme, B., Tullus, K., Tuvemo, T., Wallensteen, M., Westphal, O., Dahlquist, G. and Aman, J. (2007). SUMO4 M55V polymorphism affects susceptibility to type I diabetes in HLA DR3- and DR4-positive Swedish patients. *Genes and Immunity, 8,* 518-521.

[128] Kawasaki, E., Awata, T., Ikegami, H., Kobayashi, T., Maruyama, T., Nakanishi, K., Shimada, A., Uga, M., Kurihara, S., Kawabata, Y., Tanaka, S., Kanazawa, Y., Lee, I. and Eguchi, K. (2006). Systematic search for single nucleotide polymorphisms in a lymphoid tyrosine phosphatase (PTPN22) gene: Association between promoter polymorphism and type 1 diabetes in Asian populations. *American Joournal of Medical Genetics, 140,* 586–593.

[129] Tsurumaru, M., Kawasaki, E., Ida, H., Migita, K., Moriuchi, A., Fukushima, K., Fukushima, T., Abiru, N., Yamasaki, H., Noso, S., Ikegami, H., Awata, T., Sasaki, H., Eguchi, K. (2006). Evidence for the role of small ubiquitin-like modifier 4 as a general autoimmunity locus in the Japanese population. *Journal of Clinical Endocrinology and Metabolism, 91,* 3138–3143.

[130] Gibbons, L.J., Thomson, W., Zeggini, E., Worthington, J., Barton, A., Eyre, S., Donn, R. and Hinks, A. (2005). The type 1 diabetes susceptibility gene SUMO4 at IDDM5 is not associated with susceptibility to rheumatoid arthritis or juvenile idiopathic arthritis. *Rheumatology, 44,* 1390–1393.

[131] Costas, J., Perez-Rampin, E., Ferreidos-Vidal, I., Torres, M., Phillips, C., Vicario, J.L., Pablos, J.L., Carracedo, A., Gomez-Reino, J.J. and Gonzales, A. (2006). SUMO4 and MAP3K7IP2 single nucleotide polymorphisms and susceptibility to rheumatoid arthritis. *Journal of Rheumatology, 33,* 10048-1051.

[132] Orozco, G., Sanchez, E., Gonzalez-Gay, M.A., Lopez-Nevot, M.A., Torres, B., Pascual-Salcedo, D., Balsa, A., Pablos, J.L., Garcia, A., Gonzales-Escribano, M.F., Martin, J. (2006). SLC22A4, RUNX1, and SUMO4 polymorphisms are not associated with rheumatoid arthritis: a case-control study in a Spanish population. *Journal of Rheumatology, 33,* 1235–1239.

[133] Orozco, G., Sanchez, E., Gomez, L.M., Gonzalez-Gay, M.A., Lopez-Nevot, M.A., Torres, B., Ortego-Centeno, N., Jimenez-Alonso, J., de Ramon, E., Sanchez Roman, J., Anaya, J.M., Sturfelt, G., Gunnarsson, I., Svennungsson, E., Alarcon-Riquelme, M., Gonzalez-Escribano, M.F. and Martin, J. (2006). Study of the role of functional variants of SLC22A4, RUNX1, and SUMO4 in systemic lupus erythematosus. *Annals of Rheumatoid Disease, 65,* 791-795.

[134] Bohren, K.M., Nadkarni, V., Song, J.H., Gabbay, K.H. and Owerbach, D. (2004). A M55V polymorphism in a novel SUMO gene (SUMO-4) differentially activates heat shock transcription factors and is associated with susceptibility to type I diabetes mellitus. *Journal of Biological Chemistry, 279,* 27233–27238.

[135] Ehninger, A., Mziaut, H. and Solimena, M. (2007). Emerging role of SUMO in pancreatic beta-cells. *Hormone Metabolism Research, 39,* 658-664.

[136] Li, M., Guo, D., Isales, C.M., Eizirik, D.L., Atkinson, M., She, J.X. and Wang, C.Y. (2005). SUMO wrestling with type 1 diabetes. *Journal of Molecular Medicine, 83,* 504–513.

[137] Mabb, A.M. and Miyamoto, S. (2007). SUMO and NF-kappaB ties. *Cell Molecular and Life Sciences, 64,* 1979-1996.

[138] Eizirik, D.L. and Mandrup-Poulsen, T. (2001). A choice of death–the signal transduction of immune-mediated beta-cell apoptosis. *Diabetologia, 44,* 2115–2133.

[139] Lee, C.H., Olson, P., Evans, R.M. (2003). Minireview: lipid metabolism, metabolic diseases, and peroxisome proliferator-activated receptors. *Endocrinology, 144,* 2201–2207.

[140] Blaschke, F., Caglayan, E. and Hsueh, W.A. (2006). Peroxisome proliferator-activated receptor damma agonists: their role as vasoprotective agents in diabetes. *Endocrinology and Metabolism Clinics of North America, 35,* 561–574.

[141] Florez, J.C., Hirschhorn, J. and Altshuler, D. (2003). The inherited basis of diabetes mellitus: implications for the genetic analysis of complex traits. *Annual Reviews in Genomics and Human Genetics, 4,* 257–291.

[142] Deeb, S.S., Fajas, L., Nemoto, M., Pihlajamaki, J., Mykkanen, L., Kuusisto, J., Laakso, M,, Fujimoto, W. and Auwerx, J. (1998). A Pro12Ala substitution in PPARgamma2 associated with decreased receptor activity, lower body mass index and improved insulin sensitivity. *Nature Genetics, 20,* 284–287.

[143] Eftychi, C., Howson, J.M.M., Barratt, B.J., Vella, A., Payne, F., Smyth, D.J., Twells, R.C.J., Walker, N.M., Rance, H.E., Tuomilehto-Wolf, E., Tuomilehto, J., Undlien, D.E., Ronningen, K.S., Guja, C., Ionescu-Tırgovishte, C., Savage, D.A. and Todd, J.A. (2004). Analysis of the type 2 diabetes–associated single nucleotide polymorphisms in the genes IRS1, KCNJ11, and PPARG2 in type 1 diabetes. *Diabetes, 53,* 870-873.

[144] Johansen, A., Jensen, D.P., Bergholdt, R., Mortensen, H.B., Pociot, F., Nerup, J., Hansen, T., Pedersen, O. and The Danish Society of Childhood Diabetes (2006). IRS1,

KCNJ11, PPAR□2 and HNF-1□: do amino acid polymorphisms in these candidate genes support a shared aetiology between type 1 and type 2 diabetes? *Diabetes, Obesity and Metabolism, 8,* 75–82.

[145] Waden, J., Thorn, L.M., Forsblom, C., Lakka, T., Saraheimo, M., Rosengard-Barlund, M., Heikkila, O., Wessman, M., Turunen, J.A., Parkkonen, M., Tikkanen, H. and Groop, P.-H. (2007). Leisure-time physical activity is associated with the metabolic syndrome in type 1 diabetes. Effect of the PPAR□ Pro12Ala polymorphism: the FinnDiane Study. *Diabetes Care, 30,* 1618-1620.

[146] Bennett, S.T. and Todd, J.A. (1996). Human type 1 diabetes and the insulin gene: principles of mapping polygenes. *Annual Reviews in Genetics, 30,* 343–370.

[147] Beales, P.E. and Pozzilli, P. (2002). Thiazolidinediones for the prevention of diabetes in the non-obese diabetic (NOD) mouse: implications for human type 1 diabetes. *Diabetes Metabolism Research and Reviews, 18,* 114–117.

[148] Botolin, S., Faugere, M.-C., Malluche, H., Orth, M., Meyer, R. and McCabe, L.R. (2005). Increased bone adiposity and peroxisomal proliferator-activated receptor-□2 expression in type I diabetic mice. *Endocrinology, 146,* 3622–3631.

[149] Masugi, J., Tamori, Y., Mori, H., Koike, T. and Kasuga, M. (2000). Inhibitory effect of a proline-to-alanine substitution at codon 12 of peroxisome proliferator-activated receptor-gamma2 on thiazolidinedione-induced adipogenesis. *Biochemical and Biophysical Research Communications, 268,* 178–182.

[150] Jacob, S. (2000). The PPARgamma2 polymorphism pro12Ala is associated with better insulin sensitivity in the offspring of type 2 diabetic patients. *Hormone Metabolism Research, 32,* 413–416.

[151] Ek, J. (2001). Studies of the Pro12Ala polymorphism of the peroxisome proliferator-activated receptor-gamma2 (PPAR-gamma2) gene in relation to insulin sensitivity among glucose tolerant Caucasians. *Diabetologia, 44,* 1170–1176.

[152] Ricote, M., Li, A.C., Willson, T.M., Kelly, C.J. and Glass, C.K. (1998). The peroxisome proliferator-activated receptorgamma is a negative regulator of macrophage activation. *Nature, 391,* 79–82.

[153] Augstein, P., Dunger, A., Heinke, P., Wachlin, G., Berg, S., Hehmke, B., Salzsieder, E. (2003). Prevention of autoimmune diabetes in NOD mice by troglitazone is associated with modulation of ICAM-1 expression on pancreatic islet cells and IFN-gamma expression in splenic T cells. *Biochemical and Biophysical Research Communications, 304,* 378–384.

[154] Mein, C.A., Esposito, L., Dunn, M.G., Johnson, G.C., Timms, A.E., Goy, J.V., Smith, A.N., Sebag-Montefiore, L., Merriman, M.E., Wilson, A.J., Pritchard, L.E., Cucca, F., Barnett, A.H., Bain, S.C. and Todd, J.A. (1998). A search for type 1 diabetes susceptibility genes in families from the United Kingdom. *Nature Genetics, 19,* 297-300.

[155] Nishimura, M., Obayashi, H., Maruya, E., Ohta, M., Tegoshi, H., Fukui, M., Hasegawa, G., Shigeta, H., Kitagawa, Y., Nakano, K., Saji, H. and Nakamura, N. (2000). Association between type 1 diabetes age-at-onset and intercellular adhesion molecule-1 (ICAM-1) gene polymorphism. *Human Immunology, 61,* 507-510.

[156] Kristiansen ,O.P., Nolsoe, R.L., Holst, H., Reker, S., Larsen, Z.M., Johannesen, J., Nerup, J., Pociot, F. and Mandrup-Poulsen, T. (2000). The intercellular adhesion molecule-1 K469E polymorphism in type 1 diabetes. *Immunogenetics, 52,* 107-111.

[157] Nejentsev, S., Laine, A.P., Simell, O. and Ilonen, J. (2000). Intercellular adhesion molecule-1 (ICAM-1) K469E polymorphism: no association with type 1 diabetes among Finns. *Tissue Antigens, 55,* 568-570.

[158] Ma, J., Mollsten, A., Prazny, M., Falhammar, H., Brismar, K., Dahlquist, G., Efendic, S. and Gu, H.F. (2006). Genetic influences of the intercellular adhesion molecule 1 (ICAM-1) gene polymorphisms in development of type 1 diabetes and diabetic nephropathy. *Diabetic Medicine, 23,* 1093-1099.

[159] Guja, C., Todd, J.A., Welsh, A., Marshall, S. and Ionescu-Tirgoviste, C. (1999). Increased transmission of intracellular adhesion molecule 1 469E allele in type 1 Romanian diabetic families. *Diabetologia, 42 (Suppl. 1),* 327.

[160] Nejentsev, S., Guja, C., McCormack, R., Cooper, J., Howson, J.M.M., Nutland, S., Rance, H., Walker, N., Undlien, D., Ronningen, K.S., Tuomilehto-Wolf, E., Tuomilehto, J., Ionescu-Tirgoviste, C., Gale, E.A.M., Bingley, P.J., Gillespie, K.M., Savage, D.A., Carson, D.J., Patterson, C.C., Maxwell, A.P., Todd, J.A. (2003). The ARG241 allele of the intercellular adhesion molecule-1 is associated with a reduced risk of type 1 diabetes. *Lancet, 362,* 1723–1724.

[161] Todd, J.A., Walker, N.M., Cooper, J.D., Smyth, D.J., Downes, K., Plagnol, V., Bailey, R., Nejentsev, S., Field, S.F., Payne, F., Lowe, C.E., Szeszko, J.S., Hafler, J.P., Zeitels, L., Yang, J.H., Vella, A., Nutland, S., Stevens, H.E., Schuilenburg, H., Coleman, G., Maisuria, M., Meadows, W., Smink, L.J., Healy, B., Burren, O.S., Lam, A.A., Ovington, N.R., Allen, J., Adlem, E., Leung, H.T., Wallace, C., Howson, J.M., Guja, C., Ionescu-Tirgoviste, C.; Genetics of Type 1 Diabetes in Finland, Simmonds, M.J., Heward, J.M., Gough, S.C.; Wellcome Trust Case Control Consortium, Dunger, D.B., Wicker, L.S. and Clayton, D.G. (2007). Robust associations of four new chromosome regions from genome-wide analyses of type 1 diabetes. *Nature Genetics, 39,* 857-864.

[162] Vora, D.K., Rosenbloom, C.L., Beaudet, A.L. and Cottingham, R.W. (1994). Polymorphisms and linkage analysis for ICAM-1 and the selectin gene cluster. *Genomics, 21,* 473-477.

[163] Joling, P., Boom, S., Johnson, J., Dekker, M.E.M., van den Tweel, J.G., Schuurman, H.-J. and Bloem, A.C. (1994). Domain 5 of the intercellular adhesion molecule-1(ICAM-1) is involved in adhesion of B-cells and follicular dendritic cells. *Advances in Experimental Medicine and Biology,* 355, 131-135.

[164] Molgg, M., Schwaeble, W., Johnson, J.P. and Dierich, M.P. (1991). Generation of recombinant, carbohydrate-free intercellular adhesion molecule-1 (ICAM-1) and ICAM-1 fragments in Escherichia coli and mapping of epitopes recognized by anti-ICAM-1 monoclonal antibodies. *Immunology Letters, 28,* 237-243.

[165] Iwao, M., Morisaki, H. and Morisaki, T. (2004). Single-nucleotide polymorphism g.1548G > A (E469K) in human ICAM-1 gene affects mRNA splicing pattern and TPA-induced apoptosis. *Biochemical and Biophysical Research Communications, 7:* 729–735.

[156] Casasnovas, J.M., Stehle, T., Liu, J.H., Wang, J.H. and Springer, T.A. (1998). A dimeric crystal structure for the N-terminal two domains of intercellular adhesion molecule-1. *Proceedings of the National Academy of Sciences of USA, 95,* 4134-4139.

[157] Yang, H., Vora, D.K., Targan, S.R., Toyodam, H., Beaudet, A.L. and Rotter, J.I. (1995). Intercellular adhesion molecule 1 gene associations with immunologic subset of inflammatory bowel disease. *Gastroenterology, 109,* 440-448.

[158] van de Stolpe A. and van der Saag, P.T. (1996). Intercellular adhesion molecule-1. *Journal of Molecular Medicine, 74,* 13–33.

[159] Hanninen, A., Salmi, M., Simell, O. and Jalkanen, S. (1993). Endothelial cell-binding properties of lymphocytes infiltrated into human diabetic pancreas. Implications for pathogenesis of IDDM. *Diabetes, 42,* 1556-1562.

[170] Hanninen, A., Taylor, C., Streeter, P.R., Stark, L.S., Sarte, J.M., Shizuru, J.A., Simell, O. and Michie, S.A. (1993). Vascular addressins are induced on islet vessels during insulitis in nonobese diabetic mice and are involved in lymphoid cell binding to islet endothelium. *Journal of Clinical Investigations, 92,* 2509-2515.

[171] Yagi, N., Yokono, K., Amano, K., Nagata, M., Tsukamoto, K., Hasegawa, Y., Yoneda, R., Okamoto, N., Moriyama, H., Miki, M., Tominaga, Y., Miyazaki, J., Yagita, H., Okumura, K., Mizoguchi, A., Miki, A., Ide, C., Maeda, S. and Kasuga, M. (1995). Expression of intercellular adhesion molecule 1 on pancreatic β-cells accelerates β-cell destruction by cytotoxic T-cells in murine autoimmune diabetes. *Diabetes, 44,* 744-752.

[172] Herold, K.C., Vezys, V., Gage, A. and Montag, A.G. (1994). Prevention of autoimmune diabetes by treatment with anti-LFA-1 and anti-ICAM-1 monoclonal antibodies. *Cellular Immunology, 157,* 489-500.

[173] Martin, S., Hibino, T., Faust, A., Kleeman, R. and Kolb, H. (1996). Differential expression of ICAM-1 and LFA-1 versus L-selectin and VCAM-1 in autoimmune insulitis of NOD mice and association with both Th1 and Th2-type infiltrates. *Journal of Autoimmunity, 9,* 637-643.

[174] Martin, S. (1997). Soluble adhesion molecules in type 1 diabetes mellitus. *Hormone Metabolism Research, 29,* 639-642.

[175] Wellcome Trust Case Control Consortium. (2007). Genome-wide association study of 14,000 cases of seven common diseases and 3,000 shared controls. *Nature, 447,* 661–678.

[176] The International HapMap Consortium (2005). A haplotype map of the human genome. *Nature, 437,* 1299–1320.

[177] Parkes, M., Barrett, J.C., Prescott, N.J., Tremelling, M., Anderson, C.A., Fisher, S.A., Roberts, R.G., Nimmo, E.R., Cummings, F.R., Soars, D., Drummond, H., Lees, C.W., Khawaja, S.A., Bagnall, R., Burke, D.A., Todhunter, C.E., Ahmad, T., Onnie, C.M., McArdle, W., Strachan, D., Bethel, G., Bryan, C., Lewis, C.M., Deloukas, P., Forbes, A., Sanderson, J., Jewell, D.P., Satsangi, J., Mansfield, J.C.; Wellcome Trust Case Control Consortium, Cardon, L. and Mathew, C.G. (2007). Sequence variants in the autophagy gene IRGM and multiple other replicating loci contribute to Crohn's disease susceptibility. *Nature Genetics, 39,* 830-832.

[178] Iversen, L.F., Moller, K.B., Pedersen, A.K., Peters, G.H., Petersen, A.S., Andersen, H.S., Branner, S., Mortensen, S.B. and Moller, N.P. (2002). Structure determination of T cell protein-tyrosine phosphatase. *Journal of Biological Chemistry, 277,* 19982-19990.

[179] Galic, S., Klingler-Hoffmann, M., Fodero-Tavoletti, M.T., Puryer, M.A., Meng, T.C., Tonks, N.K. and Tiganis, T. (2003). Regulation of insulin receptor signaling by the protein tyrosine phosphatase TCPTP. *Molecular and Cellular Biology, 23,* 2096–2108.

[180] Galic, S., Hauser, C., Kahn, B.B., Haj, F.G., Neel, B.G., Tonks, N.K. and Tiganis, T. (2005). Coordinated regulation of insulin signaling by the protein tyrosine phosphatases PTP1B and TCPTP. *Molecular and Cellular Biology, 25,* 819-829.

[181] Dube, N., Tremblay, M.L. (2005). Involvement of the small protein tyrosine phosphatases TC-PTP and PTP1B in signal transduction and diseases: from diabetes, obesity to cell cycle, and cancer. *Biochimica et Biophysica Acta, 1754,* 108-117.

[182] Lembertas, A.V., Perusse, L., Chagnon, Y.C., Fisler, J.S., Warden, C.H., Purcell-Huynh, D.A., Dionne, F.T., Gagnon, J., Nadeau, A., Lusis, A.J. and Bouchard, C. (1997). Identification of an obesity quantitative trait locus on mouse chromosome 2 and evidence of linkage to body fat and insulin on the human homologous region 20q. *Journal of Clinical Investigations, 100,* 1240-1247.

[183] Bento, J.L., Palmer, N.D., Mychaleckyj, J.C., Lange, L.A., Langefeld, C.D., Rich, S.S., Freedman, B.I., Bowden, D.W. (2004). Association of protein tyrosine phosphatase 1B gene polymorphisms with type 2 diabetes. *Diabetes, 53,* 3007-3012.

[184] Simoncic, P.D., McGlade, C.J. and Tremblay, M.L. (2006). PTP1B and TC-PTP: novel roles in immune-cell signaling. *Canadian Journal of Physiology and Pharmacology, 84,* 667-675.

[185] Heinonen, K.M., Nestal, F.P., Newell, E.W., Charette. G., Seemayer, T.A., Tremblay., M.L. and Lapp, W.S. (2004). T-cell protein tyrosine phosphatase deletion results in progressive systemic inflammatory disease. *Blood, 103,* 3457-3464.

[186] Simoncic, P.D., Lee-Loy, A., Barber, D.L., Tremblay, M.L. and McGlade, C.J. (2002). The T cell protein phosphatase is a negative regulator of Janus family kinases 1 and 3. *Current Biology, 12,* 446-453.

[187] Van Vliet, C., Bukczynska, P.E., Puryer, M.A., Sadek, C.M., Shields, B.J., Tremhlay, M.L. and Tiganis, T. (2005). Selective regulation of tumor necrosis factor-induced Erk signaling by Src family kinases and the T cell protein tyrosine phosphatase gene. *Gene, 237,* 351-360.

[188] Aoki, N. and Matsuda, T. (2002). A nuclear protein-tyrosine phosphatase TC-PTP is a potential negative regulator of the PRL-mediated signaling pathway: dephosphorylation and deactivation of signal transducerand activator of transcription 5a and 5b by TC-PTP in nucleus. *Molecular Endocrinology, 16,* 58-69.

[189] Zhu, W., Mustelin, T. and David, M. (2002). Arginine methylation of STAT1 regulates its dephosphorylation by T cell protein tyrosine phosphatase. *Journal of Biological Chemistry, 277,* 35787-35790.

[190] Smyth, D.J., Howson, J.M.M., Payne, F., Maier, L.M., Bailey, R., Holland, K., Lowe, C.E., Cooper, J.D., Hulme, J.S., Vella, A., Dahlman, I., Lam, A.C., Nutland, S., Walker, N.M., Twells, R.C.J. and Todd, J.A. (2006). Analysis of polymorphisms in 16

genes in type 1 diabetes that have been associated with other immune-mediated diseases. *BMC Medical Genetics*, *7:* 20.

[191] Holgate, S.T., Davies, D.E., Powell, R.M., and Holloway, J.W. (2005). ADAM33: a newly identified gene in the pathogenesis of asthma. *Immunology and Allergy Clinics of North America, 25,* 655-668.

[192] Del Mastro, R.G., Turenne, L., Giese, H., Keith, T.P., Van Eerdewegh, P., May, K.J. and Little, R.D. (2007). Mechanistic role of a disease-associated genetic variant within the ADAM33 asthma susceptibility gene. *BMC Medical Genetics, 8:* 46.

[193] Lesueur, F., Oudot, T., Heath, S., Foglio, M., Lathrop, M., Prud'Homme, J.F. and Fischer, J. (2007). ADAM33, a new candidate for psoriasis susceptibility. *PLos ONE, 2:* e906.

[194] Lesueur, F., Lefevre, C., Has, C., Guilloud-Bataille, M., Oudot, T., Mahe, E., Lahfa, M., Mansouri, S., Mosharraf-Olmolk, H., Sobel, E., Heath, S., Lathrop, M., Dizier, M.H., Prud'Homme, J.F. and Fischer, J. (2007). Confirmation of psoriasis susceptibility loci on chromosome 6p21 and 20p13 in French families. *Journal of Investigations in Dermatology, 127,* 1403-1409.

[195] Simpson, A., Maniatis, N., Jury, F., Cakebread, J.A., Lowe, L.A., Holgate, S.T., Woodcock, A., Ollier, W.E., Collins, A., Custovic, A., Holloway, J.W. and John, S.L. (2005). Polymorphisms in a disintegrin and metalloprotease 33 (ADAM33) predict impaired early-life lung function. *American Journal of Respiration and Critical Care Medicine, 172,* 55-60.

[196] Van Eerdewegh, P., Little, R.D., Dupuis, J., Del Mastro, R.G., Falls, K., Simon, J., Torrey, D., Pandit, S., McKenny, J., Braunschweiger, K., Walsh, A., Liu, Z., Hayward, B., Folz, C., Manning, S.P., Bawa, A., Saracino, I., Thackston, M., Benchekroun, Y., Capparell, N., Wang, M., Adair, R., Feng, Y., Dubois, J., FitzGeralad, M.G., Huang, H., Gibson, R., Allen, K.M., Pedan, A., Danzig, M.R., Umland, S.P., Egan, R.W., Guss, F.M., Rorke, S., Clough, J.B., Holloway, J.W., Holgate, S.T. and Keith, T.P. (2002). Association of the ADAM33 gene with asthma and bronchial hyperresponsiveness. *Nature, 418,* 426–430.

[197] Powell, R.M., Wicks, J., Holloway, J.W., Holgate, S.T. and Davies, D.E. (2004). The splicing and fate of ADAM33 transcripts in primary human airways fibroblasts. *American Journal of Respiratory Cell Molecular Biology, 31,* 13–21.

[198] Zou, J., Zhang, R., Zhu, F., Liu, J., Madison, V. and Umland, S.P. (2005). ADAM33 enzyme properties and substrate specificity. *Biochemistry, 44,* 4247-4256.

[199] Zou, J., Zhu, F., Liu, J., Wang, W., Zhang, R., Garlisi, C.G., Liu, Y.H., Wang, S., Shah, H., Wan, Y. and Umland, S.P. (2004). Catalytic activity of human ADAM33. *Journal of Biological Chemistry, 279,* 9818-9830.

[200] Shibuya, A., Campbell, D., Hannum, C., Yssel, H., Franz-Bacon, K., McClanahan, T., Kitamura, T., Nicholl, J., Sutherland, G.R., Lanier, L.L. and Phillips, J.H. (1996). DNAM-1, a novel adhesion molecule involved in the cytolytic function of T lymphocytes. *Immunity, 4,* 573-581.

[201] Shibuya, K., Shirakawa, J., Kameyama, T., Honda, S., Tahara-Hanaoka, S., Miyamoto, A., Onodera, M., Sumida, T., Nakauchi, H., Miyoshi, H. and Shibuya, A. (2003). CD226 (DNAM-1) is involved in lymphocyte function–associated antigen 1

costimulatory signal for naive T cell differentiation and proliferation. *Journal of Experimental Medicine, 198,* 1829–1839.

[202] Shirakawa, J., Wang, Y., Tahara-Hanaoka, S., Honda, S., Shibuya, K. and Shibuya, A. (2006). LFA-1-dependent lipid raft recruitment of DNAM-1 (CD226) in CD4+ T cell. *International Immunology, 18,* 951–957.

[203] Shibuya, K., Lanier, L.L., Phillips, J.H., Ochs, H.D., Shimizu, K., Nakayama, E., Nakauchi, H. and Shibuya, A. (1999). Physical and functional association of LFA-1 with DNAM-1 adhesion molecule. *Immunity, 11,* 615–623.

[204] Bottino, C., Castriconi, R., Moretta, L. and Moretta, A. (2005). Cellular ligands of activating NK receptors. *Trends in Immunology, 26,* 221-226.

[205] Sherrington, P.D., Scott, J.L., Jin, B., Simmons, D., Dorahy, D.J., Lloyd, J., Brien, J.H., Aebersold, R.H., Adamson, J., Zuzel, M. and Burns, G.F. (1997). TliSA (PTA1) activation antigen implicated in T cell differentiation and platelet activation is a member of the regulation of expression. *Journal of Biological Chemistry, 272,* 21735-21744.

[206] Tao, D., Shangwu, L., Qun, W., Yan, L., Wei, J., Junyan, L., Feili, G., Boquan, J. and Jinquan, T. (2005). CD226 expression deficiency causes high sensitivity to apoptosis in NK T cells from patients with systemic lupus erythematosus. *Journal of Immunology, 174,* 1281-1290.

[207] Hakonarson, H., Grant, S.F.A., Bradfield, J.P., Marchand, L., Kim, C.E., Glessner, J.T., Grabs, R., Casalunovo, T., Taback, S.P., Frackelton, E.C., Lawson, M.L., Robinson, L.J., Skraban, R., Lu, Y., Chiavacci, R.M., Stanley, C.A., Kirsch, S.E., Rappaport, E.F., Orangel, J.S., Monos, D.S., Devoto, M., Qu, H.-Q. and Polychronakos, C. (2007). A genome-wide association study identifies KIAA0350 as a type 1 diabetes gene. *Nature, 448,* 591-594.

[208] Cambi, A. and Figdor, C.G. (2005). Levels of complexity in pathogen recognition by C-type lectins. *Current Opinion in Immunology, 17,* 345–351.

[209] Robinson, M.J., Sancho, D., Slack, E.C., Leibundgut-Landmann, S. and Reis e Sousa, C. (2006). Myeloid C-type lectins in innate immunity. *Nature Immunology, 7,* 1258-1265.

[210] Kanazawa, N. (2007). Dendritic cell immunoreceptors: C-type lectin receptors for pattern recognition and signaling on antigen-presenting cells. *Journal of Dermatological Science, 45,* 77-86.

[211] Gullick, W.J. (1996). The c-erB3/HER3 receptor in human cancer. *Cancer Surveys, 27,* 339-349.

[212] Lee, H., Alita, R.W., Sliwkowski, M.X. and Maihle, N.J. (2001). A naturally occurring secreted human ErB3 receptor isoform inhibits heregulin-stimulated activation of ErbB2, ErbB3, and ErbB4. *Cancer Research, 61,* 4467-4473.

[213] Carver, R.S., Mathew, P.M. and Russell, W.E. (1997). Hepatic expression of ErbB3 is repressed by insulin in a pathway sensitive to PI-3 kinase inhibitors. *Endocrinology, 38,* 5195-5201.

[214] Soh, J., Katsuyama, M., Ushijima, S., Mizutani, Y., Kawauchi, A., Yabe-Nishimura, C. and Miki, T. (2007). Localization of increased insulin-like growth factor binding

protein-3 in diabetic rat penis: implications for erectile dysfunction. *Urology, 70,* 1019-1023.

[215] Britsch, S. (2007). The neuregulin-I/Erb signaling system in development and disease. *Advances in Anatomy, Embriology and Cell Biology, 190,* 1-65.

[216] Lord, C.J., Bohlander, S.K., Hopes, E.A., Montague, C.T., Hill, N.J., Prins J.-B., Peterson L.B., Wicker, L.S., Todd, J.A. and Denny, P. (1995) Mapping of the diabetes polygene Idd3 on mouse chromosome 3 using novel congenic strains. *Mammalian Genome, 6,* 563–570.

[217] Schumacher, J.M., Lee, K., Edelholf, S. and Braun, R.E. (1995). Distribution of Tenr, an RNA-binding protein, in a lattice-like within the spermatid nucleus in the mouse. *Biology of Reproduction, 52,* 1274-1283.

[218] Zhernakova, A., Alizadeh, B.Z., Bevova, M., van Leeuwen, M.A., Coenen, M.J., Franke, B., Franke, L., Posthumus, M.D., van Heel, D.A., van der Steege, G., Radstake, T.R., Barrera, P., Roep, B.O., Koeleman, B.P. and Wijmenga, C. (2007). Novel association in chromosome 4q27 region with rheumatoid arthritis and confirmation of type 1 diabetes point a general risk locus for autoimmune diseases. *American Journal of Human Genetics, 81,* 1284-1288.

[219] Van Heel, D.A., Franke, L., Hunt, K.A., Gwilliam, R., Zhernakova, A., Inouye, M., Wapenaar, M.C., Barnardo, M.C., Bethel, G., Holmes, G.K., Feighery, C., Jewell, D., Kelleher, D., Kumar, P., Travis, S., Walters, J.R., Sanders, D.S., Howdle, P., Swift, J., Playford, R.J., McLaren, W.M., Mearin, M.L., Mulder, C.J., McManus, R., McGinnis, R., Gardon, L.R., Deloukas, P. and Wijmenga, C. (2007). A genome-wide association study for celiac disease identifies risk variants in the region harboring IL2 and IL21. *Nature Genetics, 39,* 827-829.

[220] Mattuzzi, S., Barbi, S., Carletto, A., Ravagnani, V., Moore, P.S., Bambara, L.M. and Scarpa, A. (2007). Association of polymorphisms in the IL1B and IL2 genes with susceptibility and severity of systemic sclerosis. *Journal of Rheumatology, 34,* 997-1004.

[221] Leonard, W.J. and Spolski, R. (2005). Interleukin-21: a modulator of lymphoid proliferation, apoptosis and differentiation. *Nature Reviews Immunology, 5,* 688-698.

[222] King, C., Alic, A., Koelsch, K. and Sarvetnick, N. (2004). Homeostatic expansion of T cell during immune unsufficiency generates autoimmunity. *Cell, 117,* 265-277.

[223] Asano, K., Ikegami, H., Fujisawa, T., Kawabata, Y., Noso, S., Hiromine, Y. and Ogihara, T. (2006). *Annals of the New York Academy of Sciences, 1079,* 47-50.

[224] Asano, K., Ikegami, H., Fujisawa, T., Nishino, M., Nojima, K., Kawabata, Y., Noso, S., Hiromine, Y., Fukai, A. and Ogihara, T. (2007). Molecular scanning of interleukin-21 gene and genetic susceptibility to type 1 diabetes. *Human Immunology, 68,* 384-391.

[225] Halleux, P., Schurmans, S., Schiffman, S.N., Lecocq, R., Concreur, J.L., Dumont, J. and Vanderhaeghen, J.J. (1998). Calcium-binding protein calcyphosine in dog central astrocytes and ependymal cells and in peripheral neurons. *Journal of Chemical Neuroanatomy, 15,* 239-250.

[226] Gregory, S.G., Schmidt, S., Seth, P., Oksenberg, J.R., Hart, J., Prokop, A., Gallier, S.J., Ban, M., Goris, A., Barcellos, L.F., Lincoln, R., McCauley, J.L., Sawcer, S.J., Compston, D.A., Dubois, B., Hauser, S.L., Garcia-Blanco, M.A., Perisak-Vance, M.A.

and Haines, J.L. (2007). Interleukin 7 receptor alpha chain (IL7R) shows allelic and functional association with multiple sclerosis. *Nature Genetics, 39,* 1083-1091.

[227] Booth, D.R., Arthur, A.T., Teutsch, S.M., Bye, C., Rubio, J., Armati, P.J., Pollard, J.D., Heard, R.N. and Stewart, G.J. (2005). Gene expression and genotyping studies implicate the interleukin receptor gene in the pathogenesis of primary progressive multiple sclerosis. *Journal of Molecular Medicine, 83,* 822-830.

[228] Hafler, D.A., Compston, A., Sawcer, S., Lander, E.S., Daly, M.J., De Jager, P.L., de Bakker, P.I., Gabriel, S.B., Mirel, D.B., Ivinson, A.J., Perisak-Vance, M.A., Gregory, S.G., Rioux, J.D., McCauley, J.L., Haines, J.L., Barcellos, L.F., Cree, B. Oksenberg, J.R. and Hauser, S.L. (2007). Risk alleles for multiple sclerosis identified by a genomewide study. *New England Journal of Medicine, 357,* 851-862.

[229] Lundmark, F., Duveleft, K., Iacobaeus, E., Kockum, I., Wallstrom, E., Khademi, M., Otirai, A., Ryder, L.P., Saarela, J., Harbo, H.F., Celius, E.G., Salter, H., Olsson, T. and Hillert, J. (2007). Variation in interleukin 7 receptor alpha chain (IL7R) influences risk of multiple sclerosis. *Nature Genetics, 39,* 1108-1113.

[230] Kittipatarin, C. and Khaled, A. (2007). Interlinking interleukin-7. *Cytokine, 39,* 75-83.

[231] Noguchi, M., Nakamura, Y., Russell, S.M., Ziegler, S.F., Tsang, M., Cao, X. and Leonard, W.J. (1993). Interleukin-2 receptor gamma chain: a functional component of the interleukin-7 receptor. *Science, 262,* 1877-1880.

[232] Hofmeister, R., Khaled, A.R., Benbernou, N., Rajnavolgyi, E., Muegge, K. and Durum, S.K. (1999). Interleukin-7: physiological roles and mechanisms of action. *Cytokine and Growth Factors Reviews, 10,* 41-60.

[233] Roifman, C.M., Zhang, J., Chitayat, D. and Sharfe N. (2000). A partial deficiency of interleukin-7R alpha is sufficient to abrogate T-cell development and cause severe combined immunodeficiency. *Blood, 96,* 2803-2807.

[234] Harnaha, J., Machen, J., Wright, M., Lakomy, R., Styche, A., Trucco, M., Makaroun, S. and Giannoukakis, N. (2006). Interleukin-7 is a survival factor for CD4+CD25+ T-cells and is expressed by diabetes-suppressive dendritic cells. *Diabetes, 55,* 158-170.

[235] Yates, J., Rovis, F., Mitchell, P., Afzali, B., Tsang, J.Y., Garin, M., Lechler, R.I., Lombardi, G. and Garden, O.A. (2007). The maintenance of human CD4+CD25+ regulatory T cell function: IL-2, IL-4, IL-7 and IL-15 preserve optimal suppressive potency in vitro. *International Immunology, 19,* 785-799.

In: Autoimmunity: Role, Regulation and Disorders
Editor: Fynn L. Vogel and L. F. Zimmermann
ISBN 978-1-60456-833-2

Chapter 2

Subclinical Atherosclerosis in Patients with Rheumatoid and Psoriatic Arthritis

***Elisabetta Profumo*[*]*, Brigitta Buttari*[*]*, Maria Elena Tosti*[**]*, Rossana Scrivo*[†]*, Antonio Spadaro*[†]*, Chiara Tesori*[‡]*, Manuela Di Franco*[†] *and Rachele Riganò*[*]**

[*]Department of Infectious, Parasitic and Immune-mediated Diseases
[**]National Centre of Epidemiology, Surveillance and Health Promotion,
Istituto Superiore di Sanità, Rome
[†] Rheumatology Unit
[‡] Department of Surgical Sciences, University Sapienza, Rome, Italy.

Abstract

Accelerated development of atherosclerosis has been observed in patients with rheumatic diseases such as rheumatoid arthritis (RA) and psoriatic arthritis (PsA). It may be related to the inflammatory overload accompanied to the combination of an excessive production of reactive oxygen species with an impaired antioxidant defence capacity, leading to oxidative stress that may facilitate the development and progression of atherosclerosis. Compared with the general population, patients with RA die prematurely, mainly because of cardiovascular diseases but the mechanism by which premature atherosclerosis develops in RA is unknown. Recent data have demonstrated the prevalence of atherosclerosis also in patients with PsA, a chronic inflammatory autoimmune disease characterized by inflammatory arthritis and skin psoriasis. PsA shares some phenotypic characteristics with RA, even though the synovial inflammation of PsA is characterized by less macrophage infiltration and increased vascularity in comparison to RA inflammation. The increased cardiovascular risk in PsA and RA suggests the need to treat the inflammatory process and to monitor traditional atherosclerotic risk factors in these pathologies.

The aim of our study was to evaluate whether increased oxidative stress may be associated to the presence of subclinical atherosclerosis in patients with RA and in patients with PsA. For this purpose we determined the levels of oxidized low density lipoproteins (ox-LDL) and of nitric oxide (NO) in the sera obtained from 19 patients with

RA, 20 with PsA and 20 sex- and age-matched healthy controls. Patients with RA fulfilled the American College of Rheumatology criteria, and patients with PsA fulfilled the CASPAR criteria. In all patients we evaluated the activity and duration of the disease and classical risk factors for atherosclerosis. Our results showed higher levels of ox-LDL and lower levels of NO in sera from patients with RA and PsA than in sera from healthy controls. Notably, higher serum levels of ox-LDL were observed in patients with an intima-media thickness (IMT) >1 than in those with an IMT ≤1, and higher serum levels of NO in patients with an IMT ≤1 than in those with an IMT >1, in patients with RA and PsA. Our data suggest that monitoring circulating levels of ox-LDL and NO in patients with RA and PsA could give information on the development of atherosclerotic disease and therefore could be useful to the clinical management of patients.

Introduction

Rheumatoid arthritis (RA) and psoriatic arthritis (PsA) are chronic inflammatory diseases of the musculoskeletal system. In RA the inflammatory process affects the synovium and leads to joint damage and bone destruction [1]. This pathology is characterised by significant morbidity as a result of synovial inflammation and associated disability [2]; it is more frequent in women than in men with a ratio 3:1. The tissue damage is primarily caused by immune complexes and by cell-mediated immunity. In patients affected by RA the synovial joints are characterized by an inflammatory infiltrate, mainly composed by T lymphocytes and monocytes that secrete soluble factors and promote Th1 inflammation, responsible for the tissue damage. Many studies have reported an excess of cardiovascular morbidity and mortality among patients with RA [2]. Compared with the general population, patients with RA die prematurely, mainly because of cardiovascular diseases. In patients with active disease, the majority of cardiovascular deaths are caused by accelerated atherosclerosis [3-6]. Atherosclerosis is a chronic inflammatory disease caused by endothelial dysfunction and characterized by complex interactions between immune and vascular cells. The activation of endothelial cells induces the expression of adhesion molecules on these cells and the recruitment of leucocytes, thus promoting the inflammatory response. Accelerated atherosclerosis observed in patients with RA is probably due to the chronic activation of inflammatory mechanisms involved in this pathology.

Psoriatic arthritis (PsA) is an inflammatory joint disease with heterogeneous presentation and clinical course [7]. Clear evidence exists that this disease is distinct from rheumatoid arthritis and other spondyloarthropathies, based on informations derived from characteristic clinical features, and on data from histopathologic analyses, immunogenetic associations and musculoskeletal imaging. It is usually seronegative for rheumatoid factor. PsA shares some phenotypic characteristics with RA, even though the synovial inflammation of PsA is characterized by less macrophage infiltration and increased vascularity in comparison to RA inflammation. Much interest has been focused previously on the prominent role of T lymphocytes in the inflammatory process; however, many studies strongly support a major contribution of macrophages in the initiation and perpetuation of joint and skin inflammation [7]. Recent data have demonstrated the occurrence of endothelial dysfunction and the prevalence of atherosclerosis also in patients with PsA [8,9]. The occurrence of cardiovascular disease might be directly linked to the cutaneous and musculoskeletal manifestations of this disease involving subsets of circulating monocytes and tissue macrophages activated by inflammatory mediators in the skin and joint [7].

As patients with autoimmune rheumatic diseases live longer due to improved therapies and preventive measures, mortality and disability due to cardiovascular diseases are increasing [10]. The relative risk to develop atherosclerosis is approximately 1.6 in PsA and 3.0 in RA. Increased risks are found when analyzed by atherosclerotic events, causes of death, or surrogate measures of atherosclerosis, such as carotid artery plaque, intima-media thickness (IMT), or coronary artery calcification. As RA and probably PsA predispose to atherosclerosis, an important issue is how to prevent this outcome. Therefore, when considering preventive interventions, the most important question is whether patients with some particular clinical features have greater risk for atherosclerosis. This may suggest that detecting a particular clinical marker will identify patients at high risk for clinical atherosclerosis and may help in establishing a risk prediction model. In the last decade great attention has been focused on the identification of risk factors predisposing to atherosclerotic diseases [11,12]. Many studies have demonstrated correlations of atherosclerosis with clinical conditions characterized by alteration in the metabolism such as diabetes [13] and hypercholesterolemia [14]. Gender is also a risk factor for cardiovascular diseases, as men have higher risk to develop atherosclerosis than women [15], and increasing age is associated with either clinical atherosclerotic events or surrogate markers for atherosclerosis, such as the occurrence of carotid plaque. Of particular interest are the well known associations of the standard measures of acute systemic inflammation such as erythrocyte sedimentation rate (ESR) [16], with atherosclerosis. Evidence exists suggesting that C-reactive protein (CRP) is a particularly consistent predictor of increased risk for atherosclerotic disease in the general population [17]. Traditional risk factors for atherosclerosis are operational in patients with autoimmune rheumatic diseases. Increased incidence of factors such as metabolic syndrome, diabetes and hypertension has been demonstrated in these patients. Furthermore, there may be genetic and environmental risk factors that predispose an individual both to autoimmune disease and to atherosclerosis. It is probably useful to consider certain autoimmune diseases, such as RA, to be equivalent to diabetes in increasing risk for developing atherosclerosis. Of note, among patients with autoimmune diseases, the interpretation of classical risk factors as CRP can be confounded by the correlation with the systemic inflammation that occurs in these pathologies. However, several studies have identified ESR as an independent risk factor for atherosclerosis in patients with RA.

Recently, accumulating evidence has demonstrated the presence of oxidative stress in patients with rheumatic diseases and suggested a role for the use of antioxidants in prevention and treatment of these pathologies [18,19]. It is well known that the inflammatory overload accompanied to the combination of an excessive production of reactive oxygen species with an impaired antioxidant defence capacity, leading to oxidative stress may facilitate the development and progression of atherosclerosis. Furthermore pharmacological control of oxidative stress and stimulation of nitric oxide release have proved to exert beneficial effects also on vascular remodeling in experimental diabetic models [20]. In several vascular disorders, an increase in superoxide (O_2^-) has been shown to contribute to reduced NO bioavailability through its reaction with NO to form peroxynitrite [21].

Thus, it is clear that the cellular redox state is dysregulated, and the resultant generation of reactive oxygen species (ROS) may play important role in driving and possibly initiating the rheumatic disease as well as cardiovascular complications. However, the precise mechanisms of ROS metabolism, and their function in the progression of these pathologies remain largely elusive.

The increased cardiovascular risk in PsA and RA suggests the need to treat the inflammatory process and to monitor traditional atherosclerotic risk factors in these pathologies.

Seeking more information on biomarkers for atherosclerosis development in patients with RA and PsA, in our in vitro study we evaluated the possible association of oxidative stress markers in peripheral blood with the presence of subclinical atherosclerosis . For this purpose, we determined by immune enzymatic assays serum levels of oxidized low density lipoproteins (ox-LDL) and NO in patients with RA and PsA divided into two groups according to the presence of atherosclerotic disease determined by echo-color Doppler ultrasonography. As controls we used healthy subjects free of atherosclerotic disease. We also investigated whether these two serum biomarkers were correlated to traditional risk factors for atherosclerosis or to clinical features of the two autoimmune diseases.

Materials and Methods

Study Population

We enrolled 19 consecutive patients with RA fulfilling the American College of Rheumatology (ACR) criteria [22] and 20 consecutive patients with PsA fulfilling the Classification Criteria for Psoriatic Arthritis (CASPAR) [23]. We also enrolled 20 sex- and age-matched healthy subjects as controls. Exclusion criteria for patients and controls were recent infection (< 1 month), other autoimmune diseases, malignancy and inflammatory diseases. In all patients we evaluated the activity and duration of the disease and classical risk factors for atherosclerosis (Table). None of the patients and healthy subjects had a history of cardiovascular manifestations. All patients were treated with disease-modifying antirheumatic drugs. Serum samples were obtained from patients and controls and stored at -80°C until use. Informed consent was obtained from all participants.

IMT of the Common Carotid Arteries

To evaluate the presence of atherosclerosis in patients and healthy subjects, IMT of the common carotid arteries was evaluated by Echo-color Doppler. Images were acquired on an ultrasound system equipped with a 7.5 MHz frequency linear-array transducer. The radiologist of the current study was blinded to RA and PsA patients and to the control group, and measurement of the IMT was always performed at the same arterial wall 1 cm proximal to the carotid bifurcation. Two parallel echogenic lines corresponding to the lumen/intima and media/adventitia interfaces were obtained. The distance between these 2 parallel lines corresponded to the IMT. Values were expressed in millimeters.

Table. Baseline characteristics of the 19 patients with rheumatoid arthritis (RA) and of the 20 patients with psoriatic arthritis (PsA)

	Patients with RA	Patients with PsA	P[c]
N	19	20	
Age (years), median (range)	54 (30-64)	51 (35-69)	0.896
Male/female (n)	1/18	13/7	*<0.001*
Duration of the disease (years), median (range)	3 (0.5-25)	7 (1-24)	0.241
Smoking[a], n (%)	7 (37)	5 (25)	0.414
Hypertension[b], n (%)	4 (21)	2 (10)	0.374
Total cholesterol (mg/dl), median (range)	212.5 (160-257)	221 (153-296)	0.409
HDL cholesterol (mg/dl), median (range)	56.5 (45-74)	52 (30-76)	*0.028*
Triglycerids (mg/dl), median (range)	104.5 (90-166)	125 (93-566)	*0.018*
ESR, median (range)	18 (6-40)	10 (3-41)	*0.016*
CRP, median (range)	1.95 (0-43)	0 (0-16)	0.165
IMT >1, n (%)	9 (47)	11 (55)	0.271

[a] Smoking is defined as current smokers;

[b] Hypertension is defined as systolic blood pressure ≥140 mmHg, diastolic blood pressure ≥ 90 mm Hg, or need for hypertensive medication;

[c] Pearson's chi-squared test or Fisher exact test for discrete variables and Mann-Whitney test for continuous variables to evaluate the presence of a statistical significance among patients with RA and PsA;

ESR: erythrocyte sedimentation rate; CRP: C reactive protein; IMT: intima-media thickness.

Serum Ox-LDL and NO Levels

Ox-LDL and NO concentrations in serum samples from patients and healthy subjects were quantified with commercially available ELISA kits (Oxidized LDL Competitive ELISA, Mercodia, Uppsala, Sweden for ox-LDL; Nitrate/Nitrite Colorimetric Assay Kit, Cayman, Lausen Switzerland for NO), as recommended by the manufacturer. The detection limit of the assays were ≤ 0.3 U/L for ox-LDL, < 2.5 μM for NO.

Statistical Analysis

Data on serum ox-LDL and NO levels are expressed as medians and inter-quartile ranges. Mann-Whitney non parametric test was used to investigate the significance of unpaired continuous data. Pearson's chi-squared test or Fisher's exact test, when necessary, was used to evaluate the differences in discrete baseline characteristics between groups of patients. Correlations were explored by Spearman rank correlation coefficient. P values less than 0.05 were considered statistically significant.

All the statistical procedures were performed by STATA 8.1 statistical package.

Results

Serum Ox-LDL Levels in RA and PsA Patients

Patients with RA and PsA showed higher ox-LDL concentrations in serum compared to healthy subjects (Figure 1). No differences were observed between patients with RA and PsA in the ox-LDL mean level. When patients with RA and PsA were divided according to the IMT value obtained by Echo-color Doppler images, patients with IMT >1 showed higher levels of ox-LDL compared to patients with IMT ≤1 and to healthy subjects (Figure 2).

Serum NO Levels in RA and PsA Patients

Patients with RA and PsA showed lower NO levels in serum compared to healthy subjects (Figure 3). The difference resulted statistically significant for PsA (PsA, P = 0.0155; RA, P = 0.0655). In patients with RA and particularly with PsA, divided according to the IMT value by Echo-color Doppler images, NO levels were lower in patients with IMT >1 compared to patients with IMT ≤1 and to healthy subjects (Figure 4).

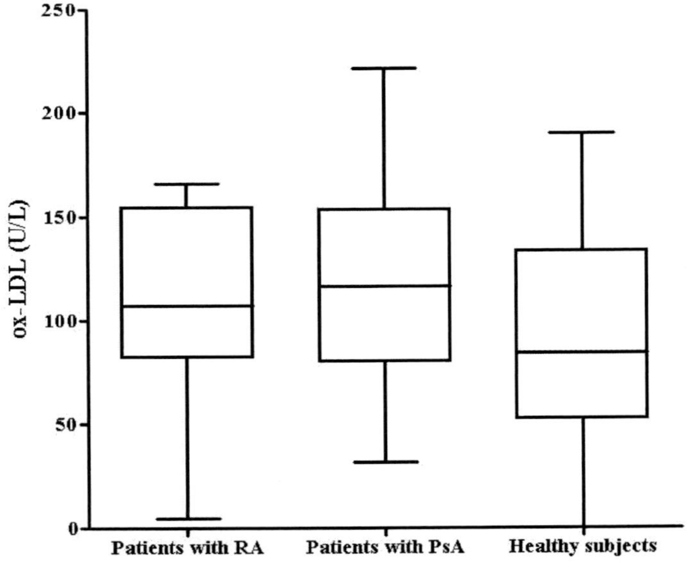

Figure 1. Box plot graphs showing oxidized LDL (ox-LDL) concentrations in serum samples from the 19 patients with rheumatoid arthritis (RA), the 20 patients with psoriatic arthritis (PsA) and the 20 healthy subjects. Patients with RA and PsA showed higher ox-LDL serum levels when compared to healthy subjects. No differences were observed between patients with RA and PsA.

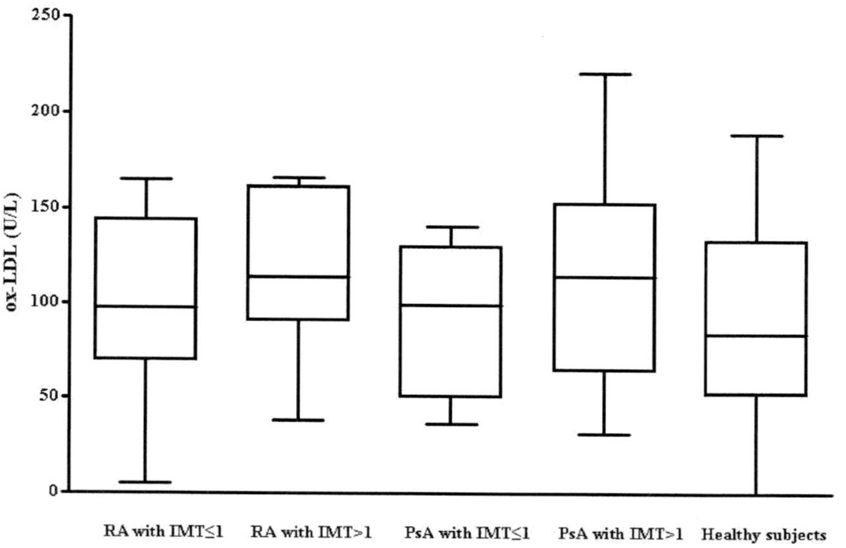

Figure 2. Box plot graphs showing oxidized LDL (ox-LDL) concentrations in serum samples from patients with rheumatoid arthritis (RA) and with psoriatic arthritis (PsA) divided according to the IMT value obtained by Echo-color Doppler images, and in serum samples from healthy subjects. Patients with RA and PsA showing an IMT >1 had higher levels of ox-LDL when compared to patients with IMT ≤1 and to healthy subjects.

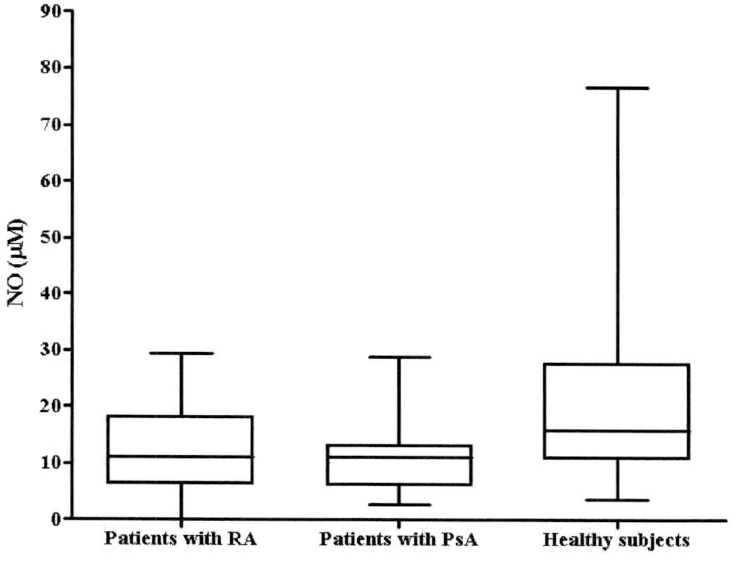

Figure 3. Box plot graphs showing nitric oxide (NO) concentrations in serum samples from the 19 patients with rheumatoid arthritis (RA), the 20 patients with psoriatic arthritis (PsA) and the 20 healthy subjects. Patients with RA and PsA showed lower NO serum levels when compared to healthy subjects. The difference resulted statistically significant for PsA (PsA, P =0.0155; RA, P = 0.0655).

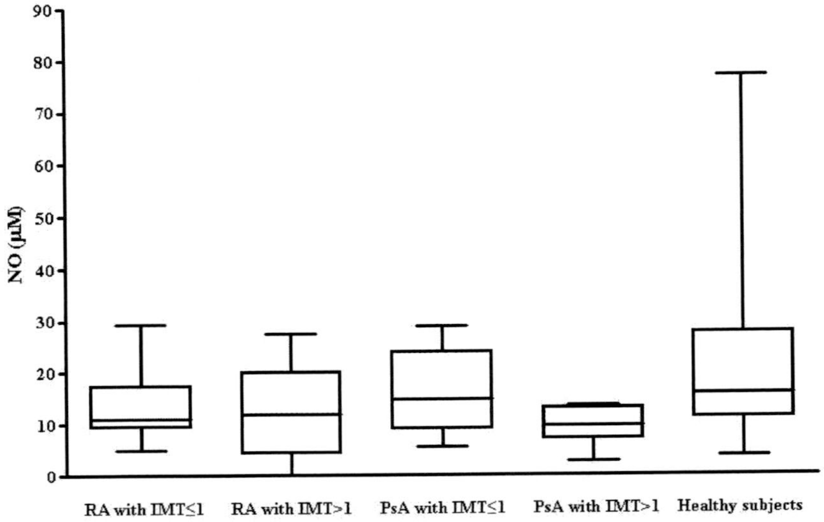

Figure 4. Box plot graphs showing nitric oxide (NO) concentrations in serum samples from patients with rheumatoid arthritis (RA) and with psoriatic arthritis (PsA) divided according to the IMT value obtained by Echo-color Doppler images, and in serum samples from healthy subjects. Patients with RA and PsA showing an IMT >1 had lower levels of NO when compared to patients with IMT ≤1 and to healthy subjects.

Association of Serum Ox-LDL and NO Levels with Baseline Characteristics of Patients

It is well known that there is a correlation among baseline clinical characteristics of patients and that these characteristics can be associated also to disease presentation. Analysis of association between risk factors and the autoimmune disease showed a significantly higher mean value of ESR and HDL-cholesterol in patients with AR than in patients with PsA ($P = 0.01$ and $P = 0.02$) (Table). In contrast the triglycerides value was significantly higher in patients with PsA than in patients with RA ($P = 0.0177$). In patients with RA, comparative analysis of risk factors with serum ox-LDL and NO levels showed a significant negative correlation between HDL-cholesterol and NO mean level ($r = -0.6$, $P = 0.013$) and a positive correlation near to the statistical significance between ox-LDL and cholesterol ($r = 0.5$, $P = 0.0528$). We did not find any correlation between traditional risk factors and the presence of subclinical atherosclerosis in patients with RA and PsA.

Conclusion

Our preliminary findings reported in this chapter indicate that serum levels of ox-LDL and NO are putative biomarkers for atherosclerosis development in patients with RA and PsA. We found that serum ox-LDL levels, higher in patients with RA and PsA than in healthy subjects, were particularly higher in patients with subclinical atherosclerosis evaluated as

IMT increase by Echo-color Doppler. In contrast serum NO levels resulted lower in patients with RA and PsA than in healthy subjects, particularly in patients with an increase in the IMT value (IMT >1). Our results of a negative association between ox-LDL and NO in patients are in line with previous findings indicating that ox-LDL impairs NO signaling and endothelial function thus contributing to the pathogenesis of atherosclerosis [24]. The endothelium plays a central role in overall vascular homeostasis by regulating vasoreactivity, platelet activation, leukocyte adhesion, and smooth muscle cell proliferation and migration. Endothelial NO, an important vasoprotective molecule, is a major modulator of these effects, and impaired NO signaling with associated endothelial activation is considered an early marker of the atherogenic process. Nitric oxide is produced by the action of endothelial NO synthase (eNOS), which uses L-arginine as its substrate [25]. However, L-arginine is also a substrate for arginase, which converts L-arginine to L-ornithine and urea [26]. Thus, substrate availability to, and thereby enzymatic products of either enzyme may be influenced by the activity and substrate utilization of the other. In human aortic endothelial cells, ox-LDL stimulation increases arginase enzyme activity in a time- and dose-dependent manner [27]. Thus, ox-LDLs increase arginase activity by a sequence of regulatory events, and this increased arginase activity contributes to ox-LDL-dependent impairment of NO production.

A limitation of our study is the low number of patients that probably does not allow to reach the statistical significance between the observed differences. The low number of patients also limits the possibility to find correlation of the two biomarkers evaluated in this study with traditional risk factors for atherosclerosis or clinical features of the rheumatic disease. Of note, in our study population the only statistically significant association was the negative correlation between NO and HDL-cholesterol levels in RA. Low levels of HDL cholesterol are usually recognized as an important independent risk factor for occurrence of cardiovascular events [28]. However, Agerholm-Larsen et al. observed an association of decreased HDL cholesterol levels with a paradoxical lower risk of ischemic heart disease in women [29]. These data suggest the hypothesis that the strong inverse association between HDL cholesterol concentrations and the occurrence of cardiovascular events observed in prospective epidemiological population studies is not due to HDL cholesterol levels per se, and that individuals with low HDL cholesterol may have a reduced risk of cardiovascular event occurrence. In the light of these previous data, it is not surprising the association between decreased levels of the vasoprotective mediator NO and increased concentrations of HDL cholesterol that we observed in patients with RA.

In conclusion, our study, although very preliminary and although not establishing a causal link between ox-LDL or NO levels and accelerated atherosclerosis, suggests that ox-LDL and NO levels may be operational as markers of atherosclerotic disease in patients with RA and PsA. The detection of circulating ox-LDL and NO levels in these patients might be a useful adjunct to imaging procedures as prognostic markers for the development of atherosclerotic disease and could be useful to the clinical management of patients. Clearly these interesting possibilities await confirmation in a larger number of patients.

References

[1] Haugeberg G, Ørstavik RE, Kvien TK. Effects of rheumatoid arthritis on bone. *Curr. Opin. Rheumatol.* 2003;15(4):469-75.

[2] Lourida ES, Georgiadis AN, Papavasiliou EC, Papathanasiou AI, Drosos AA, Tselepis AD. Patients with early rheumatoid arthritis exhibit elevated autoantibody titers against mildly oxidized low-density lipoprotein and exhibit decreased activity of the lipoprotein-associated phospholipase A2. *Arthritis Res. Ther.* 2007;9(1):R19.

[3] Gabriel SE, Crowson CS, Kremers HM, Doran MF, Turesson C, O'Fallon WM, Matteson EL. Survival in rheumatoid arthritis: a population-based analysis of trends over 40 years. *Arthritis Rheum.* 2003;48:54–8.

[4] Symmons DP. Looking back: rheumatoid arthritis – aetiology, occurrence and mortality. *Rheumatology*. 2005;44:iv14–7.

[5] Goodson N. Coronary artery disease and rheumatoid arthritis. *Curr. Opin. Rheumatol.* 2002;14:115–20.

[6] Van Doornum S, McColl G, Wicks I. Accelerated atherosclerosis: an extraarticular feature of rheumatoid arthritis? *Arthritis Rheum.* 2002;46:862–73.

[7] Ritchlin C. Psoriatic disease--from skin to bone. *Nat. Clin. Pract. Rheumatol.* 2007;3:698-706.

[8] Gonzalez-Juanatey C, Llorca J, Miranda-Filloy JA, Amigo-Diaz E, Testa A,Garcia-Porrua C, Martin J, Gonzalez-Gay MA. Endothelial dysfunction in psoriatic arthritis patients without clinically evident cardiovascular disease or classic atherosclerosis risk factors. *Arthritis Rheum.* 2007;57:287-93.

[9] Kimhi O, Caspi D, Bornstein NM, Maharshak N, Gur A, Arbel Y, Comaneshter D, Paran D, Wigler I, Levartovsky D, Berliner S, Elkayam O. Prevalence and risk factors of atherosclerosis in patients with psoriatic arthritis. *Semin. Arthritis Rheum.* 2007;36(4):203-9.

[10] Hahn BH, Grossman J, Chen W, McMahon M. The pathogenesis of atherosclerosis in autoimmune rheumatic diseases: roles of inflammation and dyslipidemia. *J. Autoimmun.* 2007;28:69-75.

[11] Gállego J, Martínez Vila E, Muñoz R. Patients at high risk for ischemic stroke: identification and actions. *Cerebrovasc. Dis.* 2007;24 Suppl 1:49-63.

[12] Pearson TA. New tools for coronary risk assessment: what are their advantages and limitations? *Circulation.* 2002;105:886-92.

[13] Steiner G. Atherosclerosis in type 2 diabetes: a role for fibrate therapy? *Diab. Vasc. Dis. Res.* 2007;4:368-74.

[14] Juonala M, Viikari JS, Rönnemaa T, Marniemi J, Jula A, Loo BM, Raitakari OT. Associations of Dyslipidemias From Childhood to Adulthood With Carotid Intima-Media Thickness, Elasticity, and Brachial Flow-Mediated Dilatation in Adulthood. The Cardiovascular Risk in Young Finns Study. *Arterioscler. Thromb Vasc. Biol.* 2008 Feb 28; [Epub ahead of print].

[15] Michos ED, Vaidya D, Gapstur SM, Schreiner PJ, Golden SH, Wong ND, Criqui MH, Ouyang P. Sex hormones, sex hormone binding globulin, and abdominal aortic

calcification in women and men in the multi-ethnic study of atherosclerosis (MESA). *Atherosclerosis.* 2008 Feb 7; [Epub ahead of print].

[16] Assayag EB, Bova I, Kesler A, Berliner S, Shapira I, Bornstein NM. Erythrocyte aggregation as an early biomarker in patients with asymptomatic carotid stenosis. *Dis. Markers*. 2008;24:33-9.

[17] de Ferranti SD, Rifai N. C-reactive protein: a nontraditional serum marker of cardiovascular risk. *Cardiovasc. Pathol.* 2007;16(1):14-21.

[18] Kabuyama Y, Kitamura T, Yamaki J, Homma MK, Kikuchi S, Homma Y. Involvement of thioredoxin reductase 1 in the regulation of redox balance and viability of rheumatoid synovial cells. *Biochem. Biophys. Res. Commun.* 2008;367:491-6.

[19] Firuzi O, Fuksa L, Spadaro C, Bousová I, Riccieri V, Spadaro A, Petrucci R, Marrosu G, Saso L. Oxidative stress parameters in different systemic rheumatic diseases. *J. Pharm. Pharmacol.* 2006;58:951-7.

[20] Spinetti G, Kraenkel N, Emanueli C, Madeddu P. Diabetes and Vessel Wall Remodeling: from Mechanistic Insights to Regenerative Therapies. *Cardiovasc. Res.* 2008 Feb 15; [Epub ahead of print].

[21] Gracia-Sancho J, Laviña B, Rodríguez-Vilarrupla A, García-Calderó H, Fernández M, Bosch J, García-Pagán JC. Increased oxidative stress in cirrhotic rat livers: A potential mechanism contributing to reduced nitric oxide bioavailability. *Hepatology*. 2007 Dec 10; [Epub ahead of print].

[22] Arnett FC, Edworthy SM, Bloch DA, McShane DJ, Fries JF and Cooper NS, Healey LA, Kaplan SR, Liang MH, Luthra HS, et al. The American Rheumatism Association 1987 revised criteria fort the classification of rheumatoid arthritis. *Arthritis Rheum.* 1988;31:315–24.

[23] Taylor W, Gladman D, Helliwell Ph, Marchesoni A, Mease Ph, Mielants H, and the CASPAR Study Group. Classification criteria for psoriatic arthritis. Development of new criteria from a large international study. *Arthritis Rheum*. 2006;54:2665-73.

[24] Ryoo S, Lemmon CA, Soucy KG, Gupta G, White AR, Nyhan D, Shoukas A, Romer LH, Berkowitz DE. Oxidized low-density lipoprotein-dependent endothelial arginase II activation contributes to impaired nitric oxide signaling. *Circ. Res*. 2006;99:951-60.

[25] Flam BR, Eichler DC, Solomonson LP. Endothelial nitric oxide production is tightly coupled to the citrulline-NO cycle. *Nitric. Oxide*. 2007;17:115-21.

[26] Durante W, Johnson FK, Johnson RA. Arginase: a critical regulator of nitric oxide synthesis and vascular function. *Clin. Exp. Pharmacol. Physiol.* 2007;34:906-11.

[27] Ryoo S, Gupta G, Benjo A, Lim HK, Camara A, Sikka G, Lim HK, Sohi J, Santhanam L, Soucy K, Tuday E, Baraban E, Ilies M, Gerstenblith G, Nyhan D, Shoukas A, Christianson DW, Alp NJ, Champion HC, Huso D, Berkowitz DE. Endothelial Arginase II. A Novel Target for the Treatment of Atherosclerosis. *Circ. Res*. 2008 Feb 28; [Epub ahead of print]

[28] Nash DT. Use of vascular ultrasound in clinical trials to evaluate new cardiovascular therapies. *J. Natl. Med. Assoc*. 2008;100:222-9.

[29] Agerholm-Larsen B, Tybjaerg-Hansen A, Schnohr P, Steffensen R, Nordestgaard BG. Common cholesteryl ester transfer protein mutations, decreased HDL cholesterol, and

possible decreased risk of ischemic heart disease: The Copenhagen City Heart Study. *Circulation*. 2000;102:2197-203.

In: Autoimmunity: Role, Regulation and Disorders
Editor: Fynn L. Vogel and L. F. Zimmermann
ISBN 978-1-60456-833-2

Chapter 3

Exogenous Nucleic Acids Contribute to Joint Inflammation in Rheumatoid Arthritis by Activating an Anti-Viral Interferon Response

Mattias Magnusson and Andrej Tarkowski*
Sahlgrenska Academy at University of Gothenburg, Department of Medicine, Rheumatology and Inflammation Research, Guldhedsgatan 10A, 413 46 Göteborg, Sweden

Abstract

Viral infections may give rise to both transient arthralgias and chronic arthritides. In addition, flares in RA have been suggested to be precipitated during viral infection. Double-stranded RNA is expressed by most viruses and is one of the strongest activators of innate anti-viral immunity. In apparent absence of ongoing viral infection, such dsRNA is found at significantly higher levels in sera and synovial fluids of RA patients than in a control population of osteoarthritis patients. This dsRNA in the joint may well be pathogenic because intra-articular injection of viral dsRNA, but not eukaryotic-like ssRNA, is highly arthritogenic. The mechanisms by which dsRNA triggers inflammation potentially include the dsRNA receptors PKR, TLR3, RIG and/or MDA5, whose activation results in production of proinflammatory cytokines. The ability of dsRNA to induce experimental arthritis in mice is, however, not dependent on PKR or TLR3, because mice devoid of these receptors develop arthritis to the same extent as wt mice, indicating that other receptors including RIG and MDA-5 may be involved. Common for activation of all these signaling pathways is that they can culminate in production of type I IFN. Production of type I IFN is the immediate, anti-

* Corresponding author: Mattias Magnusson, PhD, Sahlgrenska Academy at University of Gothenburg, Department of Medicine, Rheumatology and Inflammation Research, Guldhedsgatan 10A. 413 46 Göteborg. Sweden. Tel +46 (0)31 342 4021. Fax +46 (0) 31 823925

viral immune response upon viral infection that prevents and halts further viral replication. Mice unable to respond to type I IFN (IFNAR -/-) are completely protected against dsRNA-induced arthritis and injection of type I IFN intra-articularly into the knee of healthy mice results in a pronounced, but transient joint inflammation. Thus, if the immune response to a viral infection results in accumulation of type I IFN or deposition of dsRNA in the joint, then this defence may be directly harmful for the host by causing arthritis.

Introduction

Both transient and chronic arthralgias may ensue viral infections and flares in RA have been suggested to be precipitated by viral infection (Franssila and Hedman, 2006). Therefore we have explored if and how viral constituents may contribute to joint inflammation. Many viral species are associated with arthralgias and arthritis. For example, patients infected with influenza, rubella, parvo, hepatitis B and C and alphaviruses frequently experience arthritic symptoms (Franssila and Hedman, 2006). Therefore we have focussed on components that are omnipresent across the viral species that may contribute to arthritis. One such general component is their nucleic acids. Both viral DNA and RNA induce production of cytokines in leukocytes, which may trigger an innate inflammatory response. Certain characteristics of viral nucleic acids are thought to explain these properties: (1) viral DNA (and bacterial as well) harbours nucleotide motifs containing unmethylated CpG dinucleotides and (2) viral RNA occurs in double-stranded conformation during the replication within infected cells (Weber et al., 2006). In mammalian nucleic acids these two properties are heavily repressed, which may explain why mammalian nucleic acids do not in general trigger inflammation. The ability of the innate immune system to react to these subtle differences in nucleic acid structure may represent a way of self/non self discrimination. For example, the frequency of CpG-motifs is much lower in mammalian than in prokaryotic DNA, and in most instances when CpG occurs in mammalians, the C in CpG is methylated (Bird, 1980), which renders the DNA essentially immunologically inert (Krieg et al., 1995). The mRNA of mammalian cells is primarily single-stranded, although other forms of mammalian RNA, e.g., ribosomal RNA and tRNA occur as double stranded. Also, viral single stranded RNA may in some cases in fact be immunostimulatory (Diebold et al., 2004).

Viral Nucleic Acids Induce Joint Inflammation by Activating the Inteferon Response

In RA patients, in apparent absence of ongoing clinically overt viral infection, dsRNA levels in both synovial fluids and in sera are elevated as compared to a control population of osteoarthritis patients. This may indicate an inability to efficiently clear infections, resulting in continuous production of viral RNA that may contribute to chronic inflammation. In support of this, presence of dsRNA in synovia clearly correlates to a destructive disease course of RA (Magnusson, unpublished).

Experimentally, dsRNA deposited in a healthy joint will cause a pronounced inflammation, characterized by infiltration of leukocytes to the synovium, pannus and synovial lining hyperplasia (Zare et al., 2004). In contrast, a mimick of mammalian mRNA, single stranded RNA is devoid of this property (Magnusson et al., 2006; Zare et al., 2004). Also, DNA containing bacterial unmetylated CpG-motifs is highly arthritogenic, while DNA without such motifs is not (Deng et al., 1999). Thus, the self/non self discrimination of nucleic acids by the innate immune system may also be operative in the initiation phase of joint inflammation. That the innate immune system is primarily involved is indicated by the fact that mice devoid of functional T- and B-cell (SCID-mice) are also sensitive to such an inflammatory impact (Zare et al., 2004).

Several cellular receptors are implicated in immune activation by viral RNA (Akira et al., 2006). Using knock-out mice, we observed that the two dsRNA receptors toll like receptor 3 (Zare et al., 2004) and dsRNA-dependent protein kinase (Magnusson et al., 2006) were both redundant in dsRNA-induced arthritis. Moreover, a number of other receptors for dsRNA have been identified, including the RIG-1 and MDA5 proteins. Common for TLR3, PKR, RIG-1 and the MDA5 receptors is that they may all trigger dsRNA-dependent production of interferon-alpha (Akira et al., 2006). This anti-viral cytokine may in fact be the actual culprit of dsRNA-induced arthritis because mice unable to respond to this cytokine are completely protected against dsRNA-induced arthritis. In accordance, IFN-α by itself is highly arthritogenic if deposited intra-articularly (Magnusson et al., 2006). Therefore, all dsRNA receptors mediating activation of type I IFN could theoretically be implicated in dsRNA-induced arthritis.

Viral Nucleic Acids Recruits and Activate Production of Interferons in Synovial Dendritic Cells

Some or all of these receptors are expressed by the cells with the highest capacity to release type I IFN. These cells are dendritic cells (DC), either monocytic conventional DC or plasmacytoid DC (Eisenacher et al., 2007). In RA patients, both these cell types are accumulated in the inflamed joints, concommittant with their decrease in blood (Jongbloed et al., 2006). Thus, a localized viral joint infection could result in influx of DC to synovium leading to IFN-α production in situ. This could also explain the aggravation of joint inflammation observed during viral infections in already established RA (Franssila and Hedman, 2006). Experimentally, dsRNA-induced arthritis also involves infiltration of DC into the joint (Magnusson, unpublished). Thus, dsRNA may also activate recruitment of DC to the joint, most likely through its ability to activate production of IFN-α (see below). Without activation, DC are *per se* not arthritogenic if deposited in a healthy joint. In contrast, if stimulated with dsRNA prior to intra-articular injection, they become highly arthritogenic (Magnusson, unpublished). Thus, viral dsRNA likely induces joint inflammation by both recruitment of DC and activation of IFN-α production by DC.

Interferons Induce Joint Inflammation by Activating Innate Immunity

Type I IFNs may contribute and strengthen both innate and adaptive immune responses. It exerts the immediate anti-viral response upon infection, but also affects T- and B-cell activation including antibody production. Because this model of joint inflammation is also manifested in SCID mice, IFN-α is likely to exert its arthritogenic properties by primarily activating innate immunity. For example, IFN-α will recruit cells to the synovium by upregulating the expression of chemokine receptors (CCRs) (Parlato et al., 2001) on resident cells, which will recruit cells expressing chemokine ligands such as the macrophage inflammatory proteins (MIP). The expression of the CCR6 ligand, MIP3β is heavily upregulated in the synovium of RA patients (Ruth et al., 2003), and MIP1α and MIP1β on monocytic dendritic cells (Nagorsen et al., 2004) which indicates a CCR6 and CCR7-mediated recruitment of inflammatory cells. By upregulating CCRs IFN-α may retain and recruit cells to the synovium. Monocytes may be instrumental in this recruitment due to their extremely high expression of type I IFN receptors (Pogue et al., 2004) and ability to express CCRs. Accordingly, monocytes recruited to the synovium by IFN-α are also involved in dsRNA/IFN-α-induced arthritis because depletion of monocytes completely abrogates disease (Magnusson et al., 2006).

Another effect of IFN-α is its ability to induce production of IL-6. This activation is totally dependent on the transcription factor NFκB (Magnusson et al., 2006). The in vivo levels of IL-6 at different time points after onset of dsRNA-induced arthritis clearly follows the course of arthritis (Zare et al., 2004). The arthritis is most severe after 3-4 days and declines to full remission within two weeks. Thus, as for human RA, IL-6 may be a key component in this model of arthritis, downstream of IFN-α activation by dsRNA.

Conclusion

Viral infection may contribute to chronic and transient joint inflammation. Upon infection, the virus exposes the host to viral dsRNA. Double-stranded RNA can be detected in joints of RA patients where it may induce or aggravate inflammation. Such dsRNA induces joint inflammation by activating the host's antiviral response, manifested by release of type I IFN and infiltration of dendritic cells and monocytes to the synovium. Thus, the pro-arthritogenic properties of viral nucleic acids may explain why patients with viral infections often experience arthritic symptoms.

References

Akira, S., Uematsu, S., Takeuchi, O., 2006, Pathogen recognition and innate immunity. *Cell.* 124, 783-801.

Bird, A.P., 1980, DNA methylation and the frequency of CpG in animal DNA. *Nucleic Acids Res* 8, 1499-1504.

Deng, G.M., Nilsson, I.M., Verdrengh, M., Collins, L.V., Tarkowski, A., 1999, Intra-articularly localized bacterial DNA containing CpG motifs induces arthritis. *Nat. Med.* 5, 702-705.

Diebold, S.S., Kaisho, T., Hemmi, H., Akira, S., Reis, E.S.C., 2004, Innate antiviral responses by means of TLR7-mediated recognition of single-stranded RNA. *Science* 303, 1529-1531.

Eisenacher, K., Steinberg, C., Reindl, W., Krug, A., 2007, The role of viral nucleic acid recognition in dendritic cells for innate and adaptive antiviral immunity. *Immunobiology.* 212, 701-714 Epub 2007 Nov 2009.

Franssila, R., Hedman, K., 2006, Infection and musculoskeletal conditions: Viral causes of arthritis. *Best Pract Res. Clin. Rheumatol.* 20, 1139-1157.

Jongbloed, S.L., Lebre, M.C., Fraser, A.R., Gracie, J.A., Sturrock, R.D., Tak, P.P., McInnes, I.B., 2006, Enumeration and phenotypical analysis of distinct dendritic cell subsets in psoriatic arthritis and rheumatoid arthritis. *Arthritis Res. Ther.* 8, R15.

Krieg, A.M., Yi, A.K., Matson, S., Waldschmidt, T.J., Bishop, G.A., Teasdale, R., Koretzky, G.A., Klinman, D.M., 1995, CpG motifs in bacterial DNA trigger direct B-cell activation. *Nature* 374, 546-549.

Magnusson, M., Zare, F., Tarkowski, A., 2006, Requirement of type I interferon signaling for arthritis triggered by double-stranded RNA. *Arthritis Rheum* 54, 148-157.

Nagorsen, D., Marincola, F.M., Panelli, M.C., 2004, Cytokine and chemokine expression profiles of maturing dendritic cells using multiprotein platform arrays. *Cytokine.* 25, 31-35.

Parlato, S., Santini, S.M., Lapenta, C., Di Pucchio, T., Logozzi, M., Spada, M., Giammarioli, A.M., Malorni, W., Fais, S., Belardelli, F., 2001, Expression of CCR-7, MIP-3beta, and Th-1 chemokines in type I IFN-induced monocyte-derived dendritic cells: importance for the rapid acquisition of potent migratory and functional activities. *Blood* 98, 3022-3029.

Pogue, S.L., Preston, B.T., Stalder, J., Bebbington, C.R., Cardarelli, P.M., 2004, The receptor for type I IFNs is highly expressed on peripheral blood B cells and monocytes and mediates a distinct profile of differentiation and activation of these cells. *J. Interferon.* Cytokine Res 24, 131-139.

Ruth, J.H., Shahrara, S., Park, C.C., Morel, J.C., Kumar, P., Qin, S., Koch, A.E., 2003, Role of macrophage inflammatory protein-3alpha and its ligand CCR6 in rheumatoid arthritis. *Lab. Invest* 83, 579-588.

Weber, F., Wagner, V., Rasmussen, S.B., Hartmann, R., Paludan, S.R., 2006, Double-stranded RNA is produced by positive-strand RNA viruses and DNA viruses but not in detectable amounts by negative-strand RNA viruses. *J. Virol.* 80, 5059-5064.

Zare, F., Bokarewa, M., Nenonen, N., Bergstrom, T., Alexopoulou, L., Flavell, R.A., Tarkowski, A., 2004, Arthritogenic properties of double-stranded (viral) RNA. *J. Immunol.* 172, 5656-5663.

In: Autoimmunity: Role, Regulation and Disorders
Editor: Fynn L. Vogel and L. F. Zimmermann

ISBN 978-1-60456-833-2

Chapter 4

Antigenic Complementarity in the Induction of Autoimmunity: A Review

Robert Root-Bernstein*
Department of Physiology, 2174 Biomedical and Physical Sciences Building, Michigan State University, East Lansing, MI 48824 USA

Abstract

The causes of human autoimmune diseases remain a mystery. The reason may be that current theories based on molecular mimicry are overly simplistic, relying on single agent etiologies that do not explain how immune tolerance is broken. This essay presents a novel theory of autoimmunity based on evidence that autoimmune diseases result from concomitant exposure to multiple antigens that induce molecularly complementary immune responses. As in a normal immune response, each antigen induces a complementary antibody or T-cell response, but because the antigens are molecularly complementary, the resulting antibodies or T cells are also molecularly complementary. Antibodies or T cells against each antigen therefore mimic the structure of the other (complementary) antigen resulting in confusion as to what is "self" and "nonself", and thereby producing disregulation within the immune system. Significantly, complementary antibodies or T cells recognize each other as "nonself" and attach each other. The result is that autoimmunity is always characterized primarily by a "civil war" within the immune system itself. Diagnostic symptoms of this "civil war" are the circulating immune complexes and perivascular cuffing that occur in all autoimmune diseases. If, in addition, the antigens mimic other "self" proteins, then this "civil war" extends to other body systems. Epidemiological, clinical, and experimental evidence is presented for the presence of multiple concurrent infections preceding autoimmunity, for complementary antigens within these multiple infections, and for complementary immune responses to these antigens. Case studies include thrombocytopenia purpura, myocarditis, rheumatic fever, multiple sclerosis, and AIDS. Experimentally testable differences between the molecular mimicry, antiidiotype, and antigenic complementarity

* E-mail: rootbern@msu.edu; phone 517-355-6475 ext 1101; fax 517-355-5125

theory are presented. Mechanisms explaining prevention and suppression of animal models of autoimmunity are provided and their implications of the development of novel treatments for human autoimmune diseases discussed. The etiological implications discussed with regard to changes that the theory requires in applying Koch's postulates to autoimmune diseases. And the risks of initiating autoimmune diseases by delivering more and more vaccines concomitantly are discussed.

Introduction

Living systems are characterized by molecularly complementary components. (Root-Bernstein and Dillon, 1997; Hunding, et al., 2005) "Self" can therefore be defined as whatever has molecularly matching complementary pairs within such a system (i.e., that which is functionally and structurally integrated). "Nonself" is anything that is non-paired (i.e., has no molecular complement and is non-functional and non-integrated). Such a view of living systems has direct implications for understanding the role of the immune system and its functional mechanisms. I propose that the immune system evolved to neutralize unpaired material that poses a threat to the integrity of living systems. The immune system responds to "nonself" materials ("antigens") either by excluding or destroying the material (e.g., proteolytic digestion by lysozyme, or other innate immune mechanisms) or by producing molecularly complementary pairs (antibodies, T-cell receptors) that neutralize the ability of the unpaired material to interact destructively with the organismal system. In other words, the function of the immune system is to ensure the integrity of the pairing of the components of the living system.

The key to understanding how any system works is to examine how it fails under defined conditions. Autoimmune diseases should provide an unparalleled look at how the immune system can fail, but unfortunately the conditions under which such failures occur are not well-defined. The two dominant theories of autoimmunity at present, the molecular mimicry theory and the antiidiotype theory, have both failed to explain the origins of any human autoimmune disease. When a problem as important as autoimmunity continues to puzzle investigators for more than a century, one can be sure that a new approach to the problem is required. It is therefore worth looking at the basic concepts and assumptions that underlie the molecular mimicry and anti-idiotype theories in order to identify the specific problems that remain to be resolved.

Molecular mimicry has two inter-related meanings in biology. The original one was invented by Damian (1964) to describe how natural selection has resulted in microbial proteins that mimic those of the host in order to evade an immunological response (reviewed in Tsonis and Dwivedi, 2008). In 1983, Fujinami and Oldstone (Fujinanmi, et al., 1983; Fujinami and Oldstone, 1985) recognized that a possible consequence of such molecular camouflaging would be autoimmunity: in the event of an immune response to microbial host mimics, the host itself would be attacked. The molecular mimicry theory has been applied to a wide range of autoimmune diseases (reviewed in Barzilai, et al., 2007; Libbey, et al., 2007; Kim, et al., 2006; Benoist and Mathis, 2001; Rose and Mackay, 2000). It proposes that infectious agents trigger autoimmune diseases by inducing antibody or T-cell responses that cross-react with a "self" antigen that weakly mimics the triggering agent. As an accidental by-product of targeting the triggering agent, autoimmunity against the "self" mimic is induced (Figure 1).

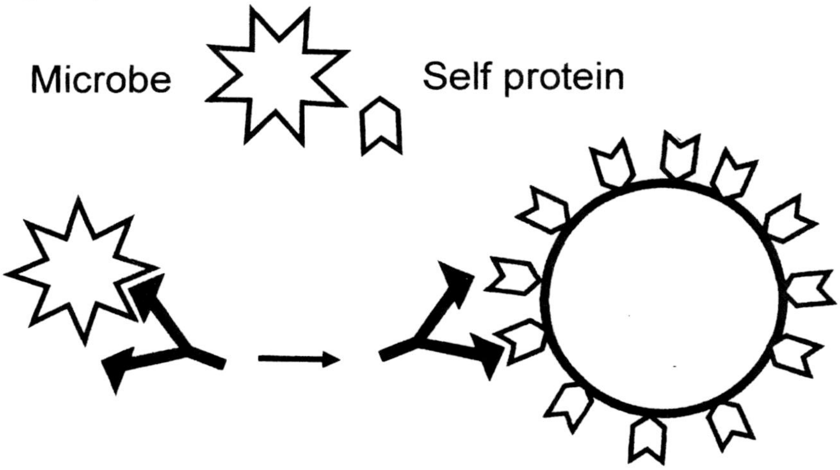

Figure 1. Fujinami and Oldstone's molecular mimicry model: an microbial antigen mimics a self antigen so that when antibodies are made against the microbial antigen, they cross-react with the self antigen resulting in autoimmunity. The theory fails to explain why everyone, or even a substantial proportion of people, infected with the same microbe do(es) not develop an autoimmune disease.

The strength of the molecular mimicry theory is that many examples of antigenic mimicry between infectious agents and human antigens have been elucidated, some of which will be described in some detail below. One key finding is that about 3.5 percent of some 600 monoclonal antibodies against viruses were found to cross-react with human organ antigens (Srinivasappa, et al, 1986). This finding strengthens the notion that molecular mimicry is certainly present between many microbial antigens and host antigens. But the molecular mimicry theory also has important limitations. First, many of the agents that mimic human antigens are virtually ubiquitous (e.g., influenza viruses, herpes viruses, streptococci, etc.) infecting huge numbers of people of whom only a very small fraction of a percent develop an autoimmune disease. No one has explained why an antigenic mimic that is present in all infected people rarely results in autoimmunity. Second, no one has managed to use a purified antigenic mimic to induce an autoimmune disease in an animal model. In order to induce autoimmunity, such antigenic mimics must always be administered along with additional antigens, most often in the form of complete (i.e., bacteria-containing) adjuvants. Finally, no one has been able to explain why the same antigenic mimics that are supposed to induce autoimmunity can, under appropriate conditions to be described below, also be used to prevent or to cure such autoimmunity in animal models. Prevention and treatment using antigenic mimics strongly suggests that there is nothing intrinsic to antigenic mimicry that results in autoimmunity, but rather that the response of the host to antigenic mimics depends upon other factors that remain to be elucidated.

The second major theory of autoimmunity is the anti-idiotype theory, which is based on the fact that many autoimmune diseases are characterized by the presence of anti-idiotype antibodies. There are two distinct versions of the anti-idiotype theory. The first version was described by Plotz in 1983 to explain how viruses could induce autoimmunity. Plotz noted that viruses and many infectious agents use cellular receptors to target particular tissues or organs for infection. The receptor-binding proteins on the infectious agent must therefore be molecularly complementary to the host receptor protein. An immune response to the triggering agent would therefore mimic the cellular receptor, but if an antiidiotype response followed, it would mimic the infectious agent, thereby targeting that cellular receptor itself. The result could be an autoimmune reaction (reviewed in Rico and Hall, 1988; Sherer and Shoenfeld, 2000; Shoenfeld, 2004) (Figure 2).

Pendergraft and Preston (Pendergraft, et al., 2004; Shoenfeld, 2004; Pendergraft et al., 2005; Preston, et al., 2005; McGuire and Holmes, 2005) have recently suggested a second mechanism in which such anti-idiotypy could result in autoimmunity. They propose that the initial autoimmune trigger is any protein that is complementary to the self antigen that will be targeted by the autoimmune reaction. This complementary protein may be self-expressed or it may be provided by an infectious agent. The initial immune response does not result in autoimmunity, but an anti-idiotypic response will mimic the initial protein, thereby targeting its complement (Figure 3). As with the molecular mimicry theory, both theories of anti-idiotypy fail to explain why everyone infected with a receptor-using pathogen, or one that contains a complementary antigen to a self protein, does not develop an autoimmune disease. Additionally, the Pendergraft-Preston version of the theory is predicated on a highly controversial form of protein complementarity called variously "hydropathic anti-complementarity" or "antisense proteins" developed by Blalock (reviewed in Weathington and Blalock, 2003; Tropsha, et al., 1992). This "hydropathic anti-complementarity" theory is not applicable to many types of antigens including glycoproteins, glycolipids, DNA,and other non-protein antigenic determinants. Moreover, there is a great deal of experimental evidence demonstrating that "hydropathic anti-complementarity" does not result in complementary peptides or proteins at all (reviewed in Root-Bernstein and Holsworth, 1999; Siemion, et al.,

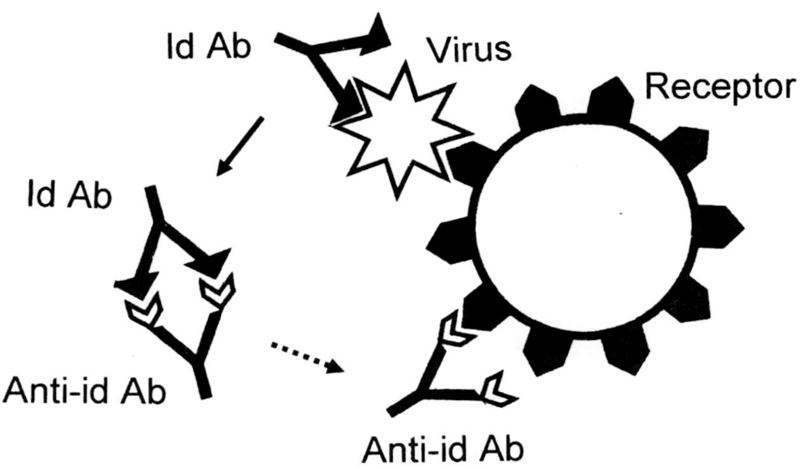

Figure 2. Plotz's anti-idiotypic model of virally-induced autoimmunity: viruses use cellular receptors to recognize and enter host cells; antibody against the virus will mimic the cellular receptor; anti-idiotypic antibodies will therefore mimic the virus, attacking the host cells bearing the appropriate receptors. As with the molecular mimicry model, this theory fails to explain why , or even a substantial proportion of people, infected with the same virus do(es) not develop an autoimmune disease.

2004). And like the molecular mimicry theory, the anti-idiotype approach has failed to yield animal models of autoimmunity induced either by a defined single antigen or by a defined anti-idiotype antibody.

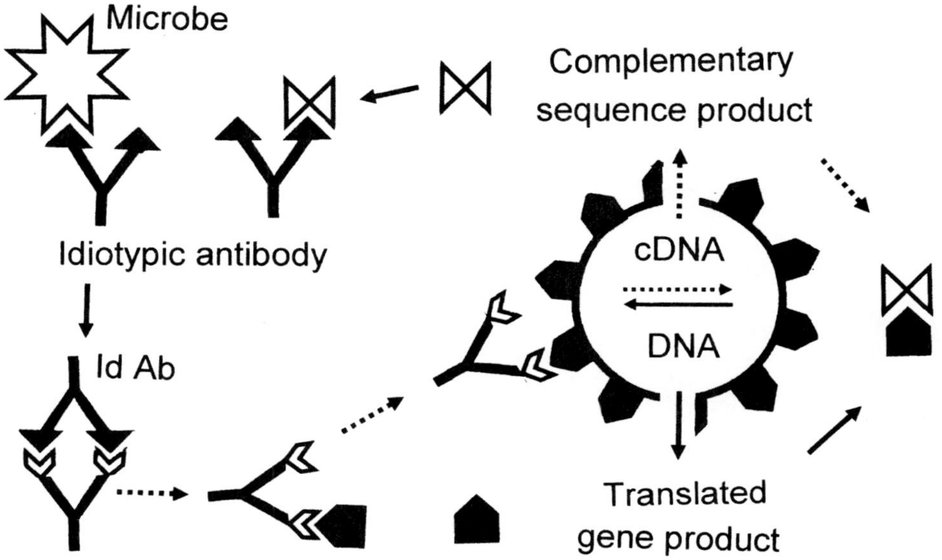

Figure 3. Pendergraft and Preston's extension of the anti-idiotype model: one strand of host DNA produces a "sense" gene product, while the other encodes a hypothetical "antisense peptide" that may or may actually be translated, but would be molecularly complementary to the "sense" peptide; if the antisense peptide is translated, then it can act as an antigen, or if it is not translated, then microbial antigens can act as mimics to this antisense peptide; in either case, antibody against the antisense peptide/microbial mimic induces an anti-idiotypic antibody that will recognize the "sense" gene product as a target, initiating autoimmunity against cells producing that "sense" peptide.

Current sentiment is that neither the molecular mimicry nor the anti-idiotype theories of autoimmunity are adequate to explain autoimmunity (reviewed in Libbey, et al., 2007; Kim, et al., 2006; Benoist and Mathis, 2001; Rose and Mackay, 2000). Westall and I proposed a very different theory of autoimmunity in 1983 that challenges the one underlying assumption shared by both the molecular mimicry and the anti-idiotype theories, which is that a single antigen initiates disease. We argue, based on both epidemiological data and evidence from animal models of autoimmune diseases, that autoimmunity results from multiple concurrent infections that present two or more molecularly complementary antigens to the immune system simultaneously (Westall and Root-Bernstein, 1983; Westall and Root-Bernstein, 1986; Root-Bernstein, 1991). I define molecular complementarity as being manifested by any pair of molecules that can bind to each other with stereochemical specificity. Antigenic complementarity results from molecularly complementary molecules that induce complementary immune responses, whether in the form of epitope-anti-epitope T-cell or B-cell receptors, or idiotype-anti-idiotype antibodies. Hoffmann, Kion and Grant (1991) have demonstrated that such antigenic complementarity would also result in MHC-anti-MHC complementarity. Such complementarity takes advantage of an "Achilles heel" in the immune system that results from its function as a moderator of systemic complementarity. *Pairs* of molecularly complementary antigens will fool the immune system into creating complementary *pairs of antibodies or T-cells* (Figures 4 and 5). These complementary antibodies or T-cells will not only pair with antigens, but with each other, resulting in confusion within the immune system between "self" and "nonself": the response to one member of a pair of complementary antigens is also an attack on the complementary immune response to the other antigen in the pair. While our multiple, complementary antigen theory (and its extension by Hoffmann, Kion and Grant [1991]) is not dependent upon Jerne's network theory of immune regulation, it is compatible with it, so that one can restate the problem posed by complementary pairs of antigens as inducing pairs of antibodies (or T-cells) that are each idiotypic, but which function as if they were idiotype-anti-idiotype pairs. According to Jerne's theory, such a situation would result in loss of network regulation of the antibody or T-cell response. Whatever theoretical basis one wants to adopt in approaching

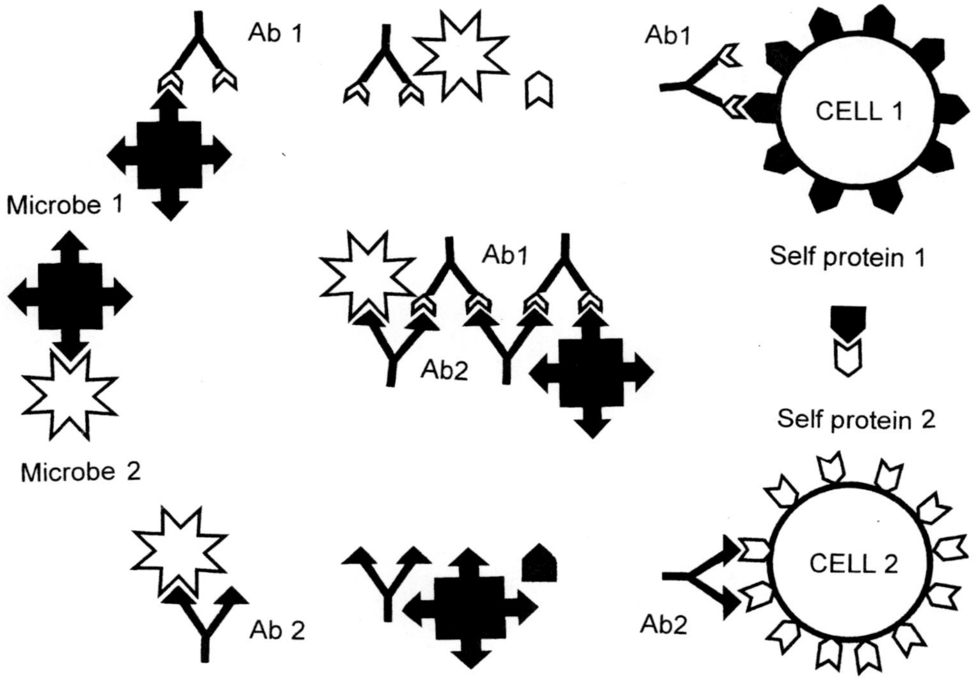

Figure 4. Westall and Root-Bernstein's complementary antigen theory: a pair of microbes (1 and 2) bearing molecularly complementary antigens infect an individual concurrently; each microbe mimics one of a pair of complementary self-antigens (1 and 2), and each microbial antigen gives rise to idiotypic antibody responses that act like idiotype-anti-idiotype pairs; the complementarity of the antibodies confuses the immune because microbe 1 mimics self-antigen 1 and antibody 2, while microbe 2 mimics self-antigen 2 and antibody 1; in this way, the immune system is tricked into having to attack itself in order to respond to the complementary microbial infections and self-tolerance is broken; in consequence, the antibodies produced by the complementary microbes attack their respective self-mimics producing autoimmunity. The theory incorporates the best elements of both the molecular mimicry and anti-idiotype models (and evidence supporting them) while also explaining how self-tolerance is broken (confusion within the immune system itself about what is self and nonself) and why microbially induced autoimmunity is relatively rare (concurrent infections with microbes bearing molecularly complementary antigens is unlikely). The same basic mechanism will produce cell-mediated autoimmune diseases as well (Figure 5). Other consequences of this theory are explored in Figures 6-8.

this problem, I assert that all autoimmune diseases are first of all, and primarily, targeted by the immune system *at itself*, and in all cases, immune system disregulation results from this intra-immunological confusion (Figures 4 and 5).

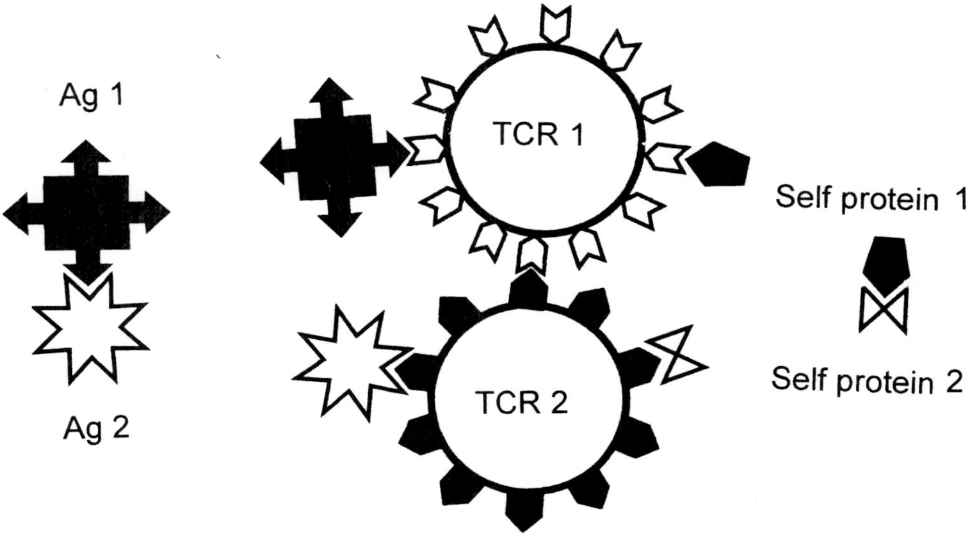

Figure 5. The complementary antigen theory of autoimmunity illustrated for cell-mediated autoimmune diseases: as in Figure 4, a pair of molecularly complementary microbial antigens that mimic a pair of molecularly complementary self-antigens induce a pair of complementary lymphocyte responses; the complementary lymphocyte responses are such that the lymphocytes against microbe 1 will also attack self-antigen 1; and the lymphocytes against microbe 2 will also attack self-antigen 2; as in Figure 4, immune tolerance is broken because each type of lymphocyte mimics one of the antigens, confusing the immune system itself as to what is self and nonself.

The specific nature of any autoimmune disease follows from the nature of the specific antigens that trigger the intra-immunological disruption. If the molecularly complementary antigens mimic one or more "self" proteins, then the disregulated immune response will also target some tissue or organ in the body. The complementary antigen theory therefore integrates the evidence gathered in support of the antigen-mimicry theories and the anti-idiotype antibody theories of autoimmunity proposed by previous investigators. To distinguish our theory from previous theories, we have called it variously the multiple-antigen-mediated autoimmunity theory (MAMA) (Root-Bernstein, 1995) or the MHC-image-anti-MHC-image theory (MIAMI) (Hoffmann, Kion, and Grant, 1991), but will use the simpler label "complementary antigen theory" (CAT) here (Root-Bernstein, 2004; Root-Bernstein and Rallo, 2004; Root-Bernstein, 2005; Root-Bernstein and Couturier, 2005; Root-Bernstein, 2007).

Unlike the molecular mimicry and anti-idiotype theories, CAT explains why autoimmune diseases are rare: it is unlikely that appropriately complementary pairs of infections will coexist in any given patient at any given time. CAT explains why multiple antigens are required (sometimes in the form of complete adjuvants) in order to induce autoimmunity in animal models. And it explains (as will be done in detail below) how molecular mimics and anti-idiotype antibodies are involved not only in the induction of autoimmunity, but can prevent and treat disease when administered alone. The purpose of this chapter is to review evidence supporting the CAT theory.

In particular, I will argue 1) that autoimmune diseases occur at much higher rates among multiply-infected individuals than among singly-infected individuals; 2) that each of the multiple infections mimics a self antigen and that the self-antigens mimicked by infectious agents are themselves molecularly complementary, so that there is *multiple* antigenic mimicry involved in autoimmunity; 3) that it is this multiple antigenic mimicry that results in pairs of simultaneous, complementary idiotypic immune responses (i.e., the equivalent of concurrent idiotype-anti-idiotype activation) confusing the immune system first into attacking itself and then into an unregulated attack on host tissues, and that such multiple antigenic mimicry can be used to identify the probable pairs of antigens required to induce any particular type of autoimmunity; and 4) and that such autoimmunity can be prevented or treated by any single component of the multiple, complementary agents, or antibodies (idiotypic or anti-idiotypic), required to induce disease. In other words, I will argue that the molecular mimicry and anti-idiotype theories are each half right, but need to be integrated in order to explain autoimmunity fully.

I will demonstrate each of these four points with regard to the following autoimmune diseases: experimental allergic encephalomyelitis; thrombocytopenia purpura; myocarditis and rheumatic fever; and lymphocytotoxic autoimminity in AIDS.

In conclusion, I will discuss three further consequences of the CAT theory for understanding autoimmune diseases in general. 5) The theory provides insight into why all autoimmune diseases (but not normal infections) are characterized by either circulating immune complexes and/or perivascular cuffing. 6) The theory requires revision of Koch's postulates in order to prove causation. Koch's postulates are based on the assumption that each disease has one causative agent. Multi-agent diseases will require a more complex set of postulates and novel *in vivo* tests and epidemiological studies that have yet to be carried out. Some of these will be outlined. 7) Finally, the complementary antigen theory suggests that while most vaccines can be safely administered together, there may be certain vaccines that will provoke complementary immune responses that could result in autoimmunity. Testing for antibody complementarity may provide a simple, fast way to ensure that many vaccine complications are avoided.

1. Autoimmune Diseases Occur Mainly among Multiply-Infected Individuals

As noted above, the molecular mimicry theory and anti-idiotype theories are predicated on single infections whereas the complementary antigen theory requires multiple concurrent infections. Current evidence suggests that autoimmunity rarely, if ever occurs, in people with single, uncomplicated infections (reviewed in Selmi, 2007).

One test of the CAT theory is that rates of autoimmunity should be significantly higher among groups of people characterized by multiple, concurrent infections than among healthier people. This is in fact that case. Patients immunosuppressed following organ transplantation and people with AIDS are both characterized by multiple concurrent infections (reviewed in Root-Bernstein, 1990; Root-Bernstein, 1993) and with rates of autoimmune diseases dozens to hundreds of times those found among the general population (Morrow, et al, 1991). These AIDS-associated autoimmune diseases include rheumatoid arthritis, myopathies, vasculitis, the sicca syndrome, systemic lupus erythematosus, Reiter's syndrome, Graves disease, anaemia, granulocytopenia, immune thrombocytopenia, Sjogren's syndrome, autoimmune demyelinization, and diabetes (Morrow, et al., 1991; Kaye, 1989; Zon et al., 1987). Among the autoantibodies reported in HIV/AIDS patients are anti-cardiolipin, anti-beta2 GPI, anti-DNA, anti-small nuclear ribonucleoproteins (snRNP), anti-thyroglobulin, anti-thyroid peroxidase, anti-myosin,, anti-erythropoietin antibodies and lymphocytotoxic autoantibodies (Zandman-Goddard and Shoenfeld, 2002). To give an example of the degree to which risk of autoimmunity increases with AIDS, while the incidence of autoimmune or lymphocytic myocarditis in the general population is about 1%, among people with AIDS it is as high as 50% (Morrow, et al., 1991; Friman, et al., 1995; Abuf, et al., 1997). Similarly, the incidence of demyelinating diseases can be as high as 60% among AIDS patients (Parry, et al., 1997), whereas the incidence is less than 0.1% in the general population (Chio, et al., 2007; McLead, et al., 1999) Perplexingly, successful treatment of T cell deficiencies in people with AIDS results in greatly pronounced expression of their underlying autoimmune conditions (Zandman-Goddard and Shoenfeld, 2002), often requiring treatment using (ironically) immunosuppressive drugs.

More particularly, specific combinations of infections are much more highly correlated with particular autoimmune diseases than are single infections. For example, various investigators have reported that cytomegalovirus (CMV) is associated with autoimmune demyelinization. Other investigators found, in contrast, a weak correlation with mycobacterial infections. I found among a group of people with AIDS that each disease was also weakly correlated with the presence of autoimmune demyelinization, but that the simultaneous presence of CMV (or a related herpes virus) with mycobacteria accounted for all of the cases of autoimmune demyelinization. No other combination of diseases was correlated with demyelinization at all (Root-Bernstein, 1990).

Since multiple sclerosis is an autoimmune demyelinating disease, it would be interesting to determine whether similar multi-agent infections are predictive of its onset. Cytomegalovirus clearly is not (Buljevac, et al., 2005; Lunnemann, et al., 2006; Barzilai, et al., 2007). Epstein-Barr virus infection, on the other hand, has consistently been correlated with multiple sclerosis in controlled studies (Ascherio and Munger, 2008; Krone, et al., 2008; Lunnemann, et al., 2006; Buljevac, et al., 2005) as have measles (Sips, et al., 2007; Krone, et al., 2008), Chlamydia pneumoniae, herpes simplex type 2, influenza A, parainfluenza 2 and vericella zoster virus (Krone, et al., 2008). Obviously none of these infections can be "the cause" of MS for the simple reason that they are all very common and in the vast majority of cases result in no autoimmunity, let alone MS. Moreover, some of these agents, such as Epstein-Barr virus, are associated with several different autoimmune diseases (Barzilai, et al., 2007), arguing against a one-agent-one-disease model. Genetics clearly plays some role in MS risk, as it does in most autoimmune diseases, but Ebers estimates that genetics accounts for only twenty percent of the risk of MS (Ebers, 2008), which means the majority of the risk must be due to environmental factors. Ebers cavalierly dismisses any role for infectious agents based on previous failures to identify *uniquely* predictive correlations with MS, but no one has ever looked at whether any *combination* of infections accounts for MS risk, and I would argue that it is premature to discount infectious triggers for MS until such a multi-agent study is carried out. Might a combination of Epstein Barr virus or measles with Chlamydia pneumonia, for example, be far more predictive than any of these agents alone?

Even in cases as apparently as straightforward as rheumatic fever, there is evidence that co-infection is necessary for disease development. It has been known for many years that infections with Chagas disease and group A streptococci (GAS) are associated with rheumatic heart disease. Prompt antibiotic treatment for GAS led to dramatic decreases in rheumatic fever. These facts led to the theory that GAS is the cause of rheumatic fever. But the vast majority of people infected with GAS, whether treated with antibiotics or not, do not develop rheumatic heart disease, suggesting that GAS may be necessary but is not sufficient to induce that autoimmune condition. Recent work suggests that, in fact, those people who develop rheumatic heart disease following a GAS infection are often, if not always, co-infected with a virus, most commonly coxsackie. Soboleva, et al., (1978) demonstrated that rheumatic fever in one group of patients followed GAS only when coxsackie virus type A was present. Pongpanich, et al. (1983; Boonpuchnavig, et al., 1984) found in another group of patients that coxsackie virus could invariably be isolated from the hearts of acute rheumatic fever patients. Active infection was not present, however, in the chronic form of the disease, in which autoantibodies become the pathogenic agents. Antibody studies in rheumatic fever have therefore yielded similar evidence for co-infection in chronic cases. Suresh, et al. (1981) found that among 21 cases of rheumatic fever, 19 had definitive evidence of coxsackie viral infection (types 1 through 6) and 14 of concurrent streptococcal infection. Vikerfors, et al. (1988) found that 65% of rheumatic fever patients were co-infected. And Zaher, et al. (1993) reported that over 80 percent of 200 patients with rheumatic fever had evidence of coxsackie virus infection in addition to a history of streptococcal infection. Higgins (1992) found that such co-infections caused more severe and prolonged disease than uncomplicated coxsackie or GAS infections.

Notably, autoimmune myocarditis has presented the inverse picture to rheumatic fever. The onset of autoimmune myocarditis has been correlated with coxsackie B viruses, cytomegalovirus, adenovirus, parvovirus B19, Chlamydia pneumoniae, and Borrelia burgdorferi infection (reviewed in Pankuweit, et al., 2004; Friman, et al., 1995). Given this diversity of possible initiating agents, it is striking that Vikerfors, et al. (1988) reported that 75% of patients with acute myocarditis had streptococcal infections and 48% also had simultaneous coxsackie virus infections. Additional studies of co-infections in myocarditis are therefore warranted.

Idiopathic thrombocytopenia purpura (ITP) presents a similar picture of multiple causative agents present concurrently. Epidemiological studies have identified HIV-1, rubella, Vericella zoster, the herpes viruses (including cytomegalovirus, herpes simplex type II, and Epstein-Barr virus), group A *Streptococcus*, *Mycobacterium*, *Mycoplasma,* and *Helicobacter pyelori.* (Kehane, et al., 1981; Bar-Meir, et al., 2000; Candelli, et al., 2003; Wright, et al., 1996; Yenicesu, et al., 2002; Kooter, et al., 2002; Gural, et al., 1998). The fact that thrombocytopenia occurs more frequently among people with AIDS than any other group of people, but the relevant antibodies are not elicited by HIV nor directed at it (Stricker, et al., 1985), strongly suggests that other concurrent infections that characterize this syndrome, such as Epstein-Barr virus and cytomegalovirus, are responsible for the thrombocytopenia (Scaradavou, 2002; Stricker, et al., 1985).

2. Autoantigens Are Complementary and Mimic Complementary "Self" Determinants

One of the unique features of CAT is its prediction that autoimmunity is triggered by combinations of molecularly complementary antigens each of which mimics a "self" determinant. In this way, the results of the molecular mimicry theory are all incorporated into the CAT theory, as are the data supporting the anti-idiotype theory, which is predicated on the presence of "self"-complementary antigens.

A multitude of evidence exists for the presence of sets of complementary antigens in many autoimmune diseases. Such evidence is particularly clear in AIDS. People with AIDS almost invariably develop lymphocytotoxic autoantibodies (LCTA) as part of their disease process (reviewed in Russo and Lopalco, 2006). These LCTA target both CD4-bearing cells, such as T-helper cells (e.g., Stricker, et al., 1987a; Stricker, et al., 1987b, Zarling, et al., 1990; Morrow, et al., 1991; Caporossi, et al, 1998), and also MHC II-bearing cells, such as antigen-presenting cells, macrophages, and dendritic cells (see references next paragraph). CD4 and MHC II are molecularly complementary proteins that bind to each other in the presence of antigen to initiate an immune response. One would therefore expect that the antigens that elicited these LCTA would also be molecular complementary, with one antigen mimicking CD4 and the other mimicking MHC II, and this is, in fact, the case.

It is well established that the gp120 coat protein of HIV mimics MHC II and that antibody to gp120 recognized MHC II as a target as well (Fraziano, et al., 1997; Wilson, et al., 1997; Metlas, et al., 1994; Bisset, 1994; Golding, et al., 1988; Silvestris, Williams and Damacco, 1995; Muller, et al., 1992; Argov, et al., 1991). The apparent difficulty with these observations is that the cells that are most adversely affected in HIV infection are not MHC-bearing cells but CD4-bearing cells. In consequence, various possible mechanisms have been proposed to explain how CD4 cells become targets in HIV-associated autoimmunity. Kennedy (1992) suggested that complementarity between HIV's gp120 and the CD4 protein of T helper cells would lead to anti-CD4 autoantibodies through an anti-idiotype mechanism of the type Plotz (1983) had proposed earlier (Figure 2). Susal, et al. (1993; 1996) and Serres (2001) have proposed more complicated mechanisms in which both idiotypic and anti-idiotypic antibodies to MHC proteins result in complementary immune responses that disturb the immune system in much the same way predicted by complementary antigen theories. Hoffmann, Kion and Grant (1991; and Hoffmann, 1994) have refined and developed this idiotype-anti-idiotype theory.

Notably, Kion and Hoffmann (1991) developed an HIV-free model of AIDS in mice that produces just the sort of idiotype-anti-idiotype LCTA their theory predicts. Alloimmune mice exposed to parental lymphocytes developed not only anti-MHC antibodies, but also anti-anti-MHC antibodies (i.e., anti-CD4 antibodies). These antibodies caused immune suppression. The antibodies also recognized the gp120 and gp24 antigens of HIV, thus proving that anti-

MHC antibodies act like anti-HIV antibodies. The results of Kion and Hoffmann (1991) have been reproduced and extended by other investigators including Stott (1991) and Ter-Grigorov, et al., (1997). Thus, it is well-established that HIV in conjunction with the cells it infects induce complementary antibodies that target MHC and CD4 cells. And equally notably, the presence of such complementary antibodies against lymphocytes are characteristic of people at risk for AIDS (Witkin and Sonnabend, 1983; Kiprov, et al., 1985).

I have demonstrated that the presence of anti-CD4 antibodies in AIDS can also be explained by the fact that most of the co-factor infections in AIDS have proteins that mimic CD4 directly. These include a wide range of mycoplasmas, Mycobacteria species, cytomegalovirus, and the hepatitis viruses (Root-Bernstein and Hobbs, 1991; Root-Bernstein and Hobbs, 1993; Root-Bernstein and Dewitt, 1994). In addition to infectious cofactors, some people who develop AIDS are immunologically exposed to semen antigens, which also mimic CD4 protein (Root-Bernstein and Dewitt, 1995). It has been proven that HIV binds directly to CD4-like proteins on the cell surfaces of sperm (Bagasra, et al., 1999), that anti-CD4 antibodies cross-react with sperm (Gobert et al., 1990), and that anti-sperm antibodies act as lymphocytotoxic autoantibodies (LCTA) (Mathur, et al., 1981; Witkin and Sonnabend, 1983; James and Hargreave, 1984; Mavligit et al., 1984; Kiprov et al., 1985; Adams et al., 1988; Bagasra et al., 1988). Thus a combination of HIV, which mimics MHC II, with sperm, which mimics CD4, would result the simultaneous presentation of a pair of complementary antigens to the immune system.

During the initial phases of the AIDS pandemic, a similar risk of encountering complementary antigens existed for whole blood transfusion and blood clotting factor recipients. Such patients received not only HIV-contaminated blood or blood products mimicking MHC II, but also CD4-bearing cells or CD4 proteins (Root-Bernstein, 1993).

Since one or more antigenically complementary cofactors is found along with HIV in every person who develops AIDS, every such person would have to either produce immune responses cross-reactive with both CD4 and MHC II or fail to respond adequately to their exposure to infections and alloantigens. It should be noted that one of the consequences of the production of complementary antibodies that cross-react with both MHC II and CD4 cells is not only down-regulation of the immune response, which is typical of AIDS, but also specific inhibition of the responses to HIV and its CD4-like cofactors by antibody-antibody neutralization. Two of the most puzzling aspects of AIDS are the fact that it is characterized by hypergammaglobulinemia and immune suppression directed not against all infectious agents (responses to influenza, cold viruses, and most vaccines is not affected), but specifically against those infections defined as opportunistic ones. The hypergammaglobulinemia can be explained by complementary antibodies attacking each other leading to an ever-escalating immunological civil war, while the specific defects in immunity to opportunistic infections can be explained by the co-neutralization of antibodies against HIV and its cofactor infections.

A similarly well-defined complementary mixture of antigens occurs in experimental allergic encephalomyelitis, an animal model sometimes used to study multiple sclerosis, but actually more appropriate to studying acute demyelinating processes. The minimal agents required to induce EAE in various animal species have been defined at the molecular level. In guinea pigs, for example, EAE induction requires a combination of a nonapeptide derived from myelin basic protein along with "adjuvant peptide", N-actyl-muramyl-D-ala-L-isoGln, a cell-wall derivative from mycobacteria or B. pertussis. EAE cannot be produced by any dose of either of these agents alone and they must be present in approximately equimolar concentrations simultaneously. Notably, the two antigens bind to each other quite specifically as demonstrated by nuclear magnetic resonance spectroscopy (Root-Bernstein and Westall, 1990). Equally compelling is the fact that a number of viruses associated with demyelinating autoimmune diseases, including cytomegalovirus, measles, and the hepatitis viruses, are highly homologous to the encephalitigenic regions of myelin basic protein (Fujinami and Oldstone, 1985). Thus, the fact that demyelinizing autoimmunity is associated with a combination of CMV with mycobacterial infections in people with AIDS (Root-Bernstein, 1990) satisfies the requirement for induction of a pair of complementary antigens.

Myocarditis and rheumatic fever are also characterized by the presence of complementary antigens that mimic "self" proteins. Cunningham and others have demonstrated using many methods that the M protein of group A streptococci (GAS) mimics cardiac myosin and that antibodies and T cells activated against one recognize the other. Antibody against myosin also appears in experimental autoimmune myocarditis induced by coxsackie virus infection, but Rose and his colleagues have demonstrated that this antibody is a secondary, possibly anti-idiotypic response to infection. Notably, actin is also a target of the immune system in both rheumatic fever and myocarditis. Actin is, of course, molecularly complementary to myosin and their complex is necessary to muscle function. Notably, coxsackie viruses have multiple and very substantial regions of homology with cardiac actin. Antibody against coxsackie virus recognizes cardiac actin and antibody against cardiac acting recognizes coxsackie virus. Thus, while the M protein of GAS mimics myosin, coxsackie proteins mimic actin and a combined infection would present molecularly complementary antigens to the immune system (Root-Bernstein, Vonck and Podufaly, in press).

The same type of antigenic complementarity is also present in the disease agents associated with induction of autoimmune thrombocytopenia. Notably, the two main targets of the autoimmune process in thrombocytopenia are platelet glycoprotein 1b and clotting factor IX (von Willebrand's factor), which are known to bind to each other as a necessary part of initiating the clotting cascade. Unfortunately, no antigen-initiated animal model of thrombocytopenia yet exists, so it is impossible to say at this time whether the antigens required to initiate autoimmunity are themselves complementary, but evidence to be presented in the next section strongly suggests that they are. In this case, we have used the fact that the targets of the autoimmunity are known and are molecularly complementary to predict and screen for infectious disease antigens that mimic the two "self" targets and are therefore themselves antigenically complementary.

The upshot of antigenic complementarity combined with antigenic mimicry is that it provides a stratagem for identifying potential co-infections that can induce autoimmunity. Whether one first identifies an infectious agent that mimics a self determinant, or one identifies an anti-idiotypic antibody associated with a self target, one can infer the nature of the autoimmune cofactor from the molecular complementarity of the self determinant or target. Thus, if a receptor is the target of autoimmunity, one can assume both that there is an infectious agent that mimics that receptor and also that there is a second infectious agent that mimics the ligand for that receptor. In the case of multiple sclerosis, for example, it is clear that myelin basic protein is a target of the autoimmune process, but it is also known that gangliosides bind to MBP and may be a target for autoimmunity as well. If so, then infectious agents that have antigens mimicking gangliosides may be critical determinants of MS initiation.

3. Antigenic Complementarity Is Reflected in Immunological Complementarity

Although it is well known that an idiotypic antibody can elicit an anti-idiotypic antibody and that such anti-idiotypic antibodies can be involved in autoimmune processes, it is only in light of the complementary antigen theory of autoimmunity that the possibility has emerged that two idiotypic antibodies might act as if they were an idiotype-anti-idiotype pair. Evidence for idiotype-idiotype complementarity has several important implications. One is that such complementarity is uniquely predicted by the complementary antigen theory. A second is that all evidence for a role of anti-idiotype antibodies in autoimmune processes may have to be re-evaluated in light of the possibility that the evidence for anti-idiotypy is actually evidence for complementarity between independently elicited idiotypes.

Two simple procedures can be used to search for idiotypic complementarity. One is a modification of Ouchterlony immunodiffusion in which antibodies replace antigens so that various idiotypic antibodies are diffused at each other. We call this method "double antibody diffusion", or DAD. Only those antibodies that are idiotypically complementary will precipitate each other resulting in observable bands of protein. The second method is a similar modification of the enzyme-linked immune-adsorption assay (ELISA) that we call "double antibody ELISA, or DA-ELISA). In DA-ELISA an idiotypic antibody is bound to the ELISA plate, a blocking agent added, followed by a second idiotypic antibody from a different species, and completed with an enzyme-linked antibody against this different species in order to determine how much of the second antibody bound to the first. DA-ELISA has the advantage of DAD that the former provides quantitative data on binding affinities, but DA-ELISA can only be used with idiotypic antibodies raised in two different species of animal, which limits its application.

We have run approximately 2000 more-or-less random combinations of viral and bacterial antibodies against each other in DAD experiments resulting in about two percent of these antibodies precipitating each other (Root-Bernstein, 1995; Root-Bernstein, 2004; Root-Bernstein, 2005; Root-Bernstein and Rallo, 2004). This figure is therefore approximately the same as Oldstone and his collaborators found for the percent of antibodies raised against viruses that cross-react with human tissue antigens (Srinivasappa, et al., 1986). Whether such antigenic complementarity, like antigenic mimicry, is a result of the selective pressures of functional co-evolution between microbes; a result of different microbes mimicking different human epitopes that are, by chance, complementary; or a consequence of one microbe being protected by mimicking the antibody or T-cell response to a previous (complementary) microbial infection remains to be determined.

In a few cases, the precipitations confirm complementarity between viral antigens that has already been established, as when antibody against hepatitis B core protein precipitates antibody against hepatitis B surface protein, as one would expect from the fact that these two proteins must bind to each other in order to form hepatitis virus particles. Also as one would expect from the antigenic complementarity of HIV and CD4 protein, antibodies against HIV gp 160 and HIV gp 120 are complementary to (and therefore precipitate) antibodies against CD4 (Root-Bernstein, 1995; Root-Bernstein, 2004; Root-Bernstein, 2005; Root-Bernstein and Rallo, 2004). In addition, antibodies against HIV gp160 and gp 120 are complementary to human sperm surface proteins, as would be predicted by the fact that HIV binds directly to sperm (Root-Bernstein and DeWitt, 1995).

As predicted by the fact that many cofactor infections mimic CD4 protein, while HIV mimics MHC II, HIV antibodies are often found to precipitate antibodies from other infections highly associated with AIDS, including cytomegalovirus (CMV), hepatitis B and C viruses, mycobacteria spp., and various mycoplasmas (Root-Bernstein, 1995; Root-Bernstein, 2004; Root-Bernstein, 2005; Root-Bernstein and Rallo, 2004). These instances of idiotypic complementarity make sense in light of the evidence presented in the previous section that these AIDS cofactors all have proteins that mimic the CD4 protein of T lymphocytes just as HIV mimics MHC II. In fact, one can take the idiotypic complementarity one step further and demonstrate that HIV antibody precipitates antibody against CD4 and that CMV, hepatitis viruses, mycobacteria and mycoplasmas often produce antibodies that precipitate antibody against MHC II. Finally, of course, antibody against CD4 protein precipitates antibody against MHC II, closing the idiotypic complementarity circle (Root-Bernstein, 1995; Root-Bernstein, 2004; Root-Bernstein, 2005; Root-Bernstein and Rallo, 2004) (Figure 4).

What such data suggest is that co-infections with complementary antigens such as HIV and CMV (or other cofactors) will elicit a pair of complementary antibodies. Since HIV mimics MHC II, the resulting antibodies to HIV mimic antibodies to CD4. Simultaneously, since CMV (or another cofactor infection) mimics CD4, the resulting antibodies will mimic antibodies to MHC II. But the further consequence is that these antibodies mimicking MHC II also mimic HIV; and the antibodies mimicking CD4 also mimic CMV (or another cofactor infection). The immune system has thus been tricked into producing antibodies that mimic microbial antigens and loses its ability to distinguish "self" from "nonself". A civil war will begin within the immune system in which these antibodies will attack each other, producing the hypergammaglobulinemia typifying AIDS. As a consequence of this "civil war", neither set of antibodies will properly neutralize their appropriate microbial targets, and both sets of the antibodies will inappropriately target the host mimic (CD4 or MHC II protein) as well, acting as lymphocytotoxic antibodies . Such a scenario suggests that AIDS pathogenesis is at least in part autoimmune in nature and results from the immune system attacking itself (Root-Bernstein, 1993).

One of the predictions that follows from the scenario just described is that what appear to be anti-idiotypic antibodies (but which are actually idiotypic antibodies against cofactor infections) should be a common concomitant of the development of AIDS. This is, in fact, the case (Shearer ,et al., 2000; Hoffmann, Kion and Grant, 1991). Thiart, et al. (1988) found anti-CD4 antibodies present in many people with AIDS, but found that these were unlikely to be anti-idiotypic in origin, suggesting that they could not have originated as anti-anti-HIV antibodies. Grant (2002) found that an anti-idiotypic antibody developed artificially against anti-HIV gp120 mimicked HCV idiotypic antibody (i.e., that idiotypic HCV antibody is complementary to idiotypic HIV antibody).

Similar networks of complementary antibodies have been found to be associated with the other autoimmune diseases discussed in this review. For example, in thrombocytopenia, antibodies are often found against both von Willebrand's factor (factor IX) and platelet glycoprotein 1b, two proteins that bind to each other during the normal blood clotting cascade. Some antibodies against cytomegalovirus recognize factor IX as an antigen, while some antibodies against group A streptococci recognize platelet glycoprotein 1b as an antigen. Strikingly, these same antibodies from CMV and GAS precipitate each other, each treating the other as an antigen (Root-Bernstein and Couturier, 2006). In consequence, a combined infection with these two infectious agents may elicit antibodies that cannot distinguish "self" from "nonself" and are themselves targets of the resulting autoimmune process. And as in the case of lymphocytotoxic autoantibodies in AIDS, the presence of what are assumed to be anti-idiotype antibodies are a common concomitant of idiopathic thrombocytopenia purpura (Balint and Jones, 1994).

The same basic story characterizes autoimmune myocarditis. The two main target of autoimmune myocarditis are cardiac myosin and cardiac actin and at least two types of infectious agents are associated with onset of the disease: group A streptococci (once again) and coxsackie viruses. Not surprisingly, antibody against cardiac myosin precipitates antibody against cardiac actin. More interestingly, some coxsackie virus antibody recognizes cardiac actin as an antigen and some group A streptococcal antibodies recognize myosin as an antigen. Most importantly, these coxsackie and group A streptococcal antibodies recognize each other as antigens and precipitate each other (Root-Bernstein, Vonck, and Podufaly, in press). Thus, once again, a complete set of complementary "self" antigens, microbial mimics, and complementary antibodies can be shown to exist at the heart of this disease.

Finally, turn to EAE, which is a cell-mediated autoimmune disease initiated by a combination of the complementary antigens adjuvant peptide and myelin basic protein. To test whether lymphocytes can be complementary in the same way that antibodies can be, we inoculated one set of strain 13 guinea pigs with saline solution, another with adjuvant peptide in incomplete Freund's adjuvant, and a third set with the tryptophan peptide of myelin basic protein in Freund's complete adjuvant. The lymphocytes from each set of animals were isolated from their mesenteric lymph nodes two weeks later. These lymphocytes were mixed. Lymphocytes from adjuvant peptide-inoculated animals mixed with those from the saline injected animals did not aggregate, nor did those from the tryptophan peptide-inoculated animals when mixed with the saline-treated ones. But when the lymphocytes from the adjuvant-peptide-inoculated animals were mixed with those from tryptophan peptide-inoculated animals, the lymphocytes formed distinct aggregates and the number of dead cells (as determined by trypan blue staining) was very significantly higher than among the other mixtures (Root-Bernstein, 1991). These data strongly suggest that lymphocytes raised against complementary antigens will, like antibodies, also be complementary to each other (Figure 5).

It is worth noting a striking feature of the data summarized in this section on immunological complementarity and autoimmunity, and that is the fact that the same microbial agent may play a role in the induction of different autoimmune diseases depending on the complementary microbe to which it is paired. For example, complete Freund's adjuvant made with mycobacteria can be used to induce adjuvant arthritis, an animal model of inflammatory arthritides such as rheumatoid arthritis. Adding myelin basic protein to this complete Freund's adjuvant, at the exact same dose, will, however, result in experimental allergic encephalomyelitis with no symptoms of arthritis whatsoever. (This observation has been used to isolate various epitopes from myelin basic protein that are shared with measles virus that are capable of preventing or treating adjuvant arthritis.) It appears that a similar story can be made for cytomegalovirus, group A streptococci, and coxsackie viruses. Cytomegalovirus is implicated above in both lymphocytotoxic autoantibodies in AIDS as well as in the induction of autoimmune thrombocytopenia purpura, but in the former case combined with HIV and in the later case with group A streptococci. Group A streptococci have also been implicated in rheumatic fever and myocarditis, but in combination with coxsackie viruses. Coxsackie viruses, in turn, have been implicated in both myocarditis and diabetes, and while there appear to be type preferences (B4 for diabetes and B3 for myocarditis), all types of coxsackie virus types have been linked to both diseases at greater or lesser rates of incidence. Such data should serve as a warning that it may be highly misleading to try to link a particular microbe exclusively with a single autoimmune disease – a point to be taken up and expanded below.

4. Individual Antigens Prevent and Suppress Complementary Antigen-Induced Autoimmunity

A further distinguishing feature of the complementary antigen theory is that it predicts that individual antigens will protect against subsequent induction of disease by pairs of complementary antigens, and also that large doses of one antigen can disrupt already existing autoimmunity caused by complementary antigens, thereby restoring normal functioning of the immune system (Westall and Root-Bernstein, 1983; Root-Bernstein, 1991; Root-Bernstein and Couturier, 2006; Root-Bernstein, 2007).

A mechanism by which prevention of complementary antigen-induced autoimmunity can occur is illustrated in Figure 6. By presenting an antigen to the immune system in the absence of that antigen's complement, the immune system is stimulated to produce antibody or T-cells (or both) against the antigen. Once the antibody or T cells have proliferated (a process that takes about two weeks), then the presentation of the complementary antigen to the immune system results in tolerance to the complementary antigen because it mimics "self" antibody and/or T-cells. In consequence, it is not possible for the immune system to launch a complementary attack on the second antigen and the distinction between "self" and "nonself" remains intact.

Suppression of an already existing autoimmune disease can also be prevented by inoculating the host with a large dose (or repeated doses) of one of the two initiating antigens. In this case (Figure 7), a complementary pair of T cells or antibodies that cross-react with "self" determinants are present. One of the key features of the complementary antigen theory is that it postulates that a relative balance must be retained between the complementary immune responses responsible for the autoimmune disease. Otherwise, one set of T cells (or antibodies) will predominate and neutralize or eliminate the other set. Variations in the relative populations of complementary T cells (or antibodies) may explain why many autoimmune diseases wax and wane with time. The requirement for a balance between the complementary immune responses can be exploited to create suppression of one of the responses by inoculating the host with a large amount (or repeated amounts) of the complementary antigen (Figure 7). This antigen will induce a greatly increased immune response to itself, causing selective proliferation of the relevant T cells (or antibodies). This selective proliferation will overwhelm the complementary immune response, resulting in either the neutralization or elimination of the complementary immune response.

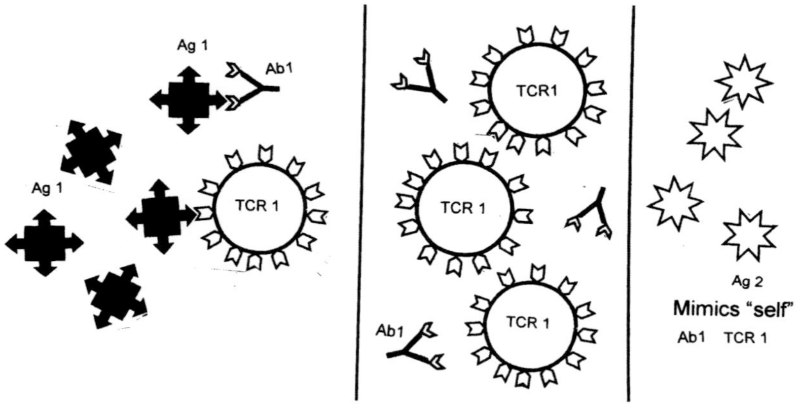

Figure 6. An explanation of prevention of autoimmunity according to the complementary antigen theory: a microbial antigen, Ag1, induces either T-cell or antibody response (or both); this immune response expands and becomes part of the self repertoire or proteins in the body; at some later time, the introduction of a microbial antigen (Ag2) that is complementary to the first microbial antigen (Ag1) is recognized as self because it mimic the antibody or T-cells against Ag1; in consequence, no immune response is mounted against the complementary antigen, Ag2. Even if the immune system did attempt to mount a response to Ag2, the pre-existing immunity to complementary antigen, Ag1, would neutralize or destroy the response to Ag2 before it became effective. Note that timing is crucial in this model. Complementary antigens must be present in a host within a couple of weeks of each other to mount effective pairs of complementary immune responses; beyond that window of time, tolerance for one antigen will be induced by the preceding complementary infection.

The distinction between "self" and "nonself" will be restored, and tolerance to the complementary antigen induced. Note, however, that an active T cell (or antibody) response will remain against the suppressing antigen. The complementary antigen theory maintains that it is not the presence of potentially auto-reactive T cells or antibodies that induces autoimmunity, but rather the immunologically confusing presence of a pair of complementary auto-reactive responses. Thus, suppressing an autoimmune disease should not eliminate all potentially auto-reactive T cells or antibodies, but should result in the continued presence of one of these along with restoration of immune regulation.

Perhaps the best characterized example of how prevention and tolerance are induced by the single agents of multi-antigen mixtures that induce autoimmune diseases is found in experimental allergic encephalomyelitis (EAE). EAE, as noted above, is induced by combinations of myelin basic protein (or its encephalitogenic peptides) with adjuvant peptide

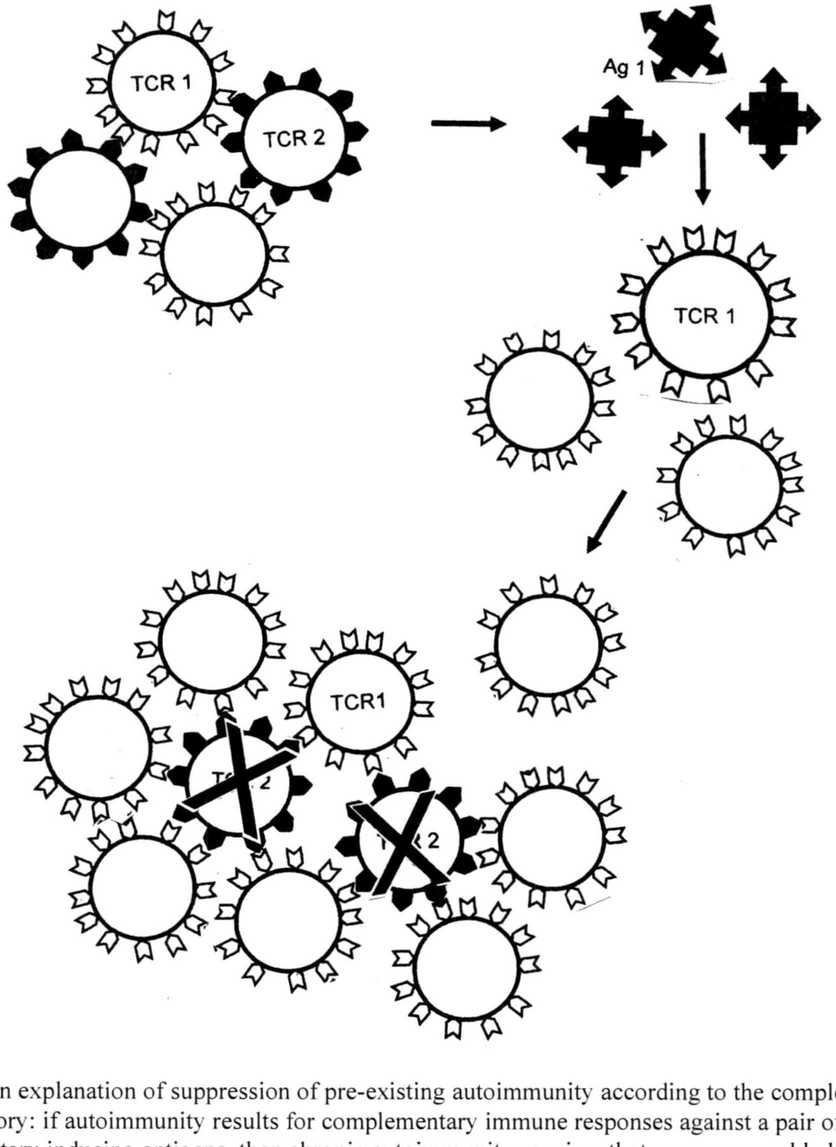

Figure 7. An explanation of suppression of pre-existing autoimmunity according to the complementary antigen theory: if autoimmunity results for complementary immune responses against a pair of complementary inducing antigens, then chronic autoimmunity requires that some reasonable balance between the pair of complementary immune response be maintained; disrupting this balance far enough should result in one of the two immune responses "winning" the immunological "civil war" that is at the heart of autoimmunity; thus, inoculating a host organism with a large dose of one of the inducing antigens should increase the antibody or cell-mediated response to that antigen to a great enough degree to overwhelm the complementary immune response, thereby reestablishing normal immune function and a proper sense of what is self and nonself. Whether the "winning" immune response actually eliminates the "losing" one or simply inactivates it by blocking all available antibody or lymphocytes, the result will be the same. Note, however, that the "winning" immune response will remain at a significant level even after the autoimmunity has been vanquished. The complementary antigen theory

predicts that the "losing" immune response will disappear, and that the host will be tolerant to the corresponding inducing antigen. Note also that the model illustrated here will work equally well in antibody-mediated autoimmune diseases.

to a complete Freund's adjuvant containing Mycobacteria or B. pertussis. The complementary antigen theory predicts that EAE should be preventable by inoculations of either the myelin basic protein (or its encephalitogenic peptides) alone or the so-called "adjuvant" alone. Both predictions are correct. Both myelin basic protein and its encephalitogenic peptides protect against induction of EAE when inoculated in incomplete Freund's adjuvant (Liu et al., 1998; Bai, et al., 1997; Marusic and Tonegawa, 1997; Guar, et al., 1992; Rauch and Einstein, 1968). MBP also suppresses existing EAE when inoculated alone after disease has begun to manifest itself (Willenborg and Higgins, 1981; Eylar, et al., 1979; Raine, et al., 1977). As predicted by the complementary antigen theory, cellular immunity against MBP remains after suppression of the disease (ibid.).

Conversely, pretreating animals with the mycobacterial or pertussis antigens used in "complete adjuvants" also prevents EAE induction by an MBP-complete "adjuvant" combination. The mycobacterial components of complete Freund's adjuvant prevent EAE (Weber and Hempel, 1989; Lehmann and Ben-Nun, 1992). Mitsuzawa, et al., (1984) showed that the muramyl dipeptide component alone was sufficient for this prevention.

Similarly, Ben-Nun et al., (1997, 1993; and Lehmann and Ben-Nun, 1992) demonstated that B. pertussis and its toxin prevent EAE. Perhaps even more interesting is the fact that both T-cells against Mycobacteria (Englert and Hempel, 1981) and antibody against B. pertussis can prevent EAE (Brenner and Abramsky, 1997), arguing that both the antigen and its complement are protective.

Finally, not only can the bacterial antigens prevent EAE, they can also suppress it. Root-Bernstein, et al. (1986) demonstrated that muramyl dipeptide can suppress existing EAE, eliminating clinical symptoms of the disease.

These data are very difficult to reconcile either with "adjuvants" being non-specific immune potentiators in these experimental autoimmune diseases or with them playing a secondary role in disease induction. The complementary antigen theory explicitly posits that "adjuvants" are in fact required complementary antigens for the induction of autoimmune diseases and play a different role immunologically than do adjuvants for vaccines or other antigens.

Another prediction made by the complementary antigen theory is that T cells against the protective or tolerizing agent should continue to be present without causing disease. Thus, Conant and Swanborg (2004) , Bai, et al., (1997) and Stepeniak, et al. (1996) have demonstrated the presence of autoreactive T cells as well as antibody against myelin basic protein in animals protected against and treated for EAE using myelin basic protein. MBP-activated T cells along with MBP-reactive B cells can even be used to adoptively transfer protection against EAE to naïve animals (Karpus and Swanborg, 1991; Hashim, 1981). There appear to be no studies of what happens to MBP reactivity in adjuvant prevention or adjuvant suppression of EAE, but such studies would represent crucial experiments for testing the complementary antigen theory.

The same sort of protection by individual inducing antigens that has been found for EAE has also been demonstrated in experimental myocarditis. As noted above, the main experimental models of myocarditis involve inoculating animals with cardiac myosin, the M protein from group A streptoccoci (which mimics cardiac myosin), or some peptide fragment of M protein, in combination with coxsackie virus or a complete Freund's adjuvant containing Mycobacteria or B. pertussis. Inoculating animals with cardiac myosin or its fragments, the M protein from GAS, or some fragment of M protein in incomplete Freund's adjuvant or linked to splenocytes not only does not induce myocarditis, but protects against subsequent induction of myocarditis (Li, et al., 2005; Godsel, et al., 2001; Wang, et al., 2000; Huber and Cunningham, 1996). Conversely, antibodies against coxsackie virus (presented in the absence of myosin) protect against induction of experimental myocarditis by the combination of virus and myosin (Job, et al., 1986; Estrin, et al., 1986).

Similar tolerance and suppression effects induced have also been demonstrated in many other experimental autoimmune diseases requiring complex mixtures of antigens, including experimental myasthenia gravis, experimental diabetes, collagen- and adjuvant-induced arthritis, and experimental thyroiditis (reviewed in Whitacre, et al., 1996).

Because of the novel explanation it provides for preventing and suppressing autoimmunity in animal models, the complementary antigen theory has important implications for the future development of treatments for human autoimmune diseases. In essence, the theory suggests that the elucidation of the complementary antigens responsible for inducing autoimmunity will provide the materials for preventing and suppressing the autoimmune diseases in question. Either of the two antigens should, at high enough doses, be capable of either preventing the disease in genetically susceptible individuals, or of suppressing it in people already afflicted with the disease. One caveat, however, is that there may be multiple pairs of antigens that can cause the same autoimmune disease symptoms. B. pertussis and M. tuberculosis can be both be used as "adjuvants" in EAE; HIV has many potential CD4-like cofactors; etc. These similarly acting agents may, or may not, be interchangeable in preventing or suppressing any given autoimmune disease. So proper understanding of the initiating antigens (as indicated, perhaps, by increased antibody levels to specific infectious agents) may be required to implement effectively the use of any initiating agent as a toleragen or treatment.

Further Tests and Consequences of CAT

The CAT theory of autoimmunity suggests a number of implications that can be used to further test the theory. The first concerns the origins and nature of circulating immune complexes and perivascular cuffing in autoimmune diseases; the second, the need for a revised version of Koch's postulates for the elucidation of the etiologies of autoimmune diseases; and third, the possibility of inducing autoimmunity in an animal using T cells or antibodies transferred to it from two healthy animals, one immunized against each of two, complementary antigens. Each of these further implications, and their associated tests, is unique to the CAT theory.

5. A Novel Explanation of Circulating Immune Complexes and Perivascular Cuffing in Autoimmune Diseases

Circulating immune complexes (CIC) are found in all autoimmune diseases and are often cited as possible contributors to the pathogenesis of these diseases. For example, CIC levels predict increased progression towards death in people with AIDS (Schechter, et al., 1989; Schechter, et al., 1990). CIC are associated with autoimmune forms of myocarditis (Cristea, et al., 1986; Radhakrishnan, 1996; Tincani, et al., 2006; Fairweather, et al., 2006) and also in idiopathic thrombocytopenia (reviewed in Root-Bernstein and Couturier, 2005). In contrast, EAE, which is a cell-mediated disease, is characterized by perivascular cuffing (reviewed in Root-Bernstein, 1991).

Circulating immune complexes (CIC) and perivascular cuffing are often diagnostic symptoms of autoimmune diseases. Very low levels of CIC exist transiently in all normal people (Simpson, Myles and Smith, 1983; Morgan, Rossman and Twomey, 1979) but since antibodies and antigens always bind to each other during any antibody-mediated immune response, it is not clear from any existing description of CIC why high levels these complexes are only seen in autoimmune diseases. Similarly, perivascular cuffing is found in T-cell mediated autoimmune diseases and consists of the massive aggregation of lymphocytes around vasculature near, but not actually at, the sites at which immunological destruction is occurring. Once again, there is no good explanation for why perivascular cuffing occurs around the vasculature rather than at the actual site of tissue destruction, nor is it clear why a massive accumulation of lymphocytes should be present in autoimmune phenomena but not in other instances of tissue destruction. The complementary antigen theory provides novel explanations for both CIC and perivascular cuffing in terms of the interaction of complementary antibodies and lymphocytes. CIC are usually described as complexes of antibodies with their antigens and this is often the case when they are present in acute infection. In autoimmune diseases, however, the inducing antigens are not present after the initial infection, yet CIC persist throughout the chronic course of autoimmunity. Thus, CIC in autoimmunity must involve something other than antigen-antibody complementarity.

The fact that CIC persist in autoimmune diseases long after the initiating antigens have disappeared provides strong evidence that something other than antibody-antigen pairs must be involved in CIC formation. I propose instead that CIC are a necessary result of antigenic complementarity. The antibodies against complementary antigens will themselves be complementary, therefore forming antibody-antibody aggregates (Figure 8). These antibody aggregates will also bind up the complementary antigens, resulting in CIC that contain two complementary antibodies as well as each of their antigens.

Perivascular cuffing has a similar origin according to the complementary antigen theory. In T-cell mediated autoimmune diseases, antigens will elicit complementary lymphocyte responses resulting in lymphocyte-lymphocyte aggregation. Lymphocytes attracted to sites of tissue destruction will migrate through nearby vascular walls attracted by the breakdown products of the tissue destruction. The lymphocytes are likely to run into, and be delayed by interaction with, complementary lymphocytes migrating through the vascular walls

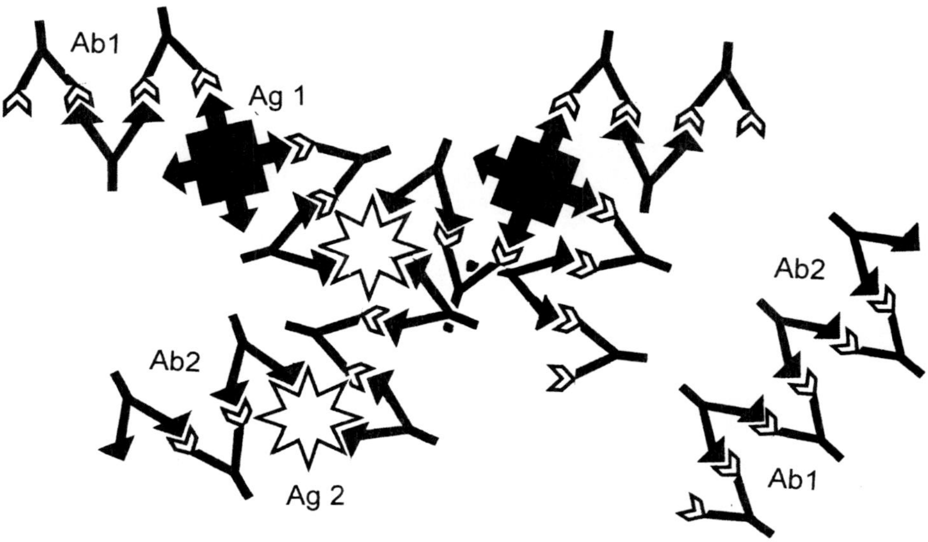

Figure 8. An explanation for the formation of circulating immune complexes (CIC) in antibody-mediated autoimmune diseases according to the complementary antigen theory: complementary antigens induce pairs of idiotypic complementary antibodies that self-aggregate into idiotype-anti-idiotype-like complexes. Such complexes will contain two different antibodies as well as their respective antigens.

The result of the co-migration of pairs of complementary lymphocytes will therefore be the accumulation of lymphocyte complexes around the vasculature near tissue destruction (Figure 9). Such perivascular cuffs will produce huge concentrations of chemokines and related lymphocyte molecules which will fuel the further attraction of even more lymphocytes. If antibodies also play a role in the autoimmune disease, these may also interact with the lymphocyte aggregates within perivascular cuffs.

There is no direct evidence at present that perivascular cuffs are composed of complementary sets of lymphocytes, so this particular aspect of the complementary antigen theory stands as a testable prediction.

There is, however, substantial evidence that antibody-antibody complexes are part of CIC (Simpson, Myles and Smith, 1983; Morgan, Rossman and Twomey, 1979) as well as those associated with autoimmune pathologies (Rose, Goldman and Lambert, 1982; Morgan, Rossman and Twomey, 1987; Nordstrom, et al., 2000).

Notably, Jackson (1988) found just such antibody-antibody complexes made up of antibody-anti-antibody complexes associated with IgA nephropathy, noting that such antibody-anti-antibody complexes are also very common in people with AIDS (Jackson, Dawson and Kotler, 1988).

Finally, such antibody-antibody complexes have also been documented in other autoimmune diseases, most notably rheumatoid arthritis (in which "rheumatoid factor" is composed of antibody-antibody immune complexes [Morgan, Rossman and Twomey, 1987; Nordstrom, et al., 2000]), Sjogren's syndrome (Bergonzi, et al., 1987), systemic lupus erythematosus (Tincani, et al., 2006), and myasthenia gravis (Lebrun-Grandie, et al., 1987).

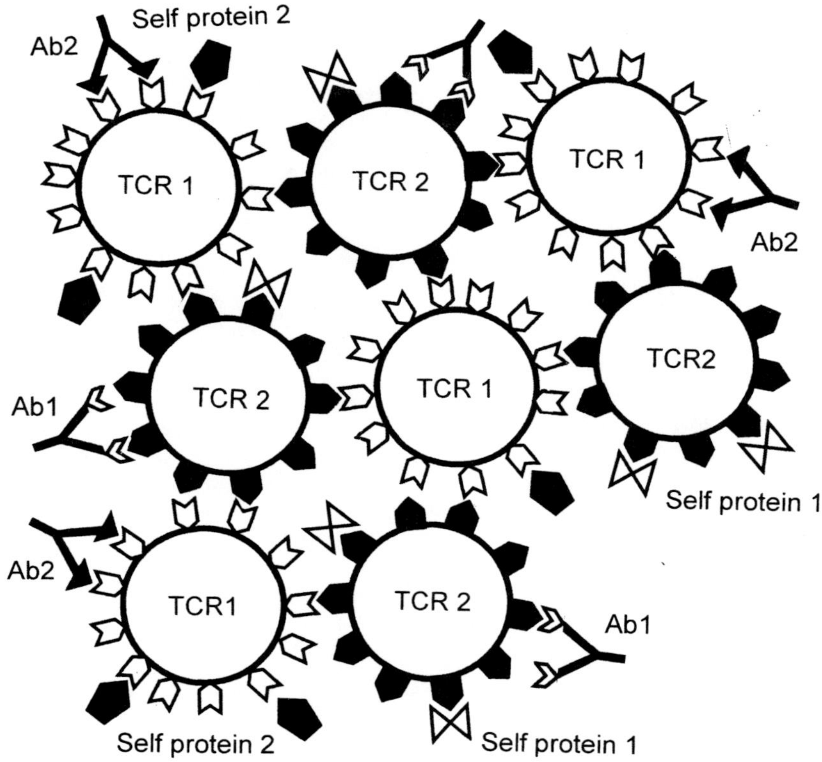

Figure 9. An explanation for the formation of perivascular cuffs in cell-mediated autoimmune diseases according to the complementary antigen theory: complementary antigens induce pairs of complementary lymphocyte cell lines that self-aggregate into cellular complexes. These complexes will form as the cells meet each other exiting the vasculature near antigen sources, and thus will contain antigen as well. It is also possible that antibodies participate in complex formation if the autoimmune disease has both cellular and antibody components.

Further research needs to be done to determine whether the antibodies involved in CIC, and the lymphocytes involved in perivascular cuffing, are not only complementary to one another, but represent pairs of idiotypic antibody responses to complementary precipitating antigens rather than idiotype-anti-idiotype pairs.

6. Multiple Antigen Diseases Require Modifaction of Koch's Postulates

The presence of multiple, complementary antigens in the induction of experimental and human autoimmune diseases suggests that the usual approaches to disease etiology need to be revised. Disease eitiology is generally predicated on the concept of one disease agent causing one disease. If, however, pathogens are indeed triggers for autoimmune diseases, then clearly each such pathogen can cause more than one disease: the acute disease resulting from infection and the chronic autoimmunity that may follow. Theories of autoimmunity based on single agents (such as the molecular mimicry and anti-idiotype theories) have so far failed to demonstrate how a single agent can create two different diseases. One of the explicit conditions upon which the complementary antigen theory is predicated is that individual antigens are not sufficient to cause autoimmunity. Autoimmune diseases can only be triggered by specific, chronologically concurrent, *combinations* of antigens. In other words, pairs of infections may result in outcomes different than single infections. If the complementary antigen theory is correct, then Koch's postulates need to be modified in significant ways before the autoimmune disease etiologies will become clear.

Koch proposed that one could prove an agent was the cause of a disease by: 1) demonstrating a correlation between the presence of an agent and its corresponding disease; 2) isolating and purifying the agent; 3) exposing a healthy animal to the purified agent resulting in the disease; 4) re-isolating the disease agent from the diseased animal. But if a disease requires multiple, concurrent agents for its induction, then Koch's postulates will not yield its cause. No single agent will produce the desired disease state – a fact that may explain why no human autoimmune disease has yet been elucidated.

Multi-agent diseases require a more complex set of postulates (Table 1) observation of two or more agents correlated with a an autoimmune disease; 2) demonstration using Koch's four postulates that none of the agents alone causes the autoimmune disease in question (they may cause *other* acute diseases, however); 3) exposure of a healthy animal to a combination of the agents resulting in the disease; and 4) demonstrating that animals exposed to the single agents are resistant to induction of the autoimmune disease by the combination of agents (Root-Bernstein, 1991; Root-Bernstein, 1993; Root-Bernstein, 2007).

The data described in previous sections are clearly more consistent epidemiologically with the multiple-antigen form of Koch's postulates than the original single-agent postulates. Unfortunately, no multi-infection autoimmune disease models have yet been attempted. All of the multiple-antigen models of autoimmune diseases thus far fall short of satisfying the modified form of Koch's postulates in utilizing a "self" antigen as one of the components. Proper satisfaction of the multiple-antigen form of the postulates will require developing and testing models that utilize combinations of infectious agents as the autoimmunity inducers. Such experiments will require a paradigm shift in the planning of experiments in this field.

For example, one of the ways that autoimmune rheumatic heart disease is induced in animal models is to inoculate animals with group A streptococci or its M protein (which

Table 1. Modifying koch's postulates for the etiology of diseases caused by multiple, concurrent infections

1. Identify a potential disease agent highly associated with the disease
2. Isolate the disease agent
3. Inoculate a healthy host with the disease agent
4. Demonstrate that the host does *NOT* develop the disease of interest
5. Repeat steps one through four with another potential disease agent
6. Inoculate a healthy host with *BOTH* of the potential disease agents simultaneously
7. Demonstrate that the host develops the desired disease

8. Re-isolate the two inducing disease agents, or in the case of an autoimmune disease, the pairs of complementary antibodies or lymphocytes responsible for the autoimmune disease (this re-isolation may be done from hosts inoculated with *individual* agents, which did not become ill!)
9. Inoculate another healthy host with the pair of disease agents (or pairs of antibodies or lymphocytes responsible for an autoimmune disease)
10. Demonstrate that the newly inoculated animal develops the disease of interest

mimics cardiac myosin) in combination with a Freund's complete adjuvant. Conversely, one of the disease models for creating autoimmune myocarditis is to inoculate animals with coxsackie virus (which mimics cardiac actin) combined with cardiac myosin. No one has thus far inoculated animals with a combination of group A streptococci (myosin mimic) and coxsackie virus (actin mimic), or even a combination of cardiac myosin with cardiac actin. Such tests would be crucial experiments for testing the complementary antigen theory.

Autoimmune diseases require another significant modification of the standard interpretation of Koch's postulates as well. If the multifactorial disease in question were infectious, then one could expect to re-isolate the infectious agents from the diseased animal. In the case of autoimmune diseases, however, it is the immune response that is responsible for the disease state. One would therefore expect to be able to isolate combinations of antibodies or T cells that are capable of transferring the disease to other, genetically identical animals. Such transfer is already carried out in many of the animal models described above (EAE, autoimmune myocarditis, etc.) But the multiple-antigen theory of autoimmunity makes the unique prediction that one could inoculate one animal with one antigen and it would remain healthy; another animal with the complementary antigen and it would stay healthy; but that a combination of either antibodies or T cells from the individual animals inoculated into a third, genetically identical animal would cause autoimmunity in this third animal. For example, with EAE, one set of animals could be inoculated with complete Freund's adjuvant; another set with myelin basic protein; and the T cells from each set of animals transferred into a third. Only the third group should develop EAE.

One should be able passively to induce antibody-mediated autoimmune diseases in the same way. In experimental myocarditis, for example, inoculating one animal with coxsackie virus (or cardiac actin), another with group A streptococci (or cardiac myosin), and transferring the antibodies from both animals to a third should be able to induce autoimmune myocarditis in the third, while the donor animals should remain healthy. Such experiments would clearly differentiate the complementary antigen theory from the molecular mimicry and anti-idiotype theories.

7. Risks of Vaccine Interactions

Each of the theories of autoimmunity suggests different risks associated with vaccines. The molecular mimicry theory, for example, suggests that current attempts to make vaccines against group A streptococci based on their M protein (myosin-mimicking protein) subunits would create a risk of inducing rheumatic heart disease in at least some vaccine recipients.

Any whole-virus vaccine should pose significant risks of autoimmune complications according to the anti-idiotype theory. The complementary antigen theory, in contrast, argues that vaccine-induced autoimmunity should be (as it is in reality) extremely rare, occurring only when a vaccine is, by chance, administered to an individual who is co-infected concurrently with just the right infectious complement to that particular vaccine (Westall and Root-Bernstein, 1986).

The complementary antigen theory also points out potential risks inherent in delivering ever-increasing numbers of vaccines concomitantly. Most vaccines will not contain complementary antigens, and so be safe to deliver together. The research summarized above, however, suggests that such safety cannot be assumed. For example, an M protein-based group A streptococcal vaccine administered concurrently with a coxsackie virus vaccine could very well induce autoimmune heart disease in many or all of the co-recipients. An HIV vaccine administered with a hepatitis, cytomegalovirus, or mycobacterial vaccine might induce lymphocytotoxic autoantibodies. A whole-virus hepatititis or cytomegalovirus or measles vaccine co-administered with a mycobacterial vaccine might induce a demyelinating disease. So far, none of these combinations have been attempted as far as I can determine, and many of these vaccines are not publically available in any case, but as progress is made on such vaccines, vaccine developers need to be aware of the possible risks.

Fortunately, the double antibody ELISAs and double antibody diffusion experiments outlined above provide extremely simple means for screening combinations of vaccines for potential interactions that might be of concern with regard to autoimmune potential. Not only would at least one of the vaccines have to induce antibodies cross-reactive with a "self" antigen, but the vaccines would have to induce antibodies (or lymphocytes) that recognized each other as antigens as well. As noted above, such complementary antibodies are found in less than two percent of randomly paired antibodies from infectious agents. Still, given the ease with which tests for antigenic complementarity can be carried out, such tests are well worth the trouble of carrying out in order to assure vaccine safety.

Conclusions

To summarize, this chapter has argued that current theories of autoimmunity, in particular the molecular mimicry and anti-idiotype theories, have failed to explain the origins of autoimmunity because they are based on single-antigen etiologies that must assume some sort of failure within the immune system. I propose instead that autoimmunity is a result of normal responses of the immune system to two or more concurrent, antigenically complementary infections that initiate a civil war within the immune system itself. Complementary antigens induce complementary antibodies or lymphocytes that attack each other. One indication of this attack is the formation of CIC and perivascular cuffs. If the initiating antigens mimic one or more "self" antigens, then the "civil war" will spread to the tissues containing these "self" antigens. Such "civil wars" can be prevented by presenting one antigen several weeks prior to the other, and ended by treating the "civil war" with large doses of only one of the initiating antigens. Evidence for all of these points from multiple autoimmune diseases has been presented and it has been pointed out how all of the data gathered during the course of testing the molecular mimicry and anti-idiotype theories is consistent with the complementary antigen theory.

The most important implication of the antigenic complementarity theory of autoimmunity is that it requires a substantial modification in the ways in which the etiology of autoimmune diseases are investigated and tested. Rather than searching for single infections to initiate autoimmune disease, we need to be looking for specific (and relatively rare) pairs of concurrent infections. Koch's postulates need to be modified appropriately to reflect the possible multi-infection nature of autoimmunity. In turn, new types of experiments must be performed involving combinations of agents, none of which will individually be capable of initiating disease. Finally, the role of "adjuvants" in the induction of autoimmunity must be reconsidered, as "adjuvants" may, in fact, represent necessary, primary antigens rather than non-specific immune potentiators in the context of autoimmunity.

Finally, I have argued that the complementary antigen theory suggests new approaches to preventing and treating autoimmune diseases, but also raises warning about blithely combining vaccines without first testing them for possible antigenic complementarity.

It is beyond the scope of this chapter to describe the application of the complementary antigen theory to autoimmune diseases other than those summarized above, but it is perhaps worth noting that several additional autoimmune diseases at least superficially appear to fit the model described here. For example, systemic lupus erythematosus is characterized by anti-DNA antibodies. Recent research has shown that circulating immune complexes in SLE are characterized not only the presence of DNA and anti-DNA antibodies, but also by the presence of HMBG1, an DNA-binding protein involved in transcription regulation, and by antibody to HMBG1. Thus, all of the criteria required by the complementary antigen theory are satisfied: two complementary "self" molecules, each of which is targeted by its own antibody, all of which aggregate to form circulating immune complexes (Pisetsky, 2007; Tian, et al., 2007). The initiating disease antigens remain unknown, but knowing the set of targets may reduce the possibilities to a manageable set that can be identified by homology searching..

Similarly, it is known that insulin is one of the main targets of type 1 diabetes mellitus (T1DM). We have demonstrated that insulin is complementary to glucagon, and that all insulin antibodies have much higher affinity for a complex of insulin plus glucagon than for insulin alone. We have demonstrated that insulin antibodies bind to glucagon antibodies (Root-Bernstein and Dobbelstein, 2001). And antibodies against a number of infectious agents associated with diabetes onset, including coxsackie virus type B4 and Epstein-Barr virus, recognize insulin and the insulin receptor as immunological targets, while others, such as Pseudomonas aeruginosa, recognize glucagon as an immunological target (work in progress). These insights may eventually identify pairs of infections capable of initiating T1DM in animal models.

Presumably, all infection-induced autoimmune diseases will be found to result from complementary antigens if the theory is correct and disease-specific preventions and treatments devised for each one based on an understanding of its initiating agents.

References

Abuaf N , Laperche S , Rajoely B , Carsique R , Deschamps A , Rouquette AM , Barthet C , Khaled Z , Marbot C , Saab N , Rozen J , Girard PM , Rozenbaum W. Autoantibodies to phospholipids and to the coagulation proteins in AIDS. *Thromb. Haemost.* 1997 May; 77(5): 856-61.

Adams LE, Donavan-Brand R, Friedman-Kien A, Ramahl K, hess EV. Sperm and seminal plasma antibodies in acquired immune deficiency (AIDS) and other associated syndromes. *Clin. Immunol. Immunopathol.* 1988; 46: 442-449.

Argov S , Schattner A , Burstein R , Handzel ZT , Shoenfeld Y , Bentwich Z . Autoantibodies in male homosexuals and HIV infection. *Immunol Lett.* 1991 Sep, 30(1): 31-5.

Ascherio A, Munger K. Epidemiology of multiple sclerosis: from risk factors to prevention. Semin Neurol 2008; 28 (1): 17-28.

Bagasra O, Freund M, Weidmann J, Harley G. Interaction of human immunodeficiency virus with human sperm in vitro. *J. Acquir Immune Defic .Syndr.* 1988; 1: 431-435.

Bai XF , Shi FD , Xiao BG , Li HL , van der Meide PH , Link H. Nasal administration of myelin basic protein prevents relapsing experimental autoimmune encephalomyelitis in DA rats by activating regulatory cells expressing IL-4 and TGF-beta mRNA. *J. Neuroimmunol.* 1997 Dec; 80(1-2): 65-75.

Balint Jr, JP., Jones FR. Detection of elevated anti-idiotypic antibody levels in immune thrombocytopenic patients expressing antiplatelet antibody. *Blood* 1994; 84: 664.

Bar Meir E, Amital H, Levy Y, Kneller A, Bar-Dayan Y, Shoenfeld Y. Mycoplasma-pneumoniae-induced thrombotic thrombocytopenic purpura. *Acta Haematol.* 2000; 103: 112.

Barzilai O ; Sherer Y ; Ram M ; Izhaky D ; Anaya JM ; Shoenfeld Y. Epstein-Barr virus and cytomegalovirus in autoimmune diseases: are they truly notorious? A preliminary report. *Ann. NY Acad Sci.* 2007; 1108: 567-77.

Barzilai O ; Ram M ; Shoenfeld Y. Viral infection can induce the production of autoantibodies. *Curr. Opin. Rheumatol*. 2007; 19(6): 636-43.

Ben-Nun A , Yossefi S , Lehmann D. Protection against autoimmune disease by bacterial agents. II. PPD and pertussis toxin as proteins active in protecting mice against experimental autoimmune encephalomyelitis. *Eur. J. Immunol.* 1993 Mar; 23(3): 689-96.

Ben-Nun A , Mendel I , Kerlero de Rosbo N. Immunomodulation of murine experimental autoimmune encephalomyelitis by pertussis toxin: the protective activity, but not the disease-enhancing activity, can be attributed to the nontoxic B-oligomer. *Proc. Assoc. Am. Physicians* 1997 Mar; 109(2): 120-5.

Benoist C ; Mathis D. Autoimmunity provoked by infection: how good is the case for T cell epitope mimicry? *Nat. Immunol.* 2001; 2(9): 797-801.

Bergonzi C , Merlini GP , Morandi S , Bianchini E , Pavesi F , Bellotti V , Montecucco CM , Ascari E. Selective bone marrow involvement of lymphoplasmacytic cells secreting monoclonal IgA rheumatoid factor in a patient with Sjögren's syndrome and serum hyperviscosity. *Ann. Rheum. Dis.* 1987 Dec; 46(12): 938-42.

Bisset LR . Molecular mimicry in the pathogenesis of AIDS: the HIV/MHC/mycoplasma triangle. *Med. Hypotheses*. 1994 Dec, 43(6): 388-96.

Blalock JE, Smith EM. Hydropathic anti-complementarity of amino acids based on the genetic code. *Biochem. Biophys. Res. Commun.* 1984; 121: 203-207.

Boonpucknavig S , Udomsangpetch R , Pongpanich B. Immunological studies on acute rheumatic fever and rheumatic heart disease. *J. Clin. Lab. Immunol.* 1984; 13(3): 133-6.

Brenner T ; Abramsky O. Natural and experimental transfer of anti-Pertussis antibodies confers resistance to experimental autoimmune encephalomyelitis. *J. Neurol. Sci.* 1993 Jan; 114(1): 13-9.

Buljevac D ; van Doornum GJ ; Flach HZ ; Groen J ; Osterhaus AD ; Hop W ; van Doorn PA ; van der Meché FG ; Hintzen RQ. Epstein-Barr virus and disease activity in multiple sclerosis. *J. Neurol. Neurosurg Psychiatry* 2005; 76(10): 1377-81.

Candelli M, Nista EC, Pignataro G, Gasbarrini G, Gasbarrini A. Idiopathic thrombocytopenic purpura and Helicobacter pylori infection. *Scand. J. Gastroenterol.* 2003; 38: 569.

Caporossi AP , Bruno G , Salemi S , Mastroianni C , Falciano M , Salotti A , Bergami N , Santilio I , Nisini R , Barnaba V . Autoimmune T-cell response to the CD4 molecule in HIV-infected patients. *Viral. Immunol.* 1998, 11(1): 9-17.

Chiò A , Cocito D , Bottacchi E , Buffa C , Leone M , Plano F , Mutani R , Calvo A. Idiopathic chronic inflammatory demyelinating polyneuropathy: an epidemiological study in Italy. *J Neurol. Neurosurg. Psychiatry* 2007 Dec; 78(12): 1349-53.

Conant SB, Swanborg RH. Autoreactive T cells persist in rats protected against experimental autoimmune encephalomyelitis and can be activated through stimulation of innate immunity. *J. Immunol.* 2004; 172:5322-5328.

Cristea A , Rus H , Niculescu F , Bedeleanu D , Vlaicu R. Characterization of circulating immune complexes in heart disease. *Immunol. Lett.* 1986 Aug; 13(1-2): 45-9.

Dalgleish AG . The pathogenesis of AIDS: classical and alternative views. *J. R Coll Physicians Lond* 1992 Apr, 26(2): 152-8.

Damien RT. Molecular mimicry: Antigen sharing by parasite and host and its consequences. *Am. Nat.* 1964; 98: 129-149.

Ebers G. 2008. Environmental factors and multiple sclerosis. *Lancet Neurol.* 7: 268-277.

Estrin M, Smith C, Huber S: Antigen-specific suppressor T cells prevent cardiac injury in Balb/c mice infected with a nonmyocarditic variant of coxsackievirus group B, type 3. *Am. J. Pathol.* 1986; 125:578-584.

Eylar EH , Jackson JJ , Kniskern PJ. Suppression and reversal of allergic encephalomyelitis in rhesus monkeys with basic protein and peptides. *Neurochem. Res.* 1979 Apr; 4(2): 249-58.

Fairweather D , Frisancho-Kiss S , Njoku DB , Nyland JF , Kaya Z , Yusung SA , Davis SE , Frisancho JA , Barrett MA , Rose NR. Complement receptor 1 and 2 deficiency increases coxsackievirus B3-induced myocarditis, dilated cardiomyopathy, and heart failure by increasing macrophages, IL-1beta, and immune complex deposition in the heart. *J. Immunol.* 2006 Mar 15; 176(6): 3516-24.

Fraziano M , Montesano C , Lombardi VR , Sammarco I , De Pisa F , Mattei M , Valesini G , Pittoni V , Colizzi V . Epitope specificity of anti-HIV antibodies in human and murine autoimmune diseases. *AIDS Res. Hum Retroviruses.* 1996 Apr 10, 12(6): 491-6.

Friman G ; Wesslén L ; Fohlman J ; Karjalainen J ; Rolf C. The epidemiology of infectious myocarditis, lymphocytic myocarditis and dilated cardiomyopathy. *Eur. Heart J.* 1995; 16 Suppl O: 36-41

Fujinami RS, Oldstone MB, Wroblewska Z, Frankel ME, Koprowski H. Molecular mimicry in virus infection: crossreaction of measles virus phosphoprotein or of herpes simplex virus protein with human intermediate filaments. *Proc. Natl. Acad. Sci USA* 1983; 80(8):2346-50.

Fujinami RS, Oldstone MB. Amino acid homology between the encephalitogenic site of myelin basic protein and virus: mechanism for autoimmunity. *Science* 1985, 230:1043-5.

Gaur A, Wiers B, Liu A, Rothbard J, Fathman CG. Amelioration of autoimmune encephalomyelitis by myelin basic protein synthetic peptide-induced anergy. *Science* 1992; 258:1491-1494.

Gobert B, Amiel S, Tang J, Barbarino P, Bene MC, Faure G. CD4-like molecules in human sperm. *FEBS Lett.* 1990; 261/2: 339-342.

Godsel LM , Wang K , Schodin BA , Leon JS , Miller SD , Engman DM . Prevention of autoimmune myocarditis through the induction of antigen-specific peripheral immune tolerance. *Circulation* 2001; 103(12): 1709-14.

Golding H , Robey FA , Gates FT 3rd , Linder W , Beining PR , Hoffman T , Golding B . Identification of homologous regions in human immunodeficiency virus I gp41 and human MHC class II beta 1 domain. I. Monoclonal antibodies against the gp41-derived peptide and patients' sera react with native HLA class II antigens suggesting a role for autoimmunity in the pathogenesis of acquired immune deficiency syndrome. *J. Exp. Med.* 1988 Mar 1, 167(3): 914-23.

Gougeon ML , Colizzi V , Dalgleish A , Montagnier L . New concepts in AIDS pathogenesis. *AIDS Res. Hum. Retroviruses* 1993 Mar, 9(3): 287-9.

Grant MD. Antibody convergence along a common idiotypic axis in immunodeficiency virus and hepatitis C virus infections. *J. Med. Virol.* 2002 Jan; 66(1): 13-21.

Gural A , Gillis S , Gafanovich A , Israel Z , Wolf D , Pomeranz S , Ben-Yehuda D. Massive intracranial bleeding requiring emergency splenectomy in a patient with CMV-associated thrombocytopenia. *Haemostasis* 1998 Sep-Oct; 28(5): 250-5.

Hashim GA. Successful immunization against experimental allergic encephalomyelitis with myelin basic protein-sensitized allogeneic lymphocytes. *Neurochem Res* 1981 Jun; 6(6): 699-718.

Herrmann M , Baur A , Nebel-Schickel H , Vornhagen R , Jahn G , Krapf FE , Kalden JR . Antibodies against p24 of HIV-1 in patients with systemic lupus erythematosus? *Viral. Immunol.* 1992 Fall, 5(3): 229-31.

Higgins PM. Splenomegaly in acute infections due to group A streptococci and viruses. *Epidemiol Infect* 1992; 109(2): 199-209.

Hoffmann GW, Kion TA, Grant MD. An idiotypic network model of AIDS immunopathogenesis. *Proc Natl Acad Sci USA* 1991; 88: 3060-3064.

Hoffmann GW . Co-selection in immune network theory and in AIDS pathogenesis. *Immunol. Cell Biol.* 1994 Aug, 72(4): 338-46.

Huber SA, Cunningham MW: Streptococcal M protein peptide with similarity to myosin induces CD4+ T cell-dependent myocarditis in MRL/++ mice and induces partial tolerance against coxsackieviral myocarditis. *J Immunol* 1996; 156:3528-3534.

Jackson S. Immunoglobulin-antiimmunoglobulin interactions and immune complexes in IgA nephropathy. *Am. J. Kidney Dis.* 1988 Nov; 12(5): 425-9.

Jackson S , Dawson LM , Kotler DP. IgA1 is the major immunoglobulin component of immune complexes in the acquired immune deficiency syndrome. *J. Clin. Immunol.* 1988 Jan; 8(1): 64-8.

James K, Hargreave TB. Immunosuppression by seminal plasma and its possible clinical significance. *Immunol Today* 1984; 5: 357.

Job LP, Lyden DC, Huber SA: Demonstration of suppressor cells in coxsackievirus group B, type 3 infected female Balb/c mice which prevent myocarditis. *Cell Immunol.* 1986; 98:104-113.

Kahane, S., A. Dvilansky, L. Estok, I. Nathan, Z. Zolotov, I. Sarov.. Detection of anti-platelet antibodies in patients with idiopathic thrombocytopenic purpura (ITP) and in patients with rubella and herpes group viral infections. *Clin. Exp. Immunol.* 1981; 44: 49.

Karpus WJ, Swanborg RH. Protection against experimental autoimmune encephalomyelitis requires both CD4+ T suppressor cells and myelin basic protein-primed B cells. *J. Neuroimmunol.* 1991 Aug; 33(2): 173-7.

Kaye BR. Rheumatologic manifestations of infection with human immunodeficiency virus (HIV). *Ann Intern Med* 1989 Jul 15; 111(2): 158-67.

Kennedy JR . AIDS--an autoimmune model. *Med. Hypotheses* 1992, 37(1): 16-9.

Kim B , Kaistha SD , Rouse BT. Viruses and autoimmunity. *Autoimmunity* 2006, 39(1): 71-7.

Kion TA, Hoffman GW. Anti-HIV and anti-anti-MHC antibodies in alloimmune and autoimmune mice. *Science* 1991; 253: 1138-1140.

Kiprov DD, Anderson RD, Morand P, Simpson DM, Chermann JC, Levy JA, Ross AR. Antilymphocyte ntibodies and seropositivity for retroviruses in groups at high risk for AIDS. *N.Engl. J. Med.* 1985; 312: 1517.

Kogut EP , Levashova NV , Bondarenko AP , Zherdeva AI , Shuvalova IA. Eksperimental'noe izuchenie koksaki-streptokokkovoi infektsii. Translated Title: [Experimental study of Coxsackie-streptococcal infection]. *Voprosy virusologii* 1978 (6): 690-5.

Kooter AJ , Van der Linden PW , De Klerk C. Acute idiopathic thrombocytopenic purpura in adults following viral infection: report of two cases. *Neth. J. Med.* 2002 May; 60(4): 174-6.

Krone B , Pohl D , Rostasy K , Kahler E , Brunner E , Oeffner F , Grange JM , Gärtner J , Hanefeld F. Common infectious agents in multiple sclerosis: a case control study in children. *Multiple Sclerosis* 14(1): 136-139.

Lebrun-Grandie P , Souan ML , Geffard M , Dartigues JF , Mauricet B , Orgogozo JM. Anticorps anti-acétylcholine et anti-récepteur dans la myasthénie. [Anti-acetylcholine and anti-receptor antibodies in myasthenia]. *Presse Med.* 1987 Oct 3; 16(32): 1577-80.

Lehmann D, Ben-Nun A. Bacterial agents protect against autoimmune disease. I. Mice pre-exposed to Bordetella pertussis or Mycobacterium tuberculosis are highly refractory to induction of experimental autoimmune encephalomyelitis. *J. Autoimmun.* 1992 Dec; 5(6): 675-90.

Lemieux R , Bazin R. Autoantibody-induced formation of immune complexes in normal human serum. *Curr. Pharm. Des.* 2006, 12(2): 173-9.

Li Y , Heuser JS , Kosanke SD , Hemric M , Cunningham MW. Protection against experimental autoimmune myocarditis is mediated by interleukin-10-producing T cells that are controlled by dendritic cells. *Am. J. Pathol.* 2005; 167(1): 5-15.

Libbey JE , McCoy LL , Fujinami RS. Molecular mimicry in multiple sclerosis. *Int. Rev. Neurobiol.* 2007, 79: 127-47.

Liu JQ , Bai XF , Shi FD , Xiao BG , Li HL , Levi M , Mustafa M , Wahren B , Link H. Inhibition of experimental autoimmune encephalomyelitis in Lewis rats by nasal administration of encephalitogenic MBP peptides: synergistic effects of MBP 68-86 and 87-99. *Int. Immunol.* 1998; 10(8): 1139-48.

Lünemann JD, Edwards N, Muraro PA, Hayashi S , Cohen JI , Münz C , Martin R . Increased frequency and broadened specificity of latent EBV nuclear antigen-1-specific T cells in multiple sclerosis. *Brain* 2006, 129(Pt) 6: 1493-506.

Marusic S, Tonegawa S. Tolerance induction and autoimmune encephalomyelitis amelioration after administration of myelin basic protein-derived peptide. *J. Exp. Med.* 1997; 186:507-515.

Mathur S, Goust JM, Williamson HO, Fudenberg HH. Cross-reactivity of sperm and T-lymphocyte antigens. *Am J Reprod Immunol* 1981; 1: 113-118.

McGuire KL, Holmes DS. Role of complementary proteins in autoimmunity. *Trends Immunol.* 2005, 26: 367-372.

McLeod JG , Pollard JD , Macaskill P , Mohamed A , Spring P , Khurana V. Prevalence of chronic inflammatory demyelinating polyneuropathy in New South Wales, Australia. *Ann. Neurol.* 1999 Dec; 46(6): 910-3.

Metlas R , Skerl V , Veljkovic V , Colombatti A , Pongor S . Immunoglobulin-like domain of HIV-1 envelope glycoprotein gp120 encodes putative internal image of some common human proteins. *Viral Immunol.* 1994, 7(4): 215-9.

Mitsuzawa E , Yasuda T , Tamura N , Ohtani S. Pretreatment with antigen or adjuvant, and the preventability of allergic encephalomyelitis induced by basic protein with synthetic muramyl dipeptide in comparison with Freund's complete adjuvant. *Jpn. J Exp. Med.* 1984 Jun; 54(3): 97-107.

Morgan AC Jr , Rossen RD , Twomey JJ. Naturally occurring circulating immune complexes: normal human serum contains idiotype-anti-idiotype complexes dissociable by certain IgG antiglobulins. *J. Immunol.* 1979 May; 122(5): 1672-80.

Morrow WJ , Isenberg DA , Sobol RE , Stricker RB , Kieber-Emmons T . AIDS virus infection and autoimmunity: a perspective of the clinical immunological and molecular origins of the autoallergic pathologies associated with HIV disease. *Clin. Immunol. Immunopathol.* 1991 Feb, 58(2): 163-80.

Muller S , Richalet P , Laurent-Crawford A , Barakat S , Rivière Y , Porrot F , Chamaret S , Briand JP , Montagnier L , Hovanessian A. Autoantibodies typical of non-organ-specific autoimmune diseases in HIV-seropositive patients. *AIDS* 1992 Sep, 6(9): 933-42.

Nordström E , Abedi-Valugerdi M , Möller E. Longevity of immune complexes and abnormal germinal centre formation in NZB mice. *Scand J. Immunol.* 2000 Nov; 52(5): 477-82.

Pankuweit S , Lamparter S , Funck R , Maisch B. Herzmuskelbiopsiegesteuerte Diagnostik und Therapie bei entzündlicher Kardiomyopathie.[Endomyocardial biopsy-guided diagnosis and treatment of inflammatory cardiomyopathies]. *Dtsch Med Wochenschr* 2004, 129(41): 2169-72.

Parry O , Mielke J , Latif AS , Ray S , Levy LF , Siziya S. Peripheral neuropathy in individuals with HIV infection in Zimbabwe. *Acta Neurol. Scand.* 1997 Oct; 96(4): 218-22.

Pendergraft, WF,, 3RD, Preston GA, Shah RR, Tropsha a, Carater CW Jr, Jennette JC, Falk RJ. Autoimmunity is triggered by cPR-3 (105-201), a protein complementary to human autoantigen proteinase-3. *Nat. Med.* 2004; 10: 72-79.

Pendergraft WF 3rd, Jennette JC, Ralk RJ, Preston GA. Autoantigen complementarity: a new theory implicating complementary proteins as initiators of autoimmune disease. *J. Mol. Med* 2005, 83: 12-25.

Pisetsky DS. Autoimmunity: the nuclear arsenal of autoimmunity. *Immunol Cell Biol.* 2007; 85, 344–345

Plotz PH. 1983. Autoantibodies are anti-idiotype antibodies to antiviral antibodies. *Lancet* 2: 824-826Pongpanich B , Boonpucknavig S , Wasi C , Tanphaichitr P , Boonpucknavig V. Immunopathology of acute rheumatic fever and rheumatic heart disease. The demonstration of Coxsackie group B viral antigen in the myocardium. *Clin. Rheumatol.* 1983, 2(3): 217-22.

Preston GA, Pendergraft WF 3rd, Falk RJ. New insights that link microbes with the generation of antineutrophil cytoplasmic autoantibodies: the theory of autoantigen complementarity. *Curr Opin Nephrol Hypertens* 2005, 14(3): 217-222.

Radhakrishnan VV. Experimental myocarditis in the guinea-pig. *Cardiovasc Res.* 1996 Apr; 31(4): 651-4.

Raine CS , Snyder DH , Stone SH , Bornstein MB. Suppression of acute and chronic experimental allergic encephalomyelitis in Strain 13 guinea pigs. A clinical and pathological study. *J. Neurol. Sci.* 1977 Apr; 31(3): 355-67.

Rauch HC, Einstein ER, Csejtey J, Davis WJ. Protective action of the encephalitogen and other basic proteins in experimental allergic encephalomyelitis. *Immunochemistry* 1968; 5:567-575.

Rico MJ , Hall RP. Idiotypes, anti-idiotypes, and autoimmunity. *Am. Acad. Dermatol.* 1988, 19(3): 579-85.

Root-Bernstein RS. *Rethinking AIDS. 1989;* New York: Free Press.

Root-Bernstein RS. Multiple antigen mediated autoimmunity (MAMA) in AIDS: A possible model for post infectious autoimmunity. *Res. Immunol.* 1990; 141: 321-339.

Root-Bernstein RS. Self, nonself, and the paradoxes of autoimmunity. In Tauber AI, editor. *Organism and the Development of Self* 1991; Boston: Kluwer, pp. 159-209.

Root-Bernstein RS. Preliminary evidence of idiotype antiidiotype immune complexes cross-reactive with lymphocyte antigens in aids and lupus. *Med. Hypoth.* 1995; 44: 20-27.

Root-Bernstein RS. Antigenic complementarity among AIDS-associated infectious agents and molecular mimicry of lymphocyte proteins as inducers of lymphocytotoxic antibodies and circulating immune complexes. *J. Clin. Virol.* 2004 Dec; 31 Suppl 1: S16-25.

Root-Bernstein RS. Antigenic complementarity between HIV and other AIDS-associated infections results in idiotype-antiidiotype antibody complexes that cross react with lymphocyte proteins. *Vaccine* 2005 Mar 18; 23(17-18): 2160-3.

Root-Bernstein RS. Antigenic complementarity in the induction of autoimmunity: a general theory and review. *Autoimmun. Rev.* 2007 Apr; 6(5): 272-7.

Root-Bernstein RS, Couturier J. Antigenic complementarity in the origins of autoimmunity: A general theory illustrated with a case study of idiopathic thrombocytopenia purpura. *Clin Develop Immunol* 2006; 13: 49-65.

Root-Bernstein RS, Dobbelstein C. Insulin binds to glucagon forming a complex that is hyper-antigenic and inducing complementary antibodies having an idiotype-antiidiotype relationship. *Autoimmunity* 2001; 33: 153-169.

Root-Bernstein RS, Dewitt SH. CD4 similarity to proteins of infectious agents associated with AIDS and their role in autoimmunity. *Med. Hypoth.* 1994; 43: 361-371.

Root-Bernstein RS, Dewitt SH. Semen alloantigens as possible inducers of lymphocytotoxic autoimmunity in AIDS and ICL. *Genetica* 1995; 95: 133-156.

Root-Bernstein RS, Hobbs SH. Homologies between mycoplasma adhesion peptide, CD4, and class II MHC proteins: a possible mechanism for HIV-mycoplasma synergism in AIDS. *Res Immunol* 1992; 142: 519-523.

Root-Bernstein RS, Hobbs SH. Does HIV 'piggyback' on viruses, bacteria, and sperm? Implications for transmission, synergism, and autoimmunity in AIDS. *J. Theor. Biol.* 1993; 160: 249-264.

Root-Bernstein RS, Holsworth DD. Antisense peptides: A critical review. *J. Theor. Biol.* 1998; 190: 107-119.

Root-Bernstein RS, Rallo A. Antigenic complementarity resulting in idiotype-antiidiotype immune complexes: possible contributor to AIDS pathogenesis and autoimmunity. *Autoimmunity* 2004 May; 37(3): 203-10.

Root-Bernstein RS, Vonck J, Podufaly A. Antigenic complementarity between coxsackie virus and streptococcus in the induction of rheumatic heart disease and autoimmune myocarditis. *Autoimmunity* (in press).

Root-Bernstein RS, Westall FC. Serotonin binding bites. II. Muramyl dipeptides bind to serotonin binding sites on myelin basic protein, LHRH, MSH, and ACTH. *Brain Res. Bull.* 1990; 25: 827-841.

Root-Bernstein RS, Yurochko F, Westall FC. Clinical suppression of experimental allergic encephalomyelitis by muramyl dipeptide 'adjuvant' *Brain Res Bull* 1986; 17: 473-476.

Rose LM , Goldman M , Lambert PH. The production of anti-idiotypic antibodies and of idiotype-anti-idiotype immune complexes after polyclonal activation induced by bacterial LPS. *J. Immunol.* 1982 May; 128(5): 2126-33.

Rose NR , Mackay IR. Molecular mimicry: a critical look at exemplary instances in human diseases. *Cell Mol. Life Sci.* 2000; 57(4): 542-51.

Russo S, Lopalco L. Is autoimmuinity a component of natural immunity to HIV? *Curr. HIV Res.* 2006; 4: 177-190.

Scaradavou A. HIV-related thrombocytopenia. *Blood Rev.* 2002 Mar; 16(1): 73-6.

Schechter MT , Craib KJ , Le TN , Willoughby B , Douglas B , Sestak P , Montaner JS , Weaver MS , Elmslie KD , O'Shaughnessy MV. Progression to AIDS and predictors of AIDS in seroprevalent and seroincident cohorts of homosexual men. *AIDS* 1989 Jun; 3(6): 347-53.

Schechter MT , Craib KJ , Le TN , Montaner JS , Douglas B , Sestak P , Willoughby B , O'Shaughnessy MV. Susceptibility to AIDS progression appears early in HIV infection. *AIDS* 1990 Mar; 4(3): 185-90.

Selmi C. One year in autoimmunity. *Autoimmun. Rev.* 8 2007; 7: 85-93.

Serres PF . AIDS: an immune response against the immune system. Role of a precise tridimensional molecular mimicry. *Autoimmun* 2001 May, 16(3): 287-91.

Shearer MH , Dalgleish AG , Chanh TC , Kennedy RC. Idiotype cascades associated with the CD4-HIV glycoprotein 120 interaction: immunization with anti-idiotypic antibodies induces anti-anti-idiotypic responses with anti-CD4 specificity and in vitro neutralizing activity. *AIDS Res. Hum. Retroviruses* 2000 Jan 1; 16(1): 77-86.

Sherer Y , Shoenfeld Y. The idiotypic network in antinuclear-antibody-associated diseases. *Int. Arch. Allergy Immunol.* 2000, 123(1): 10-15.

Shimizu, A., T. Matsushita, T. Kondo, Y. Inden, T. Kojima, H. Saito, M. Hirai. Identification of the amino acid residues of the platelet glycoprotein Ib (GPIb) essential for the von Willebrand Factor binding by clustered charged-to-alanine scanning mutagenesis. *J. Biol. Chem* 2004; 279:16285.

Shoenfeld Y. The idiotypic network in autommunity. *Nat. Med.* 2004; 10: 17-18.

Siemion IZ, Cebrat M, Kluczyk A. The problem of amino acid complementarity and antisense peptides. *Curr. Protein. Pept Sci.* 2004; 5: 507-27.

Silvestris F , Williams RC Jr , Dammacco F . Autoreactivity in HIV-1 infection: the role of molecular mimicry. *Clin. Immunol Immunopathol.* 1995 Jun, 75(3): 197-205.

Simpson IJ , Myles MJ , Smith GW. Immune complexes in normal subjects. *J. Clin. Lab. Immunol.* 1983 Jul; 11(3): 119-22.

Sips GJ , Chesik D , Glazenburg L , Wilschut J , De Keyser J , Wilczak N. Involvement of morbilliviruses in the pathogenesis of demyelinating disease. *Rev. Med. Virol* 2007; 17(4): 223-44.

Soboleva VD , Lozovskaya LS , Alekseveva VB , Belostotskaya NP , Bushanskaya NR , Kalinina IN. Coxsackie A 13 virus in the foci of rheumatism. *J. Hyg. Epidemiol. Microbiol. Immunol.* 1978; 22(2): 195-202.

Srinivasappa J , Saegusa J , Prabhakar BS , Gentry MK , Buchmeier MJ , Wiktor TJ , Koprowski H , Oldstone MB , Notkins AL. Multiple organ-reactive monoclonal autoantibodies. *Nature* 1983 Jul 7-13; 304(5921): 73-6.

Stepaniak JA , Gould KE , Swanborg RH. Encephalitogenic T cells are present in Lewis rats protected from autoimmune encephalomyelitis by coimmunization with MBP73-84 and its analog. *J. Neurosci Res.* 1996 Aug 15; 45(4): 447-54.

Stéphan F, Cheffi MA, Kaplan C, Maillet J-M, Novara A,. Fagon J-Y, Bonnet F. Autoantibodies against platelet glycoproteins in critically ill patients with thrombocytopenia. *Am. J. Med.* 2000; 108: 554.

Stricker RB , Abrams DI , Corash L , Shuman MA. Target platelet antigen in homosexual men with immune thrombocytopenia. *N. Engl. J. Med.* 1985 Nov 28; 313(22): 1375-80.

Stott EJ. Anti-cell antibody in macaques. *Nature* 1991 Oct 3; 353(6343): 393.

Suresh L, Chandrasekar S. Rao RS, Ravi V, Badrinath S. Coxsackie virus and rheumatic fever. A correlative study. *J. Assoc Physicians India* 1981, 37(9): 582-5.

Susal C , Daniel V , Opelz G. Does AIDS emerge from a disequilibrium between two complementary groups of molecules that mimic MHC? *Immunol. Today* 1996 Mar, 17(3): 114-9.

Süsal C , Hoffman GW , Daniel V , Grant M , Opelz G . Complementarities and network interactions in AIDS. *J. Autoimmun* 1993 Oct, 6(5): 601-10.

Takahashi T, Yujiri T, Shinohara K, Inoue Y, Sato Y, Fujii Y, Okubo M, Zaitsu Y, Ariyoshi K, Nakamura Y, Nawata R, Oka Y, Shirai M, Tanizawa Y. Molecular mimicry by Helicobacter pylori CagA protein may be involved in the pathogenesis of H. pylori-associated chronic idiopathic thrombocytopenic purpura. *Br. J. Haematol.* 2004; 124: 91.

Ter-Grigorov VS , Krifuks O , Liubashevsky E , Nyska A , Trainin Z , Toder V. A new transmissible AIDS-like disease in mice induced by alloimmune stimuli. *Nat. Med.* 1997 Jan; 3(1): 37-41.

Thiriart C , Goudsmit J , Schellekens P , Barin F , Zagury D , De Wilde M , Bruck C. Antibodies to soluble CD4 in HIV-1-infected individuals. *AIDS* 1988 Oct; 2(5): 345-51.

Tian J, Avalos AM, Mao S-Y, Chen B, Senthil K, Wu H. Toll-like receptor 9-dependent activation by DNA-containing immune complexes is mediated by HMGB1 and RAGE. *Nat. Immunol.* 2007; 8: 487–496.

Tincani A , Rebaioli CB , Taglietti M , Shoenfeld Y. Heart involvement in systemic lupus erythematosus, anti-phospholipid syndrome and neonatal lupus. *Rheumatology (Oxford)* 2006 Oct; 45 Suppl 4: iv8-13.

Titani K, Takio K, Handa M, Ruggeri ZM. Amino acid sequence of the von Willebrand factor-binding domain of platelet membrane glycoprotein Ib. *Proc. Natl. Acad. Sci. USA* 1987; 84:5610.

Trent RJ, Clancy RL, Danis V, Basten A. Immune complexes in thrombocytopenic patients: cause of effect? *Br. J. Haematol.* 1980; 44: 645.

Tropsha A, Kizer JS, Chaiken IM. Making sense from antisense: A review of experimental data and developing ideas on sense-antisense peptide recognition. *J. Mol. Recogn.* 1992; 5: 43-54.

Tsonis PA, Dwivedi B. Molecular mimicry: Structural camouflage of proteins and nucleic acids. *Biochim. Biophys. Acta* 2008, 1783(2): 177-87.

Vicente,V, Kostel PJ, Ruggeri ZM. Isolation and functional characterization of the von Willebrand Factor-binding domain located between residues His^{1}-Arg^{293} of the α-chain of glycoprotein Ib. *J. Biol. Chem.* 1988; 263:18473.

Vikerfors T, Stjerna A, Olcen P, Malmcrona R, Magnius L. Acute myocarditis. Serologic diagnosis, clinical findings and follow-up. *Acta Med. Scand.* 1988, 223(1): 45-52.

Wadenvik H, Stockelberg D, Hou M. Platelet glycoproteins as autoantibody targets in idiopathic thrombocytopenic purpura. *Acta Paediatr* 1998; Suppl. 424:26.

Wang Y, Afanasyeva M, Hill SL, Kaya Z, Rose NR: Nasal administration of cardiac myosin suppresses autoimmune myocarditis in mice. *J. Am. Coll Cardiol*. 2000, 36:1992-1999.

Weber F, Hempel K. Protection against experimental allergic encephalomyelitis with complete Freund's adjuvant is unaffected by prostaglandin synthesis inhibition. *Int. Arch Allergy Appl Immunol* 1989; 89(2-3): 242-5.

Westall FC, Root-Bernstein RS. An explanation of prevention and suppression of experimental allergic encephalomyelitis. *Mol. Immunol.* 1983; 20 : 169-177.

Westall FC, Root-Bernstein RS. The cause and prevention of post-infectious and post-vaccinal encephalopathies in light of a new theory of autoimmunity. *Lancet* August 1986; ii: 251-252.

Weathington NM , Blalock JE. Rational design of peptide vaccines for autoimmune disease: harnessing molecular recognition to fix a broken network. *Expert. Rev. Vaccines* 2003, 2(1): 61-73.

Whitacre CC , Gienapp IE , Meyer A , Cox KL , Javed N. Treatment of autoimmune disease by oral tolerance to autoantigens. *Clin. Immunol. Immunopathol.* 1996 Sep; 80(3) Pt 2: S31-9.

Willenborg DO, Higgins TJ. Liposomes containing myelin basic protein (BP) suppress but do not induce allergic encephalomyelitis in Lewis rats. *Aust. J. Exp. Biol. Med. Sci.* 1981 Apr; 59(Pt) 2: 135-41.

Wilson SE , Habeshaw JA , Addawe MA , Hounsell EF , Oxford JS . HIV type 1 envelope glycoprotein 120 carboxy-terminal peptide-induced human T cell lines selectively suppress heterogeneous proliferative T cell responses to soluble antigens. *AIDS Res. Hum. Retroviruses* 1997 Oct 10, 13(15): 1313-24.

Witkin SS, Sonnabend J. Immune response to spermatozoa in homosexual men. *Fertil Steril.* 1983; 39: 337-342.

Wright JF, Blanchette VS, Wang H, Arya N, Petric M, Semple JW, Chia WK, Freedman J. Characterization of platelet-reactive antibodies in children with varicella-associated acute immune thrombocytopenic purpura (ITP). *Br. J. Haematol.* 1996; 95: 145.

Yenicesu I , Yetgin S , Ozyürek E , Aslan D. Virus-associated immune thrombocytopenic purpura in childhood. *Pediatr Hematol. Oncol.* 2002 Sep; 19(6): 433-7.

Zaher SR, Kassem AS, Hughes JJ. Coxsackie virus infections in rheumatic fever. *Indian J. Pediatr*. 1993, 60(2): 289-98.

Zandman-Goddard G , Shoenfeld Y. HIV and autoimmunity. *Autoimmun. Rev.* 2002 Dec; 1(6): 329-37.

Zarling JM, Ledbetter JA, Sias J, Fultz P, Eichberg J, Gjerset G, Moran PA. HIV-infected humans but not chimpanzees, have circulating cytotoxic T lymphocytes that lyse uninfected CD4+ cells. *J. Immunol.* 1990; 144: 2992-2998.

Zon LI , Arkin C , Groopman JE. Haematologic manifestations of the human immune deficiency virus (HIV). *Br. J. Haematol.* 1987 Jun; 66(2): 251-6.

In: Autoimmunity: Role, Regulation and Disorders
Editor: Fynn L. Vogel and L. F. Zimmermann
ISBN 978-1-60456-833-2

Chapter 5

Autoimmune Initiation of Multiple Sclerosis: Molecular Aspects

Fred C. Westall*
Institute for Disease Research
Temecula, California, USA

Abstract

Multiple sclerosis (MS) is considered to be initiated by an autoimmune attack on myelin proteins by a mimic within a protein from some unidentified microorganism. Experimental allergic encephalomyelitis (EAE) is the model for MS. Different peptides from four myelin proteins are potent known EAE immunogens. The contribution of particular amino acids to encephalitogenicity within several immunogens and the minimum adjuvant requirements have been ascertained. Thus, the EAE initiation process at a molecular level is known. Using this EAE molecular information with known aspects of clinical MS, e.g. patient's age, variable histology, clinical immunological data, epidemiology, etc., the molecular initiation process of the autoimmune aspects of MS is defined. This definition includes: a.) type of organism providing the mimic, b.) estimation of single versus multiple immunogens, c.) location of the mimic, d.) involvement of adjuvant molecules and other inflammatory agents, e.) elucidation of magnetic resonance imaging (MRI) data, f.) dissection of confusing cellular immunology data, and g.) explanation of variable histological lesion locations. With this information various therapeutic options are discussed.

Introduction

Multiple sclerosis (MS) is a slowly progressive disease of the central nervous system (CNS) distinguished by areas of demyelination. It is characterized by unpredictable relapses,

* E-mail: fcwestallidr@roadrunner.com

remissions and stationary phases, which can last for weeks, months or even years. In latter life a more progressive form without the defined relapses usually develops (McAlpine, Lumsden and Acheson, 1972). The onset of multiple sclerosis is extremely variable. The average age of onset for women is 28 years and men 32 years. Symptoms may develop rapidly in the course of minutes, hours or days. Also the frequency of the initial symptoms of MS vary considerably: motor weakness in one or more limbs, 40%; optic neuritis, 22%; paresthesia, 21%; double vision, 12%; vertigo/vomiting, 5% and disturbance of micturation, 5%.

Allergic Encephalomyelitis

Experimental allergic encephalomyelitis (EAE), considered a model for MS, is an autoimmune attack on the central nervous system myelin. Clinical signs include paralysis, loss of balance, an incontinence of urine and feces. Lesions consist characteristically of dense infiltration of mononuclear leukocytic cells surrounding blood vessels (Kies, 1965).

Various central nervous system (CNS) myelin proteins---myelin basic protein, proteolipid protein, myelin-associated oligodendrocyte glycoproteins, and myelin-associated oligodendrocyte basic protein---are capable of inducing acute EAE in a variety of mammals when they are injected with the appropriate adjuvant (Kies and Alvord, Jr., 1959; Roboz-Einstein et al. 1962; Sakai et al., 1988; Tuohy et al., 1988; Amor et al., 1994). Linear encephalitogenic sequences within these proteins have been described (Table 1) (Westall, et al., 1971; Shapira, et al., 1971; Karkhanis et al., 1975; Westall, Thompson, and Lennon, 1977; Tuohy et al., 1988, 1989; Endoh et al., 1990; Greer et al., 1992; Amor et al., 1994; Mendel, Kerelero de Rosbo and Ben-Nun, 1995). In some cases the contribution to encephalitogenicity by the individual amino acids within a site has been elucidated. This work has centered with the encephalitogenic tryptophan peptide from myelin basic protein---phe-ser-trp-gly-ala-glu-gly-gln-arg (Eylar et al., 1970; Westall et al., 1971; Westall, 1972; Sasaki, 1974; Suzuki and Sasaki 1974; Westall and Thompson, 1977b; Khanarian et al., 1979) (Table 2). Whole brain injections also produce only EAE. Therefore, the myelin of the central nervous system appears to be unique in possessing a plethora of disease-producing immunogens.

Table 1. Major Defined Encephalitogenic Sequences[1]

Encephalitogen	Active EAE species	References
Myelin Basic Protein		
fswgaegqr-tryptophan pep.	Guinea pig, rabbit, monkey	Westall et al. 1971; Eylar, Westall andBrostoff, 1971
tthygslpqk-mid-peptide	Rabbit, DR rat	Shapira et al., 1971; Smeltz, Wolf and Swanborg, 1998
pqksqrtqdenpv-hyperacute	Lewis rat, monkey	Westall, Thompson and Lennon, 1977; Levine, 1974
fklggrdsr	Rabbit, monkey	Westall and Thompson, 1978; Eylar et al., 1972; Karkhanis et al., 1975

c-terminal	rat	Westall and Thompson, 1977
sequence 89-101	mouse	Jansson et al. 1991
sequence 1-9	mouse	Zamvil et al. 1986
Lipoprotein		
hslgkwlghpdkf	Mice	Tuohy et al, 1989
ntwttcqsiafpsk	Mice	Greer et al. 1992
yktticgkglsatv	Mice	Tuohy et al., 1988
dyeylinvihafqyv	Mice	Amor et al., 1993
Oligodendrocytic glycoprotein		
mevgwyrppfsrvvhlyrngk Also 1-22; 43-57;92-106	mice	Kerlero de Rosbo and Ben-Nun, 1996; Amor et al, 1994
Oigodendrocyte basic protein		
Residues 15-36	mice	Kerlero de Rosbo et al, 2004

[1]The decision of what should be included as a "major" encephalitogenic sequence is quite arbitrary. The result depends upon the laboratories testing the sequence and the animal being tested. The purpose of the table is primarily to show that there are several proteins which are encephalitogenic and within these proteins are numerous encephalitogenic regions.

Table 2 Encephalitogenicity in Guinea Pigs of Synthetic Variants of the Tryptophan Region Of Myelin Basic Protein (Phe Ser Trp Gly Ala Glu Gly Gln Arg)[A]

Sequence	References	Clinical Activity
PheSerTrpGlyAlaGlnGlyGlnLys	Westall et al., 1971	++
SerArgPheSerTrpGlyAlaGluGlyGlnLys	Eylar et al., 1970	++
SerArgPheSerTrpGlyAlaGluGlyGln ---	Eylar et al., 1970	-
SerArgPheSerTrpGlyAlaGluGlyGlnArg	Westall et al., 1971	++
SerArgPheSerTrpGlyAlaGluGlyGlnIle	Westall et al., 1971	-
SerArgPheSerTrpGlyAlaGluGlyIleLys	Westall et al., 1971	-
SerArgPheSerTrpGlyAlaIleGlyGlnLys	Westall et al., 1971	++
SerArgPheSerPheGlyAlaGluGlyGlnLys	Westall et al, 1971	-
SerArgPheSerValGlyAlaGluGlyGlnLys	Westall et al., 1971	-
SerArgPheAlaTrpGlyAlaGluGlyGlnLys	Westall et al., 1971	++
SerArgValSerTrpGlyAlaGluGlyGlnLys	Westall et al., 1971	+
PheSerTrpAlaAlaGluGlyGlnLys	Westall, 1972	-
GlySerTrpGlyAlaGluGlyGlnArg	Westall, 1972	+
PheSerTrpGlyAlaGluGlyGluArg	Westall, 1972	-
PheSerTrpGlyAlaGluGlySerArg	Westall and Thompson, 1977b	+
PheSerTrpGlydAlaGluGly Ser Arg	Khanarain et al, 1979	-
PheSerTrpGlyGlyGluGlyGlnArg	Suzuki and Sasaki, 1974	-
PheSerTrpGlyAlaGluGlyAsnArg	Sasaki, 1974	+
PheGlyTrpGlyAlaGluGlyGlnArg	Suzuki and Sasaki, 1974	++
PheSerTrpGlyAlaGlyGlyGlnArg	Suzuki and Sasaki, 1974	++
PheSerTrpGlyAlaGluGlyGlnGlyArg	Westall, 1972	+
PheSerTrpGlyAlaGluGlyGlyGlnArg	Westall, 1972	+

All peptides containing smaller segments of the tryptophan region were inactive (Eylar et al., 1970; Westall, 1972). However, using large amounts of synthetic adjuvant Nagai (1978a) was able to induce EAE in guinea pigs with the sequence trp-gly-glu-gly-gln-arg.

[a]The antigens were dissolved just prior to injection in normal saline and emulsified with Freund's complete adjuvant.

A. Types of EAE

There are several forms of EAE, hyperacute, acute, and chronic/relapsing. Hyperacute is induced in Lewis rats by injection of guinea pig myelin basic protein (MBP) with *B. pertussis* (Levine, 1974; Lennon et al., 1976). Clinical signs initially appear within a week. A specific peptide derived from guinea pig MBP with *B. pertussis* also induces hyperacute EAE (Westall, Thompson and Lennon, 1977) (Table 3). Acute EAE, which develops within 2 weeks, can be initiated in different mammalian species with any one of four myelin proteins as described above.

Table 3. The Effect of *B. Pertussis* on the Encephalitogen-Icity of Myelin Basic Proteins in Lewis Rats[1]

Encephalitogen	Dose	Clinical	Day of Onset	Number of Deaths
Guinea pig MBP	316	5/5	9,9,10,10,10	5/5
	100	5/5	9,10,10,10,11	5/5
	31.6	5/5	9,9,9,9,10	5/5
	10	5/5	9,10,10,10,11	5/5
	3.2	5/5	10,10,11,11,11	5/5
	1.0	5/5	11,12,12,13,14	5/5
Lewis rat MBP	316	5/5	10,11,11,11,11	4/5
	100	5/5	10,10,11,11,11	5/5
	31.6	4/4	11,12,12,12,14	0/5
	10.0	5/5	12,13,13,15,15	0/5
	3.2	4/5	14,15,17,17	0/5
	1.0	0/5	-----------------	
Human MBP	316	5/5	8,8,8,9,9	2/5
	100	5/5	8,9,10,10,10	1/5
	31.6	5/5	9,10,11,11,11	1/5
	10.0	5/5	11,12,12,12,15	0/5
	3.2	0/5	-----------------	
Monkey MBP	316	5/5	11,11,11,11,12	4/5
	100	5/5	11,11,12,13,13	3/5
	31.6	5/5	12,12,13,13,15	2/5
	10.0	5/5	12,13,15,15,19	0/5
	3.2	0/5	------------------	
Pig MBP	316	5/5	7,7,10,10,10	1/5
	100	5/5	8,9,11,11,11	2/5
	31.6	5/5	10,11,11,12,13	0/5
	10.0	3/5	12,12,13	0/5
	3.2	0/5	------------------	

Encephalitogen	Dose	Clinical	Day of Onset	Number of Deaths
Cow MBP	316	5/5	10,11,12,12,12	5/5
	100	5/5	10,12,12,12,12	5/5
	31.6	5/5	12,12,12,13,13	3/5
	10.0	2/5	12,12	0/5
	1.0	0/4	------------------	
Rabbit MBP	316	5/5	10,10,10,11,12	
	100	5/5	11,11,12,12,12	
	31.6	5/5	12,13,13,13,13	
	10.0	0/5	------------------	
Sheep MBP	316	5/5	10,11,11,12,14	1/5
	100	5/5	12,12, 13, 14,14	1/5
	31.6	1/5	14	0/5
Guinea Pig				
Peptide 70-88	0.3-4.9	33/33	Mean day 9	27/33
	0.01-0.08	13/14	Mean day 13	7/14
Peptide 73-86	1.9	12/12	Mean day 10	8/12
	0.3	8/8	Mean day 13	3/8
Rat Peptide 68-86	4.9	4/5	Mean day 13	0/5

[1]HEAE was distinguished from ordinary EAE clinically by a combination of early onset (usually 9-10 days), rapid and severe course and high incidence of mortality and cerebral signs (irritability, seizures, coma and spasticity). Histologic lesions characteristic of HEAE were found in all recipients of GPMBP. Histologic lesions in recipients of large doses (31.6-316 ug) of MBP other than guinea pig also had features of HEAE when examined on days 11-15.

Chronic relapsing EAE imitates MS more closely, both clinically and histologically (Lassmann and Wisniewski, 1979). It has been induced in monkeys, rabbits and guinea pigs by sensitization with CNS tissue and complete Freund's adjuvant. True relapsing EAE was initially observed in juvenile Hartley and strain 13 guinea pigs (Raine and Stone, 1977) and later in rats (Panitech and Ciccone, 1981) and mice. In juvenile guinea pigs, the relapsing EAE was produced with whole CNS material, but only acute disease resulted when MBP was used. MBP is the prime protein encephalitogenic for guinea pigs. Furthermore, the tryptophan peptide from MBP, phe-ser-trp-gly-ala-glu-gly-gln-arg, is by far the most significant encephalitogenic region within MBP for guinea pigs (Westall et al, 1971). If the tryptophan residue in MBP is destroyed, MBP's encephalitogenicity vanishes (Chao and Einstein, 1970). Since MBP presents only one encephalitogen to guinea pigs, it was suggested that multiple antigens, were necessary for chronic EAE and maybe MS (Raine and Traugott, 1982). However, it was shown in rats (Panitech and Ciccone, 1981) and mice (Fritz, Chou and Mc Farlin, 1983) that MBP could produce chronic/relapsing EAE. Also MOG produces relapsing EAE in mice (Kerleo de Rosbo, Mendel and Ben-Nun, 1995) and rats (Johns et al., 1995).

What is the difference between guinea pigs and the other species with respect to chronic/ relapsing EAE? In these other species a variety of myelin proteins are encephalitogenic--- MBP, lipoprotein, MOG and myelin oligodendrocyte basic protein. Furthermore, there are multiple regions (immunogens) within these proteins which are themselves encephalitogenic in these species (see Table 1).These species, unlike the guinea pig, "see" multiple immunogenic regions even when only whole protein is injected. Therefore the rule that chronic relapsing EAE requires multiple immunogens is upheld. The guinea pig work suggests that a combination of strong (from MBP) and weak (from other CNS tissue) immunogens are also necessary. Since the individual peptide encephalitogens are of varying potency, non-guinea pig test animals would also see simultaneous strong and weak immunogens, when whole protein is injected.

Are their exceptions to these "rules" for chronic relapsing EAE induction? In the case of the Lewis rat, MOG peptide 35-55 is able to induce relapsing EAE (Johns et al., 1995). However, it is known that this long sequence contains at least both T cell and B cell epitopes (Bernard et al., 1997). Therefore, this example is not an exception. Furthermore 200 ug, an enormous amount for induction, per animal were used. It is interesting that Linington et al. at lower doses (1993) were unable to detect any neurological symptoms in Lewis rats using this peptide.

The mouse, however, presents an interesting story. In recent years there has been considerable work on mouse encephalitogens. In fact not only whole protein produces relapsing EAE, but synthetic peptides from these proteins are also claimed to be active (Amor et al., 1994; Kerlero de Rosbo, Mendel, Ben-Nun, 1995). This would seem to argue against the necessity of multiple immunogens for relapsing EAE induction. However, it is very difficult to compare this work with the studies involving other species. In the mouse a) usually multiple sites of injection, b) multiple adjuvants, c) large amounts of adjuvants, considering the size of the mouse, and d) large amounts of encephalitogenic peptide are employed. This last difference is particularly disturbing. Encephalitogenic peptide dose response curves are quite sharp (Young et al., 1974) (Table 4).

Table 4. Induction of EAE in Guinea Pigs Using the Tryptophan Peptide from Myelin Basic Protein

Dose ug	Clinical	% Clinical	Histological	% Hist
10.00	11/42	26.1	25/42	59.5
3.30	17/51	34.0	29/51	56.8
1.00	30/51	58.8	34/51	66.7
0.33	6/26	23.1	18/26	69.2

A few extra microorganisms can reduce the encephalitogenicity greatly. In some mice experiments the molar ratio of peptide to whole protein used for comparison is as much as 100 fold. When 1 ug is sufficient to induce potent EAE in guinea pigs (Young et al., 1974; Westall, 1978) or rats (Westall, Thompson and Lennon, 1977), why are 150-200 ug (Amor et al., 1994) used for induction in mice or the 200 ug of peptide 35-55 in Lewis rats as mentioned above. (Johns et al.,1995)? Table 3 and 4 compare acute EAE production in guinea pigs and Lewis rats using synthetic encephalitogens. It would appear at best to this author with over 40 years of encephalitogenic peptide experience, that the mouse work is employing immunological procedures and mechanisms which are totally different from those in other test species. These results also bring into question the contribution of impurities, even with synthetic peptides. An impurity of ½ % of a 200 ug preparation is still 1 ug!

Because of the large amounts of immunogen and the use of multiple adjuvants for induction, one could easily question whether the mouse is a very good model for MS. Furthermore, it has been shown in mice that MBP inducing relapsing EAE produces not only activated lymphocytes to MBP, but also to lipoprotein (Perry, Barzaga-Gilbert and Trotter, 1991). In the mouse weak encephalitogens might "allow other encephalitogenic structures" to be processed. To ascertain the differences between mouse relapsing EAE and the relapsing EAE seen in other species, encephalitogenic dose response curves and the effects of different adjuvant combinations, need to be performed. In any event, for best results in producing relapsing EAE relevant to MS, a series of immunogens must be present and that these immunogens are of varying potency. This last point probably is crucial. For each species except guinea pig, MBP for example, presents a very potent encephalitogen and one or more weaker ones. In the case of the guinea pig, other CNS material must provide the secondary immunogen(s).

It should also be noted that many of the peptide encephalitogens described for the mouse are substantially longer, 15-20 residues, than those described for other species, 9-11 residues (see Table 1). The probability of a mimic occurring in a microbial system which would trigger an autoimmune response against human myelin is directly related to the number of residues of the immunogen, the longer the immunogen the lower the probability. While some of these peptides might serve as multi-antigens, it is highly unlikely that a single mimic could imitate these long peptides.

B. Adjuvants

In order to improve immune responses to potential immunogens, a large number of substances, mostly bacterial, were studied to find general immunostimulants. These were collectively termed "adjuvants" (Freund, Stern and Pisani, 1947; Kabat, Wolf, and Bezer, 1947; Morgan, 1947). The most popular of these is Freund's complete adjuvant, which is an oil emulsion of *Mycobacteria.* With respect to autoimmune induction, the oil emulsion may or may not be required. With EAE, it appears essential. However, artificial castration (LHRH, immunogen, Carelli et al., 1982) and experimental autoimmune orchitis (aspermatogenous protein, immunogen, Toullet et al, 1977; Hagopian et al, 1977) are induced in aqueous solution.

Freund's adjuvant has been chemically defined further. Ellouz et al (1974) reported that the minimum molecular requirement for use as an adjuvant was n-acetyl-muramyl-L-ala-D-isogln (MDP or muramyl dipeptide). This molecule is found in a wide variety of bacterial cell walls. Other studies have shown that it can act as an adjuvant, a general, immunostimulant and anti-neoplastic drug. It also has been found to be pyrogenic (Kotani et al., 1977), a naturally found sleep factor (Martin et al., 1984) and a mimic of serotonin (Root-Bernstein and Westall, 1983, 1990). The single term "adjuvant" has been used whether one is discussing antibody stimulation, delayed hypersensitivity enhancement, pyrogenicity, anti-infectious effects, mitogenic responses, or autoimmune disease induction. Actually a given adjuvant may augment one or more of these actions (for review see Chedid, Audibert and Johnson, 1978). With the chemical definition of adjuvants (Ellouz et al., 1974) and the use of synthetic modifications, the different potential actions have been chemically distinguished (Adam et al., 1981).

Much work has been performed on muramyl dipeptide's ability to assist in the production of antibody against a large number of antigens. In these cases MDP appears to be functioning as a general immunostimulant (Chedid, Audibert, Johnson, 1978; Adam et al., 1981). It also does not have to be injected with the antigen or even at the same time as the antigen (Chedid et al., 1976). Since the immunogen-adjuvant complex is required (see below) for autoimmune disease initiation, MDPs function in autoimmune disease seems to be much more than just a general immunostimulant. This is further supported by the activity of synthetic modifications of muramyl dipeptide. As can be seen in Table 5, the specificity of adjuvanticity and autoimmune disease induction are similar, but decidedly different.

EAE induction by a myelin protein or its encephalitogenic peptides is dependent upon concomitant injection of Freund's complete adjuvant (FCA) or one of a number of other adjuvants or inducer types. While the encephalitogen and the inducer may be injected separately, they must be injected at the same site and within a very limited period of time to be active in EAE induction (Waksman, Adams and Mansmann, 1957). Depending upon the particular protein or peptide used and the species of the host animal, the adjuvant may be *Mycobacterium tuberculosis* or a close relative (Freund, Stern and Pisani, 1947; Kabat, Wolf, Bezer, 1947; Morgan, 1947), an active bacterial subunit, e.g. n-acetyl muramyl dipeptide (Ellouz et al., 1974; Nagai et al, 1978a; Nagai et al., 1978b), *B. pertussis* (Levine and Wenk, 1965; Lennon et al., 1976; Westall, Thompson and Lennon, 1977) or homogenates of whole spinal cord with and without synthetic adjuvants (Levine and Wenk, 1965), usually in an oil emulsion.

Table 5. Comparison between the Specificity for Adjuvanicity and EAE Induction for MDP[1]

	Clinical EAE	Adjuvanticit
Nac-Mur-L-Ala-D-Glu-Gly	3/5	poor
Nac-Mur-Gly-D-isoGln	10/10	weak
Nac-Mur-D-Ala-D-isoGln	2/5	weak
Nac-Mur-L-Ala-D-isoGln	10/10	strong
Nac-Mur-L-Ser-D-isoGln	10/10	strong
Nac-Mur-L-Ala-D-isoGln-L-Lys-D-Ala	5/5	strong
Nac-Mur-LAla-D-isoGln-L-Lys	5/5	strong

[1]EAE data from Nagai et al., 1978b. Adjuvant activity data Chedid, Audibert, and Johnson, 1978.

Nagai et al. (1978a, b) showed that n-acetyl-muramyl dipeptide (MDP) in the oil emulsion with the whole myelin basic protein, or the encephalitogenic tryptophan peptide of myelin basic protein, would induce EAE in guinea pigs. Maeda et al (1980) produced EAE in various strains of rats using MDP and whole myelin basic protein. Carilli et al., (1982) found that n-acetyl muramyl dipeptide with LHRH in an aqueous solution could induce artificial autoimmune castration. Lee and Schneider (1962) and Shaw et al. (1962), using whole proteins, have demonstrated that the ability of the encephalitogen-adjuvant combination to induce acute EAE is dependent upon the proportion of the constituents. Encephalitogenicity disappears if the proportion of adjuvant is too great or too small (Shaw et al., 1962; Simon and Anzil, 1974).

Westall (1978) noted the interesting dose response curve for both the tryptophan peptide and n-acetyl muramyl dipeptide---the minimum dose of each required for disease induction was equal on the molar basis. This led Root-Bernstein and Westall (1990) to show with nuclear magnetic resonance that the two physically formed a complex. The tryptophan peptide alone has only a slight interaction with the emulsion, whereas both muramyl dipeptide alone or in combination with the tryptophan peptide interacts considerably with the emulsion. They also found that LHRH and n-acetyl muramyl dipeptide formed a complex. In this case the complex formed in aqueous solution. More importantly they found that those combinations, whether involving tryptophan peptide, LHRH or adjuvant modifications, which did not produce disease, also did not physically form a complex. However, with respect to artificial castration, the adjuvant could be chemically attached and still disease would ensue. This association is not required for the adjuvant to act solely as a general immunostimulant (Hosmalin et al, 1987).Thus it appeared that for the induction of autoimmune disease added restrictions are placed upon the adjuvant. The immunogen and the adjuvant work as a unit.

Walter Moore and his associates investigated the tertiary structure of myelin basic protein and the encephalitogenic peptides derived from this protein. (Mendz, Moore and Carnegie, 1982; Chapman, Littlemore and Moore, 1978; Chapman and Moore, 1976). The tryptophan peptide---phe-ser-trp-gly-ala-glu-gly-gln-arg---has a distinct bent structure in aqueous solution. The oil emulsion would aid in maintaining this structure. In fact a sequence change which alters this bent form, eliminates the molecule's EAE activity. This was seen spectacularly with two sequence changes: a.) the change of an L-alanine for glycine and b.) the D-alanine for L-alanine. These are the most minimal sequence changes that can be made in the structure. However, the glycine permits a bend at the glycine-tryptophan bond. Alanine hinders it. The D-alanine change causes the molecule to twist away from the bent form. Obviously the tertiary structure of this small peptide is crucial for its activity. (Khanarian et al, 1979; Moore et al., 1981).

The conformation of the heptadecapeptide, phe-lys-leu-gly-gly-arg-asp-ser-arg-ser-gly-ser-pro-met-ala-arg-arg, comprising the encephalitogenic sequence in Rhesus monkey and rabbit has also been studied (Price, Mendz and Martenson 1988). Mendz and Moore (1983) also studied another rabbit encephalitogenic sequence. In both cases a bent form is found. Likewise, Fermandjian et al (1987), using 1H-NMR, found evidence for a MDP structure involving two successive beta turns. As mentioned above, using nuclear magnetic resonance, Root-Bernstein and Westall (1990) extensively studied the tryptophan/n-acetyl muramyl dipeptide and LHRH/n-acetyl muramyl dipeptide interactions. They found that the combinations indeed interacted and that immunologically-inactive modifications did not form a complex. (Tables 2, 6 and 7)

Table 6. Minimum Structural Requirements for Adjuvant Activity Induction of EAE in Guinea PIGs[1]

	Encephalitogenicity
Nac-Mur-L-Ala-D-isoGln	++
Nac-Mur-L-Ala	-
Nac-Mur-L-Ala-D-isoGln-L-Lys	++
L-Ala-D-isoGln-L-Lys-D-Ala	-
Nac-Mur-L-Ala-D-isoGln-L-Lys-D-Ala –L-Lys-D-Ala	++
Nac-Mur-L-Ala-D-Glu-NH2	++
Nac-Mur-L-Ala-D-Glu-Gly	+
Nac-Mur-L-Ser-D-Glu-NH2	++
Nac-Mur-Gly-D-Glu-NH2	++
Nac-Mur-D-Ala-D-Glu-NH2	+
Nac-Mur-D-Ala	-
Nac-Mur-D-Glu-NH2	-
Nac-Mur-L-Ala-D-Glu	+
Nac-Mur-L-Ala-L-Glu	-
Nac-Mur-L-Ala-D-Asp-NH2	-
alpha-Methyl-NAc-Mur-L-Ala-D-Glu-NH2	++
beta-Methyl-NAc-Mur-L-Ala-D-Glu-NH2	+
D-Lactyl-Ala-D-Glu-NH2	+
6-o-Stearoyl-NAc-Mur-L-Ala-D-Glu-NH2	-

[1-2] Nagai et al., 1978b; Chedid, Audibert and Johnson, 1978.

Is the apparent required association between adjuvant and antigen, seen between MDP and tryptophan peptide or LHRH, an apparent requirement for adjuvanticity with other adjuvants and immunogens? While most gram-positive bacteria have an acetylated muramyl structure in their cell-walls, *Mycobacteria*, *Norcardiea,* and *Micromonospora* have an acylated muramyl structure, involving a glycolyl group (Adam et al., 1976). Westall et al. (1975), using a hydrosoluble mycobacterial fraction (Migliore-Samour and Jolles, 1973) prepared by Migliore-Samour and Jolles, induced EAE in guinea pigs using whole myelin basic protein. However, when they attempted to produce EAE using the encephalitogenic tryptophan peptide eight times the adjuvant was required for induction (Westall et al., 1974).

Table 7. Summary of NMR Results of Binding Muramyl Dipeptide and its Derivatives to Immunogens

	Active Adj	EAE Induc	Trp Pep	MSH 4-10	LHRH	LHRH 4-10	LHRH 1-3
Muramyl dipeptide	+	+	+	+	+	+,-	-
N-acetyl-nor-muramyl-L-alanyl-D-isoglutamine	+	unk	+	nd	+	nd	nd
N-acetyl-nor-muramyl-D-alanyl-D-isoglutamine	-	unk	-	nd	-	nd	nd
N-acetyl-muramyl-L-alpha-aminobutyryl-Disogln	+,-	unk	-	nd	+,-	nd	nd
N-acetyl-muramyul-L-threonyl-D-isoglutamine	+	unk	+,-	nd	+	nd	nd
N-acetyl-muramyl-D-Ala-D-isoglutamine	-	-	-	-	-	-	-
N-acetyl-muramyl-L-Ala-L-isoglutamine	-	-	-	-	-	-	-
Muramic acid	-	-	-	-	-	-	-

Since the hydrosoluble mycobaterial adjuvant was effective using whole MBP and the tryptophan peptide is the only major encephalitogenic region in guinea pig, two possible explanations can be offered. First, the normal structure of the encephalitogenic peptide compared to its structure within the whole protein is different. Second, the hydrosoluble adjuvant was responding to a much weaker determinant in the whole protein, e.g. the n-terminal region (Barton et al., 1972). In either case the hydrosoluble adjuvant is specifically interacting with a particular immunogen in a different way than is seen with MDP. As stated above the n-acetyl muramyl dipepitde combined with the tryptophan peptide to form an active complex. It is very likely that the multiple carbohydrate units comprising the Mycobacterial fraction could disrupt the complex formation. In any event, the Jolles' hydrosoluble adjuvant is not just acting as a general stimulant, responding with any encephalitogen presented to it.

The whole *Mycobacterium* adjuvant appears to be effective in those mammalian species tested. However, the *B. pertussis* adjuvant shows tremendous variability in species potency. In Lewis rat, but not the Brown Norway (BN) rat, guinea pig myelin basic protein and *B. pertussis*, without the necessity of *Mycobacteria*, will produce a hyperacute form of EAE in Lewis rats (Lennon et al., 1976). This also appears in the monkey (Levine and Wenk, 1965; Levine and Wenk 1964; Levine, 1974). However, *B. pertussis* is rather ineffectual in rabbits and guinea pigs (Westall, 1977) (Tables 8-9). Within the guinea pig myelin basic protein is an encephalitogenic seqeuence, pro-gln-lys-ser-gln-arg-ser-gln-asp-glu-asn-pro-val-val, (Westall, Thompson and Lennon, 1977) which when it is injected with *B. pertussis* produces hyperacute EAE. Modified versions of this sequence, which mimic Lewis rat, rabbit, human cow and pig sequences, only produce regular EAE at normal doses. The *Mycobacterium* adjuvant will only produce ordinary EAE with any of these sequences in Lewis rat. The hyperacute site is only active in those species which are also active to *B. pertussis* (Westall, 1977). It is not active in rabbits or guinea pigs even if the *Mycobacterium* adjuvant is used.

Also the tryptophan region, which is active with n-acetyl muramyl dipeptide and *Mycobacteria*, is not active in the species which are responsive to *B. pertussis*. These data are interpreted as showing that *B. pertussis* adjuvant has a "special association" with the hyperacute site, and the MDP has a "special association" with the tryptophan peptide.

Table 8. The Effect of *B. Pertussis* on the Encephalitogeni- City of Myelin Basic Proteins in Guinea PIGs

		Numbers of *B. pertussis*			
Encephalitogen	Dose	Organisms	Clinical	Day of Onset	Day of Death
GPmbp	33ug	0	5/5	17,13,13,14,11	18,14,14,15,14
		10^{10}	5/5	14,17,13,14,19	15,18,14,15,27
		20 x 10^{10}	4/5	26,25,14,19	20,15
Lew Rat MBP	33ug	0	4/5	--,13,17,13,13	15,20,14,14
		10^{10}	5/5	17,14,18,21,13	18,27,14,20,27
		20 x 10^{10}	2/5	18,15	
Human MBP	33ug	0	5/5	11,14,11,13,13	12,15,13,14,14
		10^{10}	5/5	13,12,14,13,14	18,12,16,14,18
		20 x 10^{10}	3/5	26,19,19	20,19
Bovine MBP	33ug	0	4/5	13,13,13,13	15,14,15,15
		10^{10}	¾	10,17,17	12,18,17
		20 x 10^{10}	4/5	19, 19,18,18	20,19,19
Porcine MBP	33ug	0	5/5	11,13,12,13,13	19,20,19
		20 x 10^{10}	4/5	27,15,19,19	19,20,19
Monkey MBP	33ug	O	5/5	11,12,14,12,11	15,14,15,14,14
		20 x 10^{10}		19,25,18,19	19,25,18,20
Rabbit MBP	33ug	0	5/5	12,12,11,12,15	15,14,16,17
		20 x 10^{10}	4/5	13,13,14,20	14,14,15,20

Table 9. The Effect of *B. Pertussis* on the Encephalitogen-Icity of Myelin Basic Proteins in Rabbits

		Number of *B. pertussis*		
Encephalitogen	Dose, ug	Organisms	Clinical	Day of Onset
Guinea Pig MBP	1000	4 x 10^{10}	1 /4	20
	1000	0	3 /4	20,20,22
Human MBP	1000	4 x 10^{10}	2 /4	22,23
	1000	0	1 /4	20

Encephalitogen	Dose, ug	Organisms	Clinical	Day of Onset
Rabbit MBP	1000	4 x 10^{10}	3 /4	19,20,23
	1000	0	1 /4	23
Bovine MBP	1000	4 x 10^{10}	1 /4	18
	1000	0	1 /4	20
GP Peptide 70-88	100	4 x 10^{10}	0/4	--

C. Simultaneous Immune Processing of the Adjuvant and Immunogen

The complex requires that both the immunogen and the adjuvant are processed by the same immune cell. Only an activated system directed against the immunogen can result. There is no chance that excess immunogen or adjuvant can "turn on" suppressor systems. There is no chance that immunogen or adjuvant will be degraded prior to immune processing. There is no chance the adjuvant activated cells will "waste" their efforts on other molecules they encounter before they encounter the immunogen. Is there any other evidence which supports these conclusions? Yes LHRH has been chemically attached to the n-acetylmuramyl dipeptide. This modification should prevent the formation of the complex by complimentary interaction, but it still maintains a 1:1 association. What affect does this have on artificial castration? It still produces disease (Hosmalin et al., 1987; Bernard et al., 1987). The crucial step is the simultaneous processing by the same immune cell of both the adjuvant and immunogen. The linked complex, however, puts both immunogen and adjuvant at risk of premature digestion. However, since both the LHRH and n-acetyl muramyl dipeptide are themselves bent structures, their linked conformation might incorporate much of the complex form, and thus be protected.

Multiple Sclerosis

While the cause is unknown, it is generally believed that MS is initiated by an autoimmune attack on the CNS myelin. A microorganism which contains a region on its surface which mimics an antigenic region on one of the myelin proteins instigates the autoimmune process (Jahnke, Fisher and Alvord, 1985; Fujinami and Oldstone, 1985)

A. Immunological Restrictions on Molecular Mimicry

With the availability of information concerning peptide encephalitogens, various investigators have searched the sequences of particularly viral coat proteins for similar structures. In some cases sequences have been synthesized and tested, with little success. While some sequences have initiated T cell activation (Ufret-Vicenty et al., 1998; Wucherpfennig and Strominger, 1995; Katz-Levy et al., 1999) only one sequence initiates clinical encephalitogencity (Lenz et al, 2001). This sequence was located "in the C-terminus of a protein specified by a gene designated Cpn0483". The protein's location within the organism (*Chlamydia*) is not known. Could the immune system even access the region of the protein during human infection? Furthermore Freund's adjuvant was required to induce disease experimentally. Recently, the validity of molecular mimicry has been questioned (Bar-Or et al., 1999).

Many believe that small peptides do not possess tertiary structures. This is not true. As stated above, the structural work on encephalitogens have shown that slight changes, i.e. a D-alanine for L-alanine, or alanine for glycine, can easily alter the encephalitogencity of a peptide. Therefore, if one is looking for a molecular mimic one should be searching for "structural mimics" and not "sequential mimics". The immune system, like hormonal systems, recognizes three dimensional shapes, and not sequences. This is, however, not enough. The contributions of the individual amino acids must be ascertained. For example, not all nine residues of encephalitogenic peptide from myelin basic protein---phe-ser-trp-gly-ala-glu-gly-gln-arg--- are equally important. The phenylalanine can be replaced by other hydrophobics, especially ring structures. The arginine can be replaced by other positive structures. The glutamine can be substituted by serine but not glutamate, etc. This presents a major problem for molecular mimicry. There are very few immunologically-active peptides which have been analyzed to this degree (See Table 2).

B. Multiple Sclerosis Initiation

The author examined (2006a) the known sequences from bacteria and viruses which infect or are normally present in humans. No distinction was made between pathogens and non-pathogens or with the location of the protein within the microorganism. Sequences within these proteins were compared to the three best chemically defined encephalitogenic regions: the tryptophan peptide (phe-ser-trp-gly-ala-glu-gly-gln-arg), hyperacute site (pro-gln-lys-ser-his-qln-arg-thr-qln-asp-glu-asn-pro-val) and the mid-region (thr-thr-his-tyr-gly-ser-leu-pro-qln-lys) from myelin basic protein. The procedure outlined in the previous section was followed and was far more rigid than any previous process to identify mimics. The bacteria contained 111 encephalitogenic mimics: 39 corresponding to the midregion, 23 to the tryptophan peptide and 49 to the hyperacute site (Table 10). Very few viruses contained mimics. Almost all the mimics were found in bacteria, rather than viruses. No one immunogen dominated the group. In fact the differences in numbers of mimics seem to reflect more how extensive the immunogen had been defined, rather than any sequential preference. Sites were found in most of the bacteria examined. Gram stain characteristics of a bacterium seem to be irrelevant. The number of mimics found in a particular species seemed to reflect more on the amount of sequence data accumulated about that species. The mimics were located in all parts of the cell and within all parts of the proteins. The majority of the mimics were located in non-pathogenic gut bacteria. Since there are from 20 to 30 potential encephalitogenic regions in four myelin proteins, one must assume that structural mimics are not rare.

Table 10. Human Microorganism Proteins which Contain Potential Mimics of Defined Encephalitogens

Organism	Mid-Region Peptide	Tryptophan Peptide	Hyperacute Peptide
Bacterium			
Burkhoderia	1	1	0
Enteroccus	1	3	8
Bacteroides	6	6	3
Esherichia	7	2	8
Streptococcus	4	3	3
Lactobacillus	6	2	8
Clostridium	3	2	6
Bifidobacteria	1	2	3
Klebsiella	1	0	0
Fusobacteria	1	0	3
Salmonella	1	0	0
Chlamydophia	1	0	1
Haemophilus	1	1	0
Bacillus	1	0	0
Pseudomonas	1	0	0
Actinobacillus	1	0	0
Helicobacter	0	1	0
Serratia	0	0	5
Virus			
Hepatitis B	4	0	0
Hepatitis C	0	1	0
Papillomona	1	0	0
Influenza C	1	0	0
Blue Tongue	0	0	1
Ecovirus	0	0	1
Herpes	0	0	1

Previous to this study it was assumed that mimics were rare, which explained why MS was rare. However, they are not rare. To make matters worse the majority of the mimics are located in normal gut bacteria. If molecular mimicry is important in MS why is MS rare? Can EAE give an explanation? EAE induction first requires two molecules, the immunogen, in the MS case the mimic, and the adjuvant. However, the gut has large concentrations of gram-positive bacteria, which contain either n-acetyl muramyl dipeptide or n-acyl muramyl dipeptide. Therefore that is not a limitation. However, a second requirement is that the adjuvant and, in this case, mimic act together. The bacteria, itself is not being processed by the immune system, but the adjuvant and mimic are. For this to happen in the gut the hydrolytic processes must be activated in such a fashion to produce high concentrations of both adjuvant and mimic, which can then be immunologically processed. Aberrations in the hydrolytic processing of the gut could account for the rarity of MS. Is there any other evidence of gut involvement in MS? Yes. Serotonin metabolism is greatly altered during MS relapses. This was observed (Westall, 200a) by longitudinal measurements of (5-HIAA)/

tryptophan ratios from MS urine. This ratio drops noticeably during relapse. The urinary serotonin reflects gut metabolism and not central nervous system metabolism. As mentioned above n-acetyl muramyl dipeptide is a potent serotonin mimic. If it is elevated one could hypothesize that it would act like serotonin and feedback inhibit serotonin production by inhibition of tryptophan hydrolase production.This would lower serotonin concentrations. However the MDP could also act in place of serotonin at other receptors.This could explain why one sees a reduction of serotonin without any clinical effects.

C. Adjuvants

The importance of adjuvants in induction of experimental autoimmune disease has been known for decades. However, their possible importance in human autoimmune diseases has been essentially ignored. The fact that post viral and vaccinal neuropathies are associated with secondary infections is suggestive (Root-Bernstein and Westall, 1986). Furthermore it appears possible that the immunogens important in MS are mimicked by gut bacterial protein fragments. Some of these same bacteria contain peptidoglycans which have been linked to adjuvanticity. Thus both immunogen mimics and adjuvant molecules are readily available from the same sources. Has there been any association between adjuvants and MS. Yes. Elevated concentrations of peptidoglycans in MS neurological cells, immunological cells and in antigen-presenting cells have been reported (Schrijver el al., 2001). They also found peptidoglycan antibodies in MS CSF. Since the brains examined for this study were from patients who had had MS for over 14 years, the significance is somewhat cloudy. One could argue that the peptidoglycan concentrations in MS cells are secondary events of a chronic process.

Several studies suggest that infections correlate with MS attacks (Sibley, Bamford and Clark, 1985; Buljevac et al., 2002). However, over 80% of the infections are identified as of viral sources and certainly not all of the bacterial infections are from gram-positive (peptidoglycan-containing) bacteria. Furthermore, MS patients have fewer infections than non-sick individuals (Buljevac et al., 2002). Therefore it would seem unlikely that the increased MS peptidoglycan concentrations are from these infections. Most likely they are from the gut. Lehonten (Lehtonen, Eerola and Toivanen, 1997; Lehtonen et al., 1995) (Table 11) found that the concentration of peptidoglycans in normal immunological cells was dependent on age. At birth there were none. This increased until after puberty and then slowly declined in latter life. Therefore, negligible concentrations of peptidoglycans were expected to be found in the MS cells discussed above. Lehonten also concluded that the peptidoglycans were from gut. In any event it would seem that there is an abnormal, i.e. hydrolytic, production of peptidoglycans in MS.

Lipopolysaccharides are the gram-negative bacterial counterpart to peptidoglycans. Lipopolysaccharides have the ability to pass the gut barrier without assistance, a property which has been used by the pharmaceutical industry for some time. These compounds have been shown to grossly affect the blood-brain barrier (Xaio et al, 2001) and cause acute inflammatory responses in CNS parenchyma (Andersson, Perryand Gordon, 1992). One of the enzyme responsible for the breakdown of lipopolysaccharides, arylesterase, has been shown to be deficient in MS myelin (Back, Broch-Moeller and Boeg-Hansen, 1976). Therefore, another bacterial component has been associated with the MS pathology.

Table 11. Age Distribution of Subjects with Muramic Acid in Peripheral Blood Leucocytes

Mean Age	% Positive Subjects	Number in Group
0	0	41
14	60	20
25	23	83
35	17	41
45	0	34
55	5	61
65	7	46
75	0	38

The muamic acid was detected by gas chromatography/ mass spectrometry by the procedure in references, Lehtonen, et al., 1995; Lehtonen, Errola and Toivanen, 1997.

D. Simultaneous Activation of the Immune System by Multiple Immunogens

There is a major difference between chronic relapsing EAE and MS. In chronic EAE, the immunogens are injected in a fixed ratio as determined by the composition of the whole tissue or protein. In the case of MS, if multiple mimics are involved, the mimics encounter the immune system in variable concentrations depending on the microorganisms and hydrolytic enzymes present. This would suggest that MS clinically would present a much more varied disease than the EAE model. Of course this is what is seen.

If chronic relapsing EAE is initiated by the action of multiple immunogens, are there any data supporting simultaneous multi-immunogenic initiation of MS? As was mentioned above mimics of encephalitogenic regions appear rather plentiful. MS' rarity appears to be the result of problems in the processing of the mimic: a) either the presentation of the mimic, through digestive processes involving hydrolytic enzymes, to the immune system or b) the activation of the immune system by the mimic. Both of these processes are under strict hormonal control. This is particularly interesting since it has been suggested (see below) that the histo-clinical variance characteristic of MS is the result of proteolytic processing of myelin antigens in the CNS (Westall, 2006b). The same hormones which control CNS proteolysis also control the gut processes. In any event, MS appears as a hormonal disease which is manifested clinically as an autoimmune attack on CNS myelin (Westall, 2000a, 2007). If the processing, and not the presence of the mimic, is determining disease initiation, why would the immune system only process as single mimic at a time? It would seem more likely that multiple mimics would simultaneously be processed. In other words, MS, like chronic relapsing EAE, its model, is an autoimmune attack on the CNS myelin by the simultaneous activation of the immune system by multiple mimics of myelin antigens. Is there any other data which would support this explanation? Yes.

Various test results on the responses of different myelin proteins to MS activated immune cells have been confusing. Different groups have found myelin basic protein (MBP) (Tejada-Simon et al., 2000), lipoprotein (Trotter et al., 1998; Correale et al., 1995) and oligodendrocyte glycoprotein (MOG) (Kerlero de Rosbo et al., 1997) responsive to the activated MS system. The MOG data is the most impressive. However, when all three immunogens were tested in the same patients, better response was seen with MOG, but the other two showed positives, which certainly presents a complicated multi-antigen activation (Kerlero de Rosbo et al., 1993). Finally, the MOG data shows positive response to multiple regions within the MOG protein. This also supports a complicated multi-antigen activation.

E. Longitudinal Appearance of Cytokines and Other Inflammatory Compounds

The work discussed in this section involves only relapsing-remitting MS. The progressive form of MS usually develops late and therefore has years of chronic overlay.

MS was generally thought to be initiated by an autoimmune attack on myelin, i.e. a form of EAE. However, recent magnetic resonance imaging (MRI) work has suggested that MS is far more complicated (Lassmann, Bruck and Lachinetti, 2007; Filippi and Rocca, 2005; Griffen et al., 2002; Silver et al., 2001, Goodwin et al., 1998). Initially a rather diffuse lesion appears. These lesions develop prior to any external immunological cell invasion. In some cases the lesions develop into the classically described MS lesions. Since the initial lesions lack the presence of bacterial and viral agents or externally-produced immunological cell infiltrates, what triggers these initial lesions?

If bacteria are involved in MS by providing immunological mimics and adjuvants molecules, they should also provide other cell wall components, such as lipo-polysaccharides, which have known inflammatory properties. These agents can pass easily through the gut barrier and tight junction cells, as they are used by the pharmaceutical industry to transport drugs (Wong and Toth, 2001). Mimics and their associated adjuvant molecules initiate an autoimmune process which requires weeks to develop. The lipopolysaccharides and other inflammatory agents can activate inflammation and other degradative processes within hours (Felts et al., 2005) This process could explain the histological picture that has emerged.

Is there evidence for non-CNS MS –related activity? Gut serotonin metabolism, as reflected by the urinary tryptophan/5-hydroxyindole acetic acid ratio, drops during MS relapses (Westall, 2006a). As already mentioned peptidoglycans, which are presumably from the gut appear in abnormal concentrations in MS immunological and neurological cells. Numerous other inflammatory and immunological agents appear in the spinal fluid, serum and urine significantly earlier than the development of the classical MS immune lesions. In fact the concentrations of these agents maximizes in some cases a month or two months prior to the MS relapse (Tables 12 and 13). To the contrary in EAE the concentrations of these compounds rise quickly within days as the clinical disabilities develop and decline rapidly. Therefore the clinical expression of these compounds is quite different in MS.

Table 12. Time-Line for the Appearance of Inflammatory and Immunological Compounds Associated with Ms Relaspse

A. Abnormal mRNA Levels in Peripheral Blood Mononuclear Cells from MS Patients[1, 2]

Weeks From Relapse

Compound	-12	-11	-10	-9	-8	-7	-6	-5	-4	-3	-2	-1	0	+1	+2	+3	+4	+5	+6	+7	+8
Elevated Values																					
Caspase-1									o	o	o	x		o	o						
IL-12p35								o			o				x			o			
IL-12p40								o			x				o			o			
IL-10								o			o				x			o			
CXCR3	o				+				+				x				-				o
TNF-alpha	o				o				x				-				-				o
Lymphotoxin	o				o				x				-				-				o
Reduced Values																					
TGF-b	o				o				x				-				o				o
IL-10	o				o				x				-				o				o

[1] X refers to maximum value. + and – means that the values are increasing or decreasing to and from the maximum. O indicates essentially baseline values.

[2] References:

Caspase-1: Furlan et al., 1999a,b

TNF-a, Il-12p35, IL-12p40, and IL-10: van Boxel-Dezaire et al. 1999

CXCR3: Mahad et al., 2003

Tumor necrosis factor-alpha, Transforming growth factor-beta, lymphotoxin, and interleukin-10:Rieckmann et al, 1995

B. Abnormal Serum Levels in MS Patients[1,2]

Compounds	-12	-8	-4	0	-4	-8
Elevated						
MMP/TIMP-1	+	+	x	-	-	-
MMP-3	o	o	o	+	x	o
Glutamate	o	+	+	x	-	o

[1] X refers to maximum value. + and – means that the values are increasing or decreasing to and from the maximum. O indicates essentially baseline values.

2References:

MMP/TIMP-1 Waubert et al., 1999.

MMP-3 Kanesaka et al., 2006.

Glutamate: Westall, Myers & Ellison, 1980.

The principal physiological pathways for metabolic degradation of the extracellular matrix in mammals consist of a family of matrix metalloproteinases (MMP's). MMP activities are controlled by gene transcription, proenzyme activation and activity of tissue inhibitors of MMPs (TIMPS). In MS MMP-9 was increased over controls in 100% of relapsing remitting cases. However, similar levels of MMP-9 were detected during relapses and clinically stable phases of disease (Leppert et al., 1998).

Table 13. Inflammatory and Immunological Compounds Related to MS Relapses

Compound	Source	Correlation with MS Relapse	Reference
Kinin B1 receptor	Rna-leucocytic cells	Up-regulated	Prat et al., 2005
Gelainase B	serum	elevated	Lee et al., 1999
PAI-1	plasma	elevated	Onodera et al., 1999
Interleukin-15	Rna-mononuclear cells	No change	Kivisakk et al., 1998
ICAM-1	Serum	Slightly elevated	Alves-Leon et al., 2001
CXCL10	CSF	Increased	Moreira et al., 2006
CCL2	CSF	Lower	Moreira et al., 2006
TNF receptor	serum	Correlates	Khoury et al., 1999
Neopterin	Serum	No correlation	Bagnato et al., 2003
Beta-2 Microglobulin	Serum	No correlation	Bagnato et al., 2003
Uric acid	Serum	Lower	Mostert et al., 2005
TNF-a converting	RNA-leucocytic cells	Up regulated	Seifert et al., 2002
sVCAM-1	Serum/ CSF	Elevated	Matsuda et al., 1995
CCL2	CSF	Decreased	Malmestrom et al., 2006

In a small longitudinal study of MS patients in acute relapse, high expression of MMP-9 in CSF coincided with gadolinium-enhancing lesions on MRI (Rosenberg et al., 1996). However in a cross-sectional study of 40 patients no correlation between the number of active MS lesions and MMP-9 could be established (K. Gijbels, personal communication). Similarly the number of hyperintense MS lesions as found in T2- and proton weighted MRI scans, does not correlate with MMP-9 in CSF (Paemen et al., 1994). Kouwehoven et al. (2002) showed differences in MMPs and TIMPs expression, production, secretion and activity between immature dendritic cells and mature dendritic cells from MS patients and healthy controls, but they were unable to find correlations with clinical variables. In MS TIMP is not upgraded. CSF MMP to TIMP ratios did not differ between MS subtypes, suggesting systemic rather than CNS-restricted changes.

The Leppert study also found MMP-2 was not upgraded and did not detect MMP-7. Table 12 presents data showing MMP-3 levels were elevated transiently within 1 month after relapse. MMP-3 with its broad specificity can degrade major components of the blood-brain barrier.

Caspase -1 cleaves IL-beta and IL-18 precursor proteins into their secretory forms and it is therefore essential in the early steps of the inflammatory process. It appears to be involved in the blood-derived CNS confined inflammatory process underlying lesion formation in MS. Furlan et al. (1999a,b) found that caspase-1 mRNA levels peak significantly only in the week preceding an acute attack, subside immediately after the beginning of an acute attack, and correlate with the number of new but not persisting enhancing lesions.

Plasminogen activators (PA) convert plasminogen into the serine protease plasmin, which degrades several components of the ECM and activates MMPs. It is significant that one of the earliest detectable signs of inflammation in MS white matter is increased expression of PAs on mononuclear cells in perivascular cuffs (Cuzner et al., 1996). The CSF plasminogen activator, tPA, activity in MS patients was significantly raised, but did not correlate with disease activity (Akenami et al., 1996). Onodera et al. (1999) found the plasma plasminogen activator inhibitor-1 level in patients with active MS 6 times higher than the controls.

Cytokines are a family of polypeptides that regulate immune responses and inflammatory reactions. Three of them, interleukin-1 beta, tumor necrosis factor alpha, and interleulin-6 are secreted mainly by monocytes, but all three can also be synthesized by other immune and non-immune cells including CNS microglia and astrocytes. Interleukin-1 beta and tumor necrosis factor alpha promote the establishment of perivascular infiltrates by increasing adhesiveness between endothelium and leukocytes (Bevilacqua et al., 1995) Interkeukin-6 induces immunoglobulin production of activated B cells. All three cytokines enhance T- and B-cell immune responses (Dinarello, 1989). Both interleukin-1 beta and tumor necrosis factor alpha stimulate the proliferation of astrocytes and promote gliosis in vivo (Giulian and Lachman, 1985). Maimone et al. (1991) found CSF interleukin-6 in 10 of 34 MS patients. There were no statistical differences between active and stable MS. Frei et al. (1991) found IL-6 concentrations in MS plasma were about 17 times higher than MS CSF. This report supports the hypothesis of a systemic B cell response in MS. The results for tumor necrosis factor were similar. Beck et al. (1988) found that tumor necrosis factor and interferon peaked approximately 2 weeks before exacerbation and then declined. As early as 4 weeks prior to a relapse, tumor necrosis factor alpha and lymphotoxin mRNA expression significantly increased whereas interleukin 10 and transforming growth factor beta mRNA decreased compared to mRNA values of these cytokines at 8 or 12 weeks prior to a relapse (Rieckmann et al., 1995). Serum concentrations decreased significantly before clinical relapse and the appearance of active lesions (Galboiz and Miller, 2002).

Increased levels of soluble intercellular adhesion molecules, sVCAM-1 and sL-selectin and tumor necrosis receptor were found in the blood of clinically active MS patients experiencing a clinical relapse (Hartung et al. 1995).

Elevated CSF glutamic acid concentrations, as much as three times normal, have been reported in active MS lesions (Stover et al., 1997). This aberration can lead to neurologic cell death (Goldsmith, 2000; Werner, Pitt and Raine, 2001). Westall et al., (1980) in a longitudinal study found that the serum glutamate concentrations are elevated in active MS as much as two times normal. The increase in glutamic acid did not occur sharply during the onset of relapse. Instead it appeared to rise gradually within a month or two prior to the onset of the clinical relapse to reach a peak during the relapse and then slowly decline. Since the absolute serum concentration observed were much higher than the CSF levels, the source of the glutamate in the serum was not the CSF. Elevated levels of endogenous glutamate and/or excessive activation of glutamate receptors can stimulate MMP-9 production through a NO synthase pathway (Manabe, Gu and Lipton, 2005). It can also interfere with cystine cellular transfers via competing with the carrier molecule on the cell (Bannai, 1986).

One problem with MS research is that there are limited numbers of longitudinal studies. Clinical researchers tend to compare active MS with inactive MS to controls. Only a few studies watch individual patients as they develop a relapse and as the relapse subsides. This is unfortunate since it tends to give an all or nothing result. This is quite misleading since many of the compounds of interest peak considerably before or after the relapse (Tables 12 and 13). This adds to the confusing nature of the results reported.

Another problem in studying individual compounds and their variance in MS is that different investigators use different techniques with varying sensitivities.

F. Histological Location

Any hypothesis of the pathology of MS must include an explanation of its peculiar variability in symptoms, which of course is reflected in its histology. The most common explanation of the histo-clinical variability is that MS is a collection of diseases, which produce essentially the same clinical result. However when one examines individual patients one sees a continuum of symptoms rather than finite groups of diseases.

For the immune system to attack the myelin or areas in the vicinity of the myelin, the immune cells have to be activated. I already have suggested that this process for MS involves the exposure to the immune system of mimics by abnormal hydrolytic digestion of microorganisms, probably gut bacteria. Once the immune cells are activated they look for the appropriate antigen. Encephalitogenic regions are short peptides. In fact they were originally isolated from proteolytic digestion. These peptides tend to be rather stable. For example the 43-88 MBP region is found in the CSF of active MS patients, even though a variety of proteases inundate the MS lesion (Whitaker, 1997). Extensive digestion of myelin proteins does not necessarily destroy its encephalitogenic and antigenic regions. In fact variable processing of myelin proteins is known to hide known regions and expose newer antigens (Matsuo, 1997). The characteristic histological feature of EAE is called perivascular cuffing. This shows the activated immune cells surrounding the blood vessel, not the myelin. This strongly suggests that the activated cells are encountering initially peptides released from the myelin, presumably due to normal protein turnover. Calculations (Westall, 1974) based on the normal turnover of myelin proteins support the release of a constant gradient of peptides from its structure. The turnover is the result of the action of both intracellular and extracellular proteases. Table 14 lists the proteases associated with oligodendrocytes including their location and specificity.

While the composition of myelin within the CNS is consistent, the concentrations of the individual proteases vary greatly within different locations of the brain. (Table 14) Furthermore, most are under strict control. Therefore the proteases' concentrations are further altered in response to these controls. An individual protein will be processed differently by altering the concentrations and availability of the CNS proteases. Therefore the availability and concentration of myelin antigens will vary with the alterations in proteases. At a specific *time* and *place*, the activated immune cells will be presented with none, one or more antigens. Therefore active immune attack will vary depending on this dynamic character of the proteolytic populations. In MS histology will vary with time in an individual and among patients. This variance in histology is mirrored in variance in clinical signs---all tied to a dynamic hydrolytic process which is constantly altering. This process does not only affect histology, clinical observations, and progression of disease, but also its initiation. Everything is tied to the abnormal function of the hydrolytic controls.

Table 14. Proteases Which Have Known Association with Oligodendrocytes

PROTEASE	CHARACTERISTICS	LOCATION
Myelencephron-Specific [A-E]	Increaed by kainic acid—regulated by protease secreted	Highest in medulla oblongata, spinal cord; lowest in corpus callosum, anterior commussure
Caspase-1 (iL-1beta convert[F-H]	Involved in inflammation	Located in oligodendrocytes
Calpain [J-L]	Membrane bound, increased by calpastatin, lipids, activator protein	Located in myelin
Cathepsin [M-N]	Acid protease, increased in MS Seen in MS lesions, degrades myelin basic protein	
MMP-9 [O-Q]	Cysteine protease Induced by liposaccharides	Up in corpus callosum
Cathepsin L[R]	Extracellular-regulated by cistatin C	Located in myelin
Neuropsin [S-T]	Serine protsese, kainite induced, injury induced secreted	Neurons---Oligodendrocytes
Plasminogen Activator [U]	Serine protease	Similar distribution to myelencephalon specific protein Except lower in medulla oblonga, temporal and frontal lobes and cerebral cortex
Cathepsin A[V]	Carbxypeptidase ---increased in MS	
Dipeptidyl peptidase II[W]		Oligodendrocytes
Carboxypeptidase M [X]	Membrane bound	Rich in corpus callosum, pyramidyl and optic tracts; low in ganglia and cortex

[A-E] Scarisbrick et al., 2000
Scarisbrick et al., 2001
Yamanaka et al., 1999
Blaber, et al., 2002
Bernett, et al., 2002
[F-H] Shibata et al., 2000
Furlan et al., 1999b
Hisahara, Okano & Miura, 2003
[J-L] Li and Banik, 1995
Shields and Banik, 1998.
Chakrabarti et al., 1993.
[M-N] Schaecher , Shield and Banik, 2001.
Snyder, et al., 1985.
[O-Q] Berlet, 1986.
Chantry & Glynn 1990
Penkowa et al., 2003
[R] Oh, et al., 1999
[S-T] Stebbins, Jaffe & Moeller, 1998
Tomizawa, et al., 1999
[U] He, et al., 2001
[V] Grynbaum & Marks, 1976
[W] Gorenstein & Sweet, 1985
[X] Nagae, et al., 1992

G. Clinical Ramifications

Because hyperacute, acute and relapsing EAE overlap histopathologically and immunologically they provide experimental evidence supporting the concept that certain human demyelinating diseases represent a spectrum of autoimmunity ranging from chronic multiple sclerosis to acute hemorrahagic necrotizing leukoencephalopathy, for which hyperacute EAE is a model (Levine and Wenk, 1964; Levine, 1974). It is generally presumed that adjuvants are only necessary for experimental autoimmune induction. However, this doesn't seem to be the case. Viral neuropathies, quite rare diseases, involve autoimmune attack of the nervous system. The viral attacks are very prevalent events even though the induction of autoimmune disease is very rare. These viral neuropathies have a significant association with secondary infections (see discussion in (Westall and Root-Bernstein, 1986). The secondary infection would provide an adjuvant molecule, not provided by the virus.

Chlamydia pneumoniae has been linked to multiple sclerosis (Swanborg, Whittum-Hudson and Hudson, 2003; Stratton and Sriram, 2003). In fact a *Chlamydia pneumoniae*-specific peptide induces EAE in rats (Lenz et al., 2001). N-acetyl muramyl dipeptide is a component of the cell walls of many bacteria especially gram positive organisms. However, *Chlamydia* is an exception. It contains no muramic acid. Therefore even though *Chlamyida* contains an encephalitogenic immunogen, its infection of an animal results in no EAE. The investigators who are looking for MS immunogens should also search for MS adjuvants.

One area of therapeutic work has involved specific antigen suppression (Mozes, Sela and Tausig, 1974). This is accomplished by either injecting multiple large doses of a suspected immunogen, for example myelin basic protein, or knocking out specific cell lines which recognize a specific immunogen. Because of the mounting data supporting multiple immunogen involvement in MS this type of therapy appears ill advised. There is an added problem with attempting antigen suppression. MBP is a very effective therapeutic agent against EAE in guinea pigs, but it did not work in a MS trial. Is this because MBP is not the immunogen in MS? Or is it because the correct immunogen within MBP was not tested? Porcine MBP was used in the Salk/ Lilly MS trial (Salk et al, 1980). In guinea pigs the major encephalitogenic region is the tryptophan peptide. With the exception of an arginine for lysine, the sequence of this peptide does not vary among mammalian species. However the MBP encephalitogenic region in Lewis rat varies greatly among mammalian species. In fact porcine is only weakly active in Lewis rats. The Lewis rat encephalitogen is also active in monkeys. If the Lewis rat encephalitogen (the HEAE site) is the region active in humans, the Salk/Lilly experiment never tested the effectiveness of MBP as a therapeutic agent in MS (Table 15).One then would suggest that human MBP should be used, at least in a small initial trial. However, here again one could have a problem. In Lewis rats, Lewis rat MBP is a potent encephalitogen. However guinea pig MBP is much more powerful. It will not only suppress acute EAE but also hyperacute EAE. Rather than looking at specific immunogens or general immunosupressant, one should examine how these immunogens are produced. This work centers on the hormonal control systems involved in hydrolytic processes in the brain, gut and other sites in the human anatomy. Compounds could be produced to specifically alter the action of these hormonal controls systems. This virgin area would certainly have an excellent potential as a MS therapeutic tool.

Table 15. Suppression of Hyperacute EAE with Myelin Basic Protein in Lewis Rats

Challenge MBP [1]	Suppressor MBP in Saline[2]	Dose (ug) daily	Clinical6 Animals/ Group
Rat (35mg)	Rat	1500	0
		750	0
		500	1
		250	1
		125	5
	Guinea Pig	1500	0
		750	0
		375	1
		187	2
		94	4
	Bovine	2000	6
		1000	6
		500	6
		250	4
		125	6
	Rabbit	1000	6
		500	5
		250	6
		125	6
Bovine	Bovine	2000	0
		1000	0
		500	0
		250	0
		125	3
		0	6
Guinea Pig	Guinea Pig	2000	0
	Bovine	2000	6

[1] The basic proteins were prepared in saline, emulsified with CFA and injected intradermally into 10 week-old female Lewis rats as described in reference Lennon et al., 1977. *B. pertussis* vaccine (2 x1010 organisms) was injected subcutaneously.

[2] The suppressive dose was given daily IP from day 4-12 after challenge.

References

Adam, A., Deyys, M., Souvannavong, V., Lefrancier, P., Choay, J. and Lederer, E. (1976) Correlation of structure and adjuvant activity o fn-acetyl-muramyl-l-alanine-d-iosglutamine, its derivatives and analogues. *Biochem. Biophys. Res. Comm. 72*, 339-346.

Adam, A., Petit, J-F., Lefrancier, P. and Lederer, E. (1981) Muramyl dipeptides. *Mol. Cell. Biol. 41*, 27-47.

Akenami, F.O.T., Siren, V., Koshiniemi, M. Simes, M.A.,Teravainen, H., Vaheri, A.,(1996) Cerebrospinal fluid activity of tissue plasminogne activator in patients with neurological diseases. *J. Clin. Pathol. 49*, 577-580.

Alves-Leon, S.V., Batista, E., Papais-Alvarenga, R. and Quirico-Santos, T. (2001) Determination of soluble ICAM-1 and TNFalphaR in the cerebrospinal fluid and serum levels in a population of Brazilian patients with relapsing-remitting MS. *Arg. Neuro-Psiquiatr 59*, 1-7.

Amor, S., Baker, D., Groome, N. and Turk, J.L. (1993). Identification of a major encephalitogenic epitope of proteolipid protein for the induction of EAE in Biozzi AB/H and non-obese diabetic mice. *J. Immunol. 150*, 5666-5672.

Amor, S., Groome, N., Linington, C., et al. (1994). Identification of epitopes of myelin oligodendrocyte glycoprotein for the induction of EAE in SJL and Biozzi AB/H mice. *J. Immunol. 153*, 4339-56.

Andersson, P-B., Perry, V.H.and Gordon, S. (1992). The acute inflammatory response to liposaccharide in CNS parenchyma differs form that in other body tissues. *Neurosci. 48,* 169-186.

Back, U., Boch-Moeller, B. and Boeg-Hansen, T. C. (1976). Host resistance to liposaccharides in the pathogenesis of MS and Membranoproliferative glomerulonephritis. *Lancet II,* 188-191.

Bagnato, F., Durstandi, V., Finamore, L., Volante, G. and Millefiorini, E. (2003) Beta-2 microglobulin and neopterin as markers of disease activity in MS. *Neurol. Sci. 24*, S301-304.

Bannai, S., (1986). Exchange of cystine and glutamate across plasma membrane of human fibroblasts. *J.Biol.Chem. 261*, 2256-2263.

Bar-Or, A. Oiveira, E.M.L., Anderson, D.E and Hafler, D. (1999). Molecular pathogenesis in MS. *J. Neuroimmunol. 100*, 252-259.

Barton, M.A., McPherson, T.A., Lemieuex, R.U.and Bain, G.O. (1972). Allergic encephalomyelitis. *Can. J. Biochem. 50*, 689-96.

Beck, J., Rondot, P., Catinot. L., Falcoff, E., Kirchner, H. and Wietzerbin, J. (1988). Increased production of interferon gamma and tumor necrosis factor precedes clinical manifestation in MS: Do cytokines trigger off exacerbations? *Acta Neurol. Scand.78*, 318-323.

Berlet, H. (1986). Acid endopeptidase activty of human myelin elicited by using exogenous MBP as enzyme substrate. *FEBS 194*, 297-300.

Bernard, J.M., Gras-Masse, H., Drobeacq, H., Tartar, A., et al. (1987). Synthesis of conjugates between luteinizing hormone releasing hormone (LHRH) and MDP models of totally synthetic vaccines. *Int. Pept. Protein Res. 29*, 455-463.

Bernett, M.J., Blaber, S.I. Scarisbrick, IA, Dhanarajan, P., Thompson S.M. and Blaber, M. (2002). Crystal structure and biochemical characterization of human kallikrein 6 reveals a trypsin-like kallikrein is expressed in the CNS. *J. Biol. Chem 277*, 24562-70.

Bevilacqua, M.P., Pobver, J.S., Wheeler, M.E., et al., (1995). Interleukin 1 acts on cultured human vascular endothelium to increase the adhesion of polymorphonuclear leukocytes, monocytes and related leukocyte cell lines. *J. Clin. Invest 76*, 2003-2011.

Blaber, S.I., Scarisbrick, I.A., Bernett, M.J. et al. (2002). Enzymatic properties of rat myelencephalon-specific protease. *Biochem. 41*,1165-73.

Buljevac, D., Flach, H.Z., Hop, W.C.J., Hijdra D., Laman, J.D., et al. (2002) Prospective study on the relationship between infections and MS exacerbations. *Brain 125*, 952-960.

Carelli, C., Audibert, F., Gailard, J. and Chedid, L. (1982). Immunological castration of female mice by a totally synthetic vaccine administered in saline. *Proc.Natl.Acad. Sci, USA 79*, 5392-5395.

Chakrabarti, A.K., Banik, N.L., Lobo, D.C.,Terry, E.C. and Hogan E.L. (1993). Calcium-activated neutral proteinase (calpain) in rat brain during development compartmentation and role in myelination. *Brain Res. Dev. 71*, 107-13.

Chantry, A. and Glynn, P. (1990). A novel metalloproteinase originally isolated from brain myelin membranes is present in many tissues.*Biochem. J. 268*, 245-8.

Chao, L.P., Einstein, E.R. (1970) Localization of the active site through chemical modification of the encephalitogenic protein. *J.Biol. Chem. 245*, 6397-6403.

Chapman, B.E., Littlemore, L.T. and Moore, W.J. (1978). Conformation of myelin basic protein and its role in myelin formation. *Adv. Exp. Med. Biol. 100*, 207-220.

Chapman, B. E. and Moore, W. J. (1976). Conformation of myelin basic protein in aqueous solution from NMR spectroscopy. *Biochem. Biophys. Res. Comm. 73*, 758-766.

Chedid, L., Audibert, F. and Johnson, A.G. (1978). Biological activities of muramyl dipeptide, a synthetic glycopeptide analogous to bacterial immunoregulating agents. *Prog. Allergy, 1978*, 63-105.

Chedid, l., Audibert, F, Lefrancier, P., Choay, J. and Lederer, E. (1976). Modulation of the immune response by a synthetic adjuvant and analogs. *Proc. Natl. Acad. Sci., USA 73*, 2472-2475.

Correale, J., McMillan, M., Carthy, K.M.C., Le, T. and Weiner, L.P. (1995). Isolation and characterization of autoreactive proteolipid protein-peptide specific T cell-clones from MS patients. *Neurology 45*, 1370-8.

Cuzner,M.L., Gveric, D., Strand, C., Loughlin, A.J., Paemen, L., Opdenakker, G.and Newcombe, J. (1996). The expression of tissue type plasminogen activator, matrix metalloproteinases and endogenous inhibitors in the CNS in MS: comparison of stages in lesion evolution. *J. Neuropath. Exp. Neurol. 55*,1194-204

Dinarello, C.A. (1989). Interleukin-1 and its biologically related cytokines. In*: Advances in Immunology, Vol 44*, (pp153-205) New York, Academic Press.

Ellouz, F., Adam, A., Ciobaru, R. andLederer, E. (1974). Minimal structural requirements for adjuvant activity of bacterial peptidoglycan derivatives. *Biochem. Biophys. Res Comm. 59*, 1317-1325.

Endoh, M., Kunishita, T., Neihei, J., Nishizawa, M. and Tabira, T. (1990). Susceptibility to proteolipidaproprotein and its encephalitogenic determinants in mice. *Int. Arch. Allergy Appl. Immunol. 92*, 433-439.

Eylar, E.H., Brostoff, S., Jackson, J. and Carter, H. (1972). Allergic encephalomyelitis in monkeys induced by a peptide from the A1 protein. *Proc. Nat. Acad. Sci., USA 69*, 617-619.

Eylar, E.H., Caccam, J., Jackson, J.J., Westall, F.C. and Robinson, A.B. (1970). EAE: synthesis of disease-inducing site of basic protein. *Science 168*,1220-1223.

Eylar, E.H., Westall, F.C. and Brostoff, S. (1971) Allergic encephalomyelitis. *J. Biol. Chem, 256*, 34318-3424.

Felts, P.A., Woolston, A-M., Fernando, H.B., Asquith, S., Gregson, N.A., Mizzi, O.J.and Smith, K.J. (2005). Inflammation and primary demyelination induced by the intraspinal injection of lipopolysaccharide. *Brain 128*, 1649-1666.

Fermandjian, S., Perly, B., Level, M. and Lefrancier, P. (1987) A comparative 1H-NMR study of MDP and its analogue, muabutide: evidence for a structure involving two successive beta turns. *Carbohydrate Res. 162*, 23-32.

Filippi, M.and Rocca, M.A. (2005). MRI evidence for MS as a diffuse disease of the centralnervous system. *J. Neurol. 252*, Suppl 5, 16-24.

Frei, K., Fredrikson,S., Fontana,A.and Link, H. (1991). Interleukin-6 is elevated in plasma in MS. *J. Neuroimmunol. 31*, 147-153.

Freund, M., Stern, E.R. and Pisani, T.M. (1947). Isoallergic encephalomyelitis and radiculitis in guinea pigs after one injection of brain and *Mycobacteria* in water –in –oil emulsion. *J. Immunol. 57* 179-194.

Furlan R., Filippi, M., Bergami, A., Rocca, M.A., et al. (1999a) Peripheral levels of caspase-1 mRNA correlate with disease activity in patients with MS; a preliminary study. *J. Neruol. Neruosrug. Psychiatry 67,* 785-788.

Furlan, R., Martino, G., Galbiati, F., et al. (1999b). Caspase-1 regulates the inflammatory process leading to autoimmune demyelination. *J. Immunol. 163*, 2403-9.

Fujinami, R.S. and Oldstone, M.B. (1985). Amino acid homology between the encephalitogenic site of MBP and virus: mechanism for autoimmunity. *Science 230* 1043-1045.

Galboiz, Y.and Miller, A. (2002). Immunological indicators of disease activity and prognosis in MS. *Curr.Opin. Neurol. 15*, 233-237.

Giuliain, D., Lachman, L.B. (1985) Interleukin-1 stimulation of astroglial proliferation after brain injury. *Science 228*, 497-499.

Goldsmith, P.C. (2000). Neurological responses to elevated glutamate in the medial basal hypothalamus of the infant mouse. *J. Nutr. 130*, 1033S-1038S.

Goodwin, D.E., Rooney, W.D., Sloan, R., Bacchetti, P., et al. (1998). A serial study of new MS lesions and the white matter from which they arise. *Neurology 51*, 1689-97.

Gorenstein, C. and Sweet, J. E. (1985). Distribution of dipeptidyl peptidase. II In rat spinal cord. *Am J. Anat. 173*, 29-35.

Greer, J.M., Kuchroo, V.K., Sobel, R. A., and Lees, M.J. (1992) Identification and characterization of a second encephalitogenic determinant of myelin proteolipid protein. *J. Immunol. 149*, 783-8.

Griffen, C.M., Chard, D.T., Parker, G.J., Barker, G.J., Thompson, A.J. and Miller, D.H. (2002). The relationship between lesion and normal appearing brain tissue abnormalties in early relapsing remitting MS. *J .Neurol. 249*, 193-9.

Grynbaum, A. and Marks, N. (1976). Characterization of a rat brain catheptic carboxypeptidase inactivating angiotensin. II. *J. Neurochem 26*, 313-8.

Hagopian, A, Jackson, J.J., Carlo, D.J., Limjuco,G.A. and Eylar, E.H. (1975). Experimental allergic aspermatogenic orchitis. III. Isolation of spermatozoal glycoproteins and their role in allergic aspermatogenic orchitis. *J. Immunol. 115*, 1731-43.

Hartung, H-P., Reiners, K., Archelos, J.J., Michels, M. et al. (1995). Circulating adhesion molecules and tumor necrosis factor receptor in MS: correlation with magnetic resonance imaging. *Ann. Neurol. 38*, 186-193.

He, X-P, Shosaka, S. and Yoshida, S. (2001). Expression of neuropsin in oligodendrocytes after injury to the CNS. *Neurosci. Res. 39*, 455-62.

Hisahara, S., Okano, H. and Miura, M. (2003). Caspase-mediated oligodendrocyte cell death in the pathogenesis of autoimmune demyelination. *Neuro Sci. 46*, 387-97.

Hosmalin, A., Carelli, C., Gaillard, J., Lefrancier, P., Drobecq, H., Leclerc, C., Amar, O., Audibert, F. and Chedid, L. (1987). Structural requirements for the induction of "immunological castration" by linear monomeric LHRH-LYS-MDP administered in saline. *Clin. Immunol. Immunopath. 45*, 447-460.

Jahnke, U., Fisher, E.D. and Alvord, E.C., Jr. (1985). Sequence homology between certain viral proteins and proteins related to encephalomyelitis and neuritis. *Science 229*, 282-284.

Jansson, L., Olsson,T., Hojeberg, B. and Holdahl, R. (1991). Chronic EAE induced by the 89-101 MBP peptide in BIORIII(H-2r) mice. *Eur. J. Immunol. 21*, 693-9.

Johns, T. G., Kerlero de Rosbo, N., Menon, K., Abo, S., Gonzales, F. and Bernard, C. C. (1995). Demyelinating encephalomyelitis resembling MS after immunization with a peptide from myelin oligodendrocyte glycoprotein. *J. Immunol. 154*, 5536-5541.

Kabat, E.A., Wolf, A. and Bezer, A.F. (1947). The rapid production of acute disseminated encephalomyelitis in Rhesus monkeys by injection of heterologous and homologous brain tissue with adjuvants. *J. Exp. Med. 85*, 11-7.

Kanesaka,T., Mori, M., Hattori, T, Oki, T. and Kuwabara, S. (2006). Serum matrix metalloproteinase-3 levels correlate with disease activity in relapsing-remitting MS. *J. Neurol. Neurosurg. Psychiatry 77*, 185-188.

Karkhanis, Y.D., Carlo, D.J., Brostoff, S.W. and Eylar, E.H. (1975). Allergic encephalomyelitis. Isolation of an encephalitogenic peptide active in the monkey. *J. Biol.Chem. 250*,1718-1722.

Katz-Levy, Y., Neville, K.L., Girvin, A.M., Vanderlugt, C.L., Pope, J.G., Tan, L.J. and Miller, S.D. (1999). Endogenous presentation of self myelin epitopes by CNS-resistant APCs in Theiler's virus-infected mice. *J.Clin. Invest. 104*, 599-607.

Kerlero,de Rosbo, N. and Ben-Nun, A. (1996). Delineation of a minimal encephalitogenic epitope within the immunodominant region of myelin oligodendrocyte glycoprotein. *Eur. J. Immunol. 26*, 2470-9.

Kerero de Rosbo, N., Hoffman, M., Mendel, I., Yust, I., Kaye, J., Bakimer, R., Fletcher, S., et al. (1997). Predominance of the autoimmune response to myelin oligodendrocyte glycoprotein in MS: reactivity to the extracellular domain of MOG is directed against three main regions. *Eur. Immunol. 27*, 3059-3069.

Kerero de Rosbo, N., Kaye, J.F., Eisentein, M., Mendel, I., Hoeftberger, R., Lassmann , H., Milo, R. and Ben-Nun, A. (2004). The myelin-associated oligodendrocyte basic proein region MOBP 15-36: Encompasses the immunodominant major enephalitogenic epitope for SJL/J mice and predicted epitope for MS-associated HLA-DRB1. *J. Immunol. 173*, 1426-1435.

Kerero de Rosbo, N, Mendel, I. and Ben-Nun, A. (1995). Chronic relapsing EAE with a delayed and an atypical clinical course, induced in PL/J mice by MOG-derived peptide: preliminary analysis of MOG T cell epitopes. *Eur. J. Immunol. 25*, 985-93.

Kerero de Rosbo, N., Milo, R., Lees, M.B., Burger, D., Bernard, C.C.A. and Ben-Nun, A. (1993) Reactivity to myelin antigens in MS. *J. Clin Invest. 92*, 2602-2608.

Khanarian, G., Margeson, S.A., Moore, W.S., Pasaribu, S.J.and Westall, F.C., (1979). Effects of substitution of D-alanine for L-alanine on activity and conformation of an encephalitogenic peptide. *BBRC 87*, 236-243.

Khoury, S.J., Orav, E.J., Guttermann, C., Kikinis, R., Jolesz, F.A. and Weiner, H.L. (1999). Changes in serum levels of ICAM and TNF-R correlate with disease activity in MS. *Neurology 53*, 758-764.

Kies, M.W. (1965) Allergic encephalomyelitis. *Ann. N.Y. Acad. Sci. 122*, 161-169.

Kies, M.W. andAlvord, E.C., Jr. (1959) In: *Allergic encephalomyelitis*.(pp239-299) Springfield, Ill., Thomas..

Kivisakk, P., Matusevicius, D., He, B., Soderstrom, M., Fredrikson, S. and Link H. (1998). IL-15 mRNA expression is up-regulated in blood and cerebrospinal fluid mononuclear cells in MS. *Clin. Exp. Immunol. 111*, 193-197.

Kotani, S., Watanabe, Y., Shimono, T., Harada, K., et al. (1976). Correlation between the immunoadjuvant activities and pyrogenicities of synthetic N-acetyl muramyl peptides or -amino acids. *Biken J. 19*, 9-13.

Kouwenhoven, M., Ozenci, V., Tjernlund, A., Pashenhov, M., Homman, M., Press, R. and Link, H. (2002). Monocyte-derived dendritic cells express and secrete matrix-degrading metalloproteinases and their inhibitors and are imbalanced in MS. *J. Neuroimmunol. 126*, 161-171.

Lassmann, H., Bruck, W.and Lucchinetti, C.F. (2007). The immunopathology of MS: an overview. *Brain Pathol. 17*, 210-8.

Lassmann, H. and Wisniewski, H.M. (1979). Chronic relapsing EAE. *Arch. Neurol. 36*, 490-497.

Lee, J.M. and Schneider, H.A. (1962). Critical relationships between constituents of the antigen-adjuvant emulsion affecting EAE in a completely susceptible mouse genotype. *J. Exp. Med. 15*, 159-168.

Lee, M.A., Palace, J., Stabler,G., Ford, J., Gearing,A. and Miller, K. (1999). Serum gelatinase B, TIMP-1 and TIMP-2 levels in MS. A longitudinal clinical and MRI study. *Brain 122*, 191-197.

Lehtonen, l., Eerola, E., Oksman, P. and Toivanen P. (1995). Muramic acid in peripheral blood leukocytes of healthy human subjects. *J. Infect. Dis. 171*, 1060-4.

Lehtonen, L., Eerola, E. and Toivanen, P. (1997). Muramic acid in human peripheral blood leucocytes in different age groups. *Eur. J. Clin. Invest. 27*, 791-92.

Lennon, V.A., Westall, F.C., Thompson, M. and Ward, E. (1976). Antigen, host and adjvant requirements for induction of hyperacute EAE. *Eur. J. Immunol. 6*, 805-810.

Lenz, D. C., Lu, L., Conant, S.B., et al. (2001). A *Chlamydia pneumoniae*-specific peptide induces EAE in rats. *J. Immunol. 167*, 1803-1808.

Leppert, D., Ford, J., Stabler, G., Grygar, C., et al. (1998). Matrix metalloproteinase-9 is selectively elevated in CSF during relapses and stable phases of MS. *Brain 121*, 2327-2334.

Levine, S. and Wenk, E. J. (1964). Allergic encephalomyelitis: a hyperacute form. *Science 146*, 1681-1682.

Levine, S. and Wenk, E.J. (1965). A hyperacute form of allergic encephalomyelitis. *Amer. J. Path. 47*, 61-88.

Levine, S. (1974). Hyperacute, neurophilic and localized forms of EAE: a review. *Acta Neuropath. 28*, 174-189.

Li, Z., and Banik, N.L. (1995). The localization of m-calpain in myelin immuno-cykotchemical evidence in different areas of rat brain and nerves. *Brain Res. 697*, 112-21.

Linington, C., Berger, T., Perry, L., Weerth, S., Hinze-Selch, D., Zwang, Y., Lu, H-C. Lassmann, H. and Wekerke, H. (1993). T cells specific for the myelin oligodendrocyte glycoprotein mediate an unusual autoimmune inflammatory response in the CNS. *Eur. J. Immunol. 23*, 1364-72.

McAlpine, D., Lumsden, C.E. and Acheson, E.D. (1972). In: *Multiple Sclerosis. A reappraisal.* (pp 8-32) Edinburgh Churchill, Livingstone.

Maeda, K., Koga, T., Sakamoto, S., Onoue, K.,Kotani, S., Kusumoto, S., Shiba, T. and Sumiyoshi, A. (1980). Structural requirements of synthetic n-acetylmuramyl dipeptides for induction of EAE in the rat. *Microbiol. Immunol. 24*, 771-776.

Mahad, D, Lawry, J., Howell, S.J.L., and Woodroofe, M.N. (2003). Longitudinal study of chemokine receptor expression on peripheral lymphocytes in MS: CXCR3 upregulation is associated with relapse. *Mult. Scler. 9*, 189-198.

Maimone, D., Gregory, S., Arnason, B. G. and Reder, A.T. (1991). Cytokine levels in the cerebrospinal fluid and serum of patients with MS. *J. Neuroimmunol., 32*, 67-74.

Malmestrom, C., Andersson, B.A., Haghighi, S. and Lycke, J. (2006). IL-6 and CCL2 levels in CSF are associated with the clinical course of MS: Implications for their possible immunopathogenic roles. *J. Neurommunol. 175*,176-182

Manabe,S., Gu, Z. and Lipton, S.A. (2005). Activation of matrix metalloproteinase-9: Neuronal nitric oxide synthase contributes to NMDA-induced retinal ganglion cell death. *Invest. Opthal. Vis. Sci. 46*, 4747-4753.

Martin, S.A., Karnovsky, M.L., Kruger, J.M., Pappenheimer, J.R. and Nieman, K. (1984). Peptiodoglycan as promoters of slow wave sleep. I. Structure of the sleep-promoting factor isolated from human urine. *J. Biol. Chem. 259*, 12652-8.

Matsuda, M., Tsukada, N., Miyagi, K. and Yanagisawa, N. (1995). Increased levels of soluble vascular cell adhesion molecule-1 (VCAM-1) in the cerebrospinal fluid and serum of patients with MS and human T lymphotrophic virus type-1-associated myelopathy. *J. Neuroimmunol 59*, 35-40.

Matsuo, A., Lee, G.C., Terai, K, Takami, K., Hickey, W.F., McGeer, E.G.and Geer, P.L.(1997). Unmasking of an unusual myelin basic protein epitope during the process of myelin degeneration in humans. *Am. J. Path. 150*, 1253-1266.

Mendel, I, Kerero de Rosbo, N. and Ben-Nun, A. (1995). A myelin oligodendrocyte glycoprotein peptide induces typical chronic EAE in H2b mice: fine specificity and T-cell receptor V beta expression of encephalitogenic cells. *J. Eur. Immunol. 25*, 1951-1959.

Mendz, G.L. and Moore, W.J. (1983). NMR studies of MBP. X. Conformation of a determinant encephalitogenic in the rabbit. *Biochim. Biophys. Acta 748*, 176-83.

Mendz, G.L., Moore, W.J. and Carnegie, P.R. (1982). Proton NMR evidence for secondary and tertiary structure in myelin basic protein. *Biochem. Biophys. Res. Comm. 105*, 1333-40.

Migliore-Samour, D. and Jolles, P. (1973). Hydrosoluble adjuvant active mycobacterial fractions of low molecular weight. *FEBS Lett. 36*, 317-21.

Moore, W.J., Chapman, B.E., James, G.E., Khanarian, G., Margetson, S.A., Pasaaribu, S.J. and Westall, F.C. (1981). Conformation of encephalitogenic proteins and peptides. *Excerta Medica No. 546*, 198-211.

Moreira, M.A., Souza, A.L.S., Lana-Peixoto, M.A., Teixeira, M.M. and Teixeira, A.L. (2006). Chemokines in he cerebrospinal fluid of patients with active and stable relapsing-remitting MS. *Braz. J. Med. Biol. Res. 39*, 441-445.

Morgan, I.M. (1947). Allergic encephalomyelitis in monkeys in response to injection of normal monkey nervous tissue. *J.Exp. Med. 85*, 131-35.

Mostert J.P., Ramsaransing, S.M., Heersema, D.J., Heerings, M., Wilczak N. and De Keyer, J. (2005). *J. Neurol. Sci. 231*, 41-44.

Mozes, E., Sela,M. and Tausig, M.J. (1974). Tolerance to thymus-independent antigens. *Immunology 27*, 641-646.

Nagae, A., Deddish, P.A., Becker, R.P., et al. (1992).Carboxypeptidase M in brain and peripheral nerves. *J. Neurochem. 59*, 2201-12.

Nagai, Y., Akiyama, K., Suzuki, K., Kotani, S., Watanabe, Y., Shimono, T., Shiba, T., Kusumota, S., Ikuta, F. and Takeda, S. (1978a). Minimum structural requirements for encephalitogen and for adjuvant in the induction of EAE. *Cell. Immunol. 35*, 158-167.

Nagai, Y., Akiyam, K., Kotani, S., Watanabe, Y., Shimono, T., Shiba, T. and Kusmoto, S. (1978b). Structural specificity of synthetic peptide adjuvant for induction of EAE. Cell *Immunol. 35*, 168-172.

Oh, L.Y.S., Larsen, P.H., Krekoski, C.A., Edwards, D.R., Donovan, F., Werb, Z, et al. (1999). Matrix metalloproteinase-9/gelatinase B is required for process outgrowth by oligodendrocytes. *J. Neurosci. 1*, 8464-75.

Onodera,H., Nakashima, I., Fujihara, K., Nagata,T. and Itoyama, Y. (1999). Elevated plasma level of plasminogen activator inhibitor-1 (PAI-1) in patients with relapsing-remitting MS. *Tohoko J. Exp. Med. 189*, 259-265.

Paeman,L., Olsson, T., Soderstrom, M. Van Damme, J. and Opdenakker, G. (1993). Evaluation of gelatinases and IL-6 in the cerebrospinal fluid of patients with optic neuritis, multiple sclerosis and other inflammatory neurological diseases. *Eur. J. Neurol. 1*, 55-63.

Panitech, H. and Ciccone, C. (1981). Induction of recurrent EAE with myelin basic protein. *Ann. Neurol. 9*, 433-438.

Penkowa, M, Espejo, C., Ortega-Aznar, A., Hidalgo, J., Montalban, X and Martinez-Caceres, E.M. (2003). Metallothionen expression in the CNS of MS patients. *CMLS Cell Mol Life Sci 60*, 1258-66.

Perry, L.L., Barzaga-Gilbert, E. and Trotter, J.L. (1991). T cell sensitization to proteolipid protein in myelin basic protein-induced relapsing EAE. *J. Neuroimmunol. 33*, 7-15.

Prat, A., Biernacki, K., Saroli, T., Orav, J. E. et al. (2005). Kinin B1 receptor expression on MS mononuclear cells. *Arch. Neurol. 62,* 795-800.

Price, W.S., Mendz, G.L. and Martenson, R.E. (1988). Conformation of a heptadecapeptide comprising the segment encephalitogenic in Rheus monkey. *Biochemistry 27*, 8990-8999.

Raine, C.S. and Stone, S.H. (1977). Animal model for MS: chronic EAE in inbred guinea pigs. *N.Y. State J. Med. 77*, 1693-1697.

Raine, C.S. and Traugott, U. (1982). The pathogenesis and therapy of MS is based upon the requirement of a combination of myelin antigens for autoimmune demyelination. *J. Neuroimmunol. 2*, 83-91.

Rieckmann, P., Albrecht, M., Kitze, B., Weber, T., et al. (1995). Tumor necrosis factor alpha messenger RNA expression in patients with relapsing-remitting MS is associated with disease activity. *Ann Neurol. 37*, 82-88.

Roboz-Einstein, E., Robertson, D.M., DiCaprio, J. and Moore W. (1962). The isolation from bovine spinal cord of a homologous protein with encephalitogenic activity. *J. Neurochem. 9*, 353-361.

Root-Bernstein, R.S. and Westall, F.C. (1990). Serotonin binding sites II. *Brain Res. Bull. 25*, 826-41.

Root-Bernstein, R. S. and Westall, F.C. (1986). Clinical suppression of EAE by muramyl dipeptide "adjuvant". *Brain Res. Bull. 17*, 473-476.

Root-Bernstein, R.S. and Westall, F.C. (1983). Do muramyl peptides activate serotonin binding sites? *Lancet I*, 653.

Rosenberg, G.A., Dencoff, J.E., Correa, N. Jr., Beiners, M. and Ford, C.C. (1996). Effect of steroids on CSF matrix metalloproteinases in MS: relation to blood-brain barrier injury. *Neurology 46*, 1626-32.

Sakai, K., Zamvil, S. S., Mitchell, D.J., Lim, M., Rothbard, J.B. and Steinman, L. (1988). Characterization of a major encephalitogenic T cell epitope in SJL/J mice with synthetic oligopeptides of myelin basic protein. *J. Neuroimmunol. 19*, 21-32.

Salk, J., Romine, J.S., Westall, F.C. and Wiederholt, W.C. (1980). Myelin basic protein studies in EAE and MS. A summary with theoretical considerations of multiple sclerosis etiology. Davison, A.N. and Cuzner, M.C. eds. In: *Proceedings of the Liversedge MS Society Symposium on the Suppression* of *MS and EAE.* (pp 141-153) London, Academic Press. London.

Sasaki, Y. (1974). Studies on encephalitogenic fragments of myelin basic protein. III. Synthesis of H-Arg-Phe-Trp-Gly-Ala-Glu-Gly-Asn-Arg-OH as an analog of encephalitogenic decapeptide. *Chem Pharm. Bull. 22*, 2199-2191.

Scarisbrick, I.A., Asakura, K., Blader, S., et al. (2000). Preferred expression of myelencephalon-specific protease by oligodendrocytes of the adult rat spinal cord white matter. *Glia 30*, 219-30.

Scarisbrick, I.A.,Isackson, P.J., Ciric, B., Windebank, A.J. and Rodriquez, M. (2001). MSP—a trypsin-like serine protease is abundantly expressed in the human nervous system. *J.Comp. Neurol. 431*, 347-61.

Schaecher, K.E., Shield, D.C. and Banik, N.L. (2001). Mechanism of myelin breakdown in experimental demyelination: a putative role for calpain. *Neurochem. Res. 26*, 731-7.

Schrijver, I.A., van Meurs, M., Melief, M-J., Ang, C.W., et al. (2001). Bacterial peptidoglycan and immune reactivity in the central nervous system in MS. *Brain 124*, 1544-1554.

Seifert T., Kieseier, B.C., Ropele, S., Strasser-Fuchs, S., Ouehenberger, F., Fazekas, F. and Hartung, H-P. (2002). TACE mRNA expression in peripheral mononuclear cells precedes new lesions on MRI in MS. *Mult. Scler. 8*, 447-451.

Shapira, R., Chou, F.C-H., McKneally, S., Uraban, E. and Kibler, R.F. (1971). Biological activity and synthesis of an enephalitogenic determinant. *Science 172*, 736-738.

Shaw, C.M., Alvord, E.C., Jr., Fahlberg, W.J., Jr. and Kies W.W. (1962). Adjuvant-antigen relationships in the production of EAE in the guinea pig. *J. Exp. Med. 115*, 169-179.

Shibata, M., Hisahara, S., Hara, H., et al. (2000). Caspases determine the vulnerability fo oligodendrocytes in the ischemic brain. *J. Clin Invest. 106*, 643-53.

Shields, D.C. and Banik, N.L. (1998). Upregulation of calpain activity and expression in EAE: a putative role for calpain in demyelination. *Brain Res. 794*, 68-74.

Sibley, W.A., Bamford, C.R. and Clark, K. (1985). Clinical viral infections and MS. *Lancet I*, 1313-1315.

Silver, N. C., Tofts, P.S., Symms, M.R., Barker, G.J., Thompson, A.J. and Miller, D.H. (2001). Quantitative contrast-enhanced magnetic resonance imaging to evaluate blood-brain barrier integrity in MS: a preliminary study. *Mult. Scler. 7*, 75-82.

Simon, J. and Anzil, A.P. (1974). Immunohistological evidence of perivascular localization of basic protein in early development of EAE. *Acta Neuopath (Berl.) 27*, 33-42.

Smeltz, R.B., Wolf, N.A. and Swanborg, R.H. (1998). Delineation of two encephalitogenic myelin basic protein epitopes for DA rats. *J. Neuroimmunol. 87*, 43-48.

Snyder, D.S., Simonis, S., Uzman, B.G. and Whitaker, J.N.(1985). Rat neural tissue cathepsin D: ultrastructural immunocytochemistry. *J. Neurocytol. 14*, 579-96.

Stebbins, J.W., Jaffe, H. and Moeller, J.R. (1998). Characterization of myelin-associated glycoprotein proteolysis in the human CNS. *Neurochem Res. 23*, 1005-10.

Stover, J.F., Pleines, U.E., Morgan-Kossmann, M.C., Lowitzsch, K. and Kempski, O.S. (1997). Neurotransmitters in cerebrospinal fluid reflect pathological activity. *Eur. J. Clin. Invest. 27*, 1038-1043.

Stratton, C.W. and Sriram, S. (2003). Association of *Chlamydia pneumoniae* with CNS disease. *Microbe Infect. 5*, 1249-1253.

Suzuki, K., Sasaki, Y. (1974). Studies on encephalitogen fragments of myelin basic protein. IV. Synthesis of glycine analogs of tryptophan containing fragments. *Chem. Pharm. Bull. 22*, 2181-2187.

Swanborg, R.H., Whittum-Hudson, J.A. and Hudson, A.P. (2003). Infectious agents of MS. *J. Neuroimmunol. 136*, 1-8.

Tejada-Simon, M.V., Zang, Y.C., Yang, D., Hong, J., Li, S., Singh, R.A. et al. (2000). Aberrant T cell responses to myelin antigens during clinical exacerbation in patients with MS. *Int. Immunol. 12*, 1641-50.

Tomizawa, K., He, X-P, Yamanaka, H., Shiosaka, S. and Yoshida, S. (1999). Injury inuces neuropsin mRNA in the CNS. *Brain Res. 824*, 308-11.

Toullet, F., Audibert, F., Voisin, G.A. and Chedid, L. (1977). Production d'orchiepididymite aspermatogenique autoimmune chez le cobaye, a l'aide de differents adjuvants hydrosolubles. *Ann Immunol. (Inst Pasteur) 128C*, 267-269.

Trotter, J.L., Perfrey, C.M., Trotter, A.L., Selvidge, J.A., Gushleff, K.C. and Mohanakumaar, T. (1998). T. cell recognition of myelin proteolipid protein and myelin proteolipid protein peptides in the peripheral blood of MS and control subjects. *J. Neuroimmunol 84*, 172-8.

Tuohy, V.K., Lu., Z., Sobel, R.A., Laursen, R.A. and Lees, M.B. (1989). Identification of an encephalitogenic determinant of myelin proteolipid protein from SJl mice. *J. Immunol.142*, 1523-1532.

Tuohy, V.K., Sobel, R.A. and Lees, M.B. (1988). Myelin proteolipid protein induced EAE. Variations of disease expression in defferent mice strains. *J. Immunol. 140*, 1868-73.

Ufret-Vincenty, R. I., Quigley. L, Tresser, N., Pak, S. H.,Gado, A.,Hausm N, S., Wucherpfennig, K.W. and Brocke, S. (1998). In vivo survival of viral antigen specific T cells that induce EAE. *J. Exp. Med. 188*, 1725-1737.

van Boxel-Dezaire, A H.H., Hoff, S.C.J., van Oosten, B.W., Verweij, C.L., et al.(1999). Decreaed Interleukin-10 and Increased Interleukin-12p40 mRNA are associated with Disease activity and characterize different disease stages in MS. *Ann Neurol. 45*, 695-703.

Waksman, B.J., Adams, R.D. and Mansmann, H.C., Jr. (1957). Experimental study of diphtheritic polymeutitis in the rabbit and guinea pig. Immunologic and histologic observations. *J. Exp. Med 105*, 591-614.

Waubert, E., Goodkin, D.E., Gee, L., Bacchetti, P., Sloan, R., et al. (1999). Serum MMP-9 and TIMP-1 levels are related to MRI activity in relapsing MS. *Neurology 53*, 1397-1401.

Werner, P., Pitt, D. and Raine, C.S.(2001). MS: altered glutamate hetrostasis in lesions correlates with oligodendrocyte and axonal damage. *Ann. Neurol. 50*, 169-180.

Westall, F.C. (2006a). Molecular mimicry revisited: Gut bacteria and multiple sclerosis. *J. Clin. Microbiol. 44*, 2099-2105.

Westall, F.C. (2006b). Histoclinical variation in MS: heterogeneous proteolytic immunogenic processing. *Med. Hypoth. 66*, 566-569.

Westall, F.C. (2007). Abnormal hormonal control of gut hydrolytic enzymes causes autoimmune attack on the CNS by production of immune-mimic and adjuvant molecules: a comprehensive explanation for the induction of MS. *Med. Hypoth. 68,* 364-368.

Westall, F.C. (1977). Hyperacute allergic encephalomyelitis: a single determinant. *Immunol.Comm. 6*, 227-237.

Westall, F.C. (1978). High dose inhibition of the tryptophan peptide induced encephalitogenicity. *Immunol. Comm. 7*, 57-67.

Westall, F.C. (1974). Released myelin basic protein: the immunogenic factor? *Immunochem. 11,* 513-515.

Westall, F.C. (1972). Solid phase peptide synthesis as applied to EAE. Field, E.J., Bell. T.M. and Carnegie, P.R., eds. *In Multiple Sclerosis: Progress in Research.* (pp72-79).Amsterdam, North-Holland, Amsterdam.

Westall, F.C., Hawkins, A., Ellison, G.W. and Myers, L.W. (1980). Abnormal glutamic acid metabolism in MS. *J. Neurol. Sci. 47*, 353-364.

Westall, F.C., Robinson, A.B., ,Caccam, J., Jackson, J. and Eylar, E.H. (1971). Essential chemical requirements for induction of allergic encephalomyelitis. *Nature 229*, 22-24.

Westall, F.C. and Root-Bernstein, R.S. (1986). Cause and prevention of post-infectious and post-vaccinal neuropathies in light of a new theory of autoimmunity. *Lancet II*, 251-253.

Westall, F.C. and Thompson, M. (1977a). Encephalitogenic region for the Lewis rat within the myelin basic protein. *Immunol. Comm. 6*, 13-21.

Westall, F.C. and Thompson, M. (1977b). Further definition of the encephalitogenic region for guinea pigs. *Immunol. Comm. 6*, 23-27.

Westall, F.C. and Thompson, M. (1978). An encephalitogenic region in rabbits. *Immunochem. 15*, 189-191.

Westall, F. C., Thompson, M. and Lennon, V.A. (1977). Hyperacute autoimmune encephalomyelitis induced by a synthetic autoantigen. *Nature 269*, 425-427.

Westall, F.C., Thompson, M., Migliore-Samour, D. and Jolles, P. (1975). Induction of allergic encephalomyelitis using hydrosoluble mycobacterial fractions. *Eur. J. Immunol. 5*, 504-505.

Westall, F.C., Thompson, M., Migliore-Samour, D. and Jolles, P. (1974). Induction of EAE using hydrosoluble adjuvants and the enephalitogenic tryptophan peptide. *Immunol. Comm. 4*, 353-9.

Whitaker, J.N. (1997). Myelin encephalitogenic protein fragments in CSF of persons with MS. *Neurology 27*, 911-20.

Wong, A. and Toth, I. (2001). Lipid, sugar and lipopolysaccharides based delivery systems. *Curr. Med. Chem. 8*, 1123-36.

Wucherpfennig, K.W. and Strominger, J.L. (1995). Molecular mimicry in T cell mediated auatoimmunity: viral peptides activate human T cell clones specific for MBP. *Cell 80*, 695-705.

Yamanaka, H. He, X-P, Matsumoto, K., Shiosak, S. and Yoshida, S. (1999). Protease M/neurosin mRNA is expressed in mature oligodendrocytes. *Mol. Brain Res. 71*, 217-24.

Xaio, H., Banks, W. A., Niehoff, M. L. and Morley, J.E. (2001). Effects of LPS on the permeability of the blood-brain barrier to insulin. *Brain Research 896*, 36-42.

Young, J.D., Tsuchiya, D., Geier, M., Geier, S., Westall, F.C., Thompson, M., Cyr, R., Ward, E. and Yurochko, F. (1974). The encephalitogenic dose-response in guinea pigs of the tryptophan region of myelin basic protein. *Immunol.Comm. 3*, 219-226.

Zamvil, S.S., Mitchell, D.J., Moore, A.C., Kitamura, K., Steinman, L. and Rothbars, J.B. (1986). T-cell epitope of the autoantigen myelin basic protein that induces encephalomyelitis. *Nature 324*, 58-67.

In: Autoimmunity: Role, Regulation and Disorders
Editor: Fynn L. Vogel and L. F. Zimmermann

ISBN 978-1-60456-833-2

Chapter 6

Potential Role of an Abnormal Proliferative, Reparative Response in Initiation and Maintenance of Sjögren's Syndrome, and the Beneficial Effects of Green Tea Polyphenols

Douglas Dickinson, Kevin Gillespie, Isamu Kodani, Amy Camba and Stephen Hsu*

School of Dentistry
Medical College of Georgia
Augusta, GA. USA

Abstract

Sjogren's syndrome (SS), one of the major autoimmune disorders, causes destruction of the salivary and lacrimal glands, leading to dry mouth and dry eyes and subsequent clinical complications. SS is also associated with rheumatic disorders such as rheumatoid arthritis. Green tea polyphenols (GTPs), a complex mixture of substances, exerts anti-inflammatory and anti-apoptotic properties, which may protect tissues from--or at least delay--the onset of auto-immune disorders. We discovered that EGCG, the most potent of the GTPs, is able to suppress epithelial expression of autoantigens. The non-obese diabetic (NOD) mouse is a model for autoimmune insulin-dependent diabetes and SS-like disease. Previously, we showed that NOD mice fed with GTPs had lowered serum autoantibody levels and decreased submandibular gland lymphocyte infiltration. EGCG has the same effect. In NOD mice, cells in lymphocyte-infiltrated areas had an elevated apototic index in comparison to the epithelium in BALB/c control mice. In NOD mice fed with EGCG, apoptosis in infiltrated areas was reduced to BALB/c levels. However, in the non-infiltrated glandular epithelium of NOD mice, apoptosis was only

* Address for correspondence: Stephen Hsu, AD1443 Department of Oral Biology, School of Dentistry, Medical College of Georgia, 1120, 15th Street, Augusta, GA 30912. USA

modestly higher than in BALB/c, and the levels were not affected by EGCG. Remarkably, in the glandular epithelium of NOD mice fed with water, there was a significant increase in expression of the proliferation markers PCNA (an autoantigen) and Ki67. In contrast, expression in EGCG-fed animals was similar to BALB/c. Proteomic profiling of acinar cell proteins demonstrated alterations in NOD mice as compared to BALB/c that could in part be changed to the BALB/c expression pattern by dietary EGCG.

Our observations are consistent with a model for SS in which early lymphocyte – independent acinar cell abberations, detectable at the protein level, preceed and prime subsequent autoimmune reactions. The elevated proliferation observed in the glandular epithelium suggests an abnormal reparative response. A subsequent autoimmune attack on the acinar cells could amplify the priming signal by activation of apoptosis and autoantigen expression in infiltrates. One possible mechanism of induction is that acinar cells cannot integrate conflicting intrinsic pro-differentiation and abberant proliferation signals, leading to cell death as the default state. The beneficial effects of GTPs/EGCG likely result from their known pro-differentiation and anti-proliferation properties preventing otherwise undamaged cells from entering the default state. Complementary and alternative approaches such as green tea polyphenols could protect secretory glands from autoimmune-induced tissue destruction, and early detection of autoimmune risk for disease might be possible by examination of protein markers in saliva and serum.

Introduction

Sjogren's syndrome (SS), one of the most common human autoimmune disorders, is characterized by loss of secretory function of the salivary and lacrimal glands in association with lymphocytic infiltration of the tissues. (reviewed in Fox and Kang 1992; Fox 2005; Fox 2007; Delaleu *et al.* 2005). Other tissues can also be affected (Fox, 2005; Kassan and Moutsopoulos 2004; Tapinos *et al.* 1999). Secondary Sjogren's syndrome involves glandular dysfunction in association with a connective tissue autoimmune disease such as systemic lupus erythmatosus. The decrease in glandular secretions leads to xerostomia (dry mouth) and xeropthalmia (dry eyes). Clinically, this is associated with a significant decline in oral and ocular health, considerable discomfort for the patient, and a decline in the quality of life (Fox and Kang 1992; Fox 2005; Kassan and Moutsopoulos 2004). Serious health consequences can result from involvement of other tissues, such as the lungs (Fox, 2005).

The pathophysiology of SS, which most likely involves environmental triggers in genetically susceptible individuals, is not fully understood (reviewed in Delaleu et al. 2005; Fox 2005; Garcia-Carrasco *et al.* 2006; Hsu and Dickinson, 2006). Here, we outline recent developments in our understanding of SS, and propose a role for an abnormal, proliferative, reparative response of the glandular epithelium in initiation and maintenance of the disease, and summarize data suggesting a beneficial role for green tea polyphenols in modulation of the pathology.

Inflammation and Apoptosis in SS

Diagnostically, in addition to the subjective feeling of dry eyes and/or dry mouth, histopathological screening of biopsied labial minor salivary glands typically shows large local periductal and perivascular lymphocytic infiltration of the glandular tissue (Fox 2005). Similar infiltrations are found in major salivary and lacrimal glands. The lymphocytes are mainly interferon-γ producing CD4+ T cells, with lower proportions of B cells, macrophages and natural killer cells (reviewed in Daniels and Fox 1992; Kassan and Moutsopoulos 2004). Onset of clinical symptoms in SS patients correlates with the production of various autoantibodies by B lymphocytes, including those in the gland infiltrates (Fox and Kang 1992; Fox and Speight 1996). Some autoantibodies are non-organ specific, such as anti-SSA/Ro and anti-SSB/La, while others are specific, such as anti-type 3 muscarinic acetylcholine receptor antibody. (Delaleu et al 2005; Gao *et al.* 2005; Ramos-Casals and Font 2005).

Previously, it was thought that SS was the result of an aberrant, destructive immune system attack against the normal exocrine epithelium. Certainly, the inflammatory infiltrates replace epithelial tissue, and in some patients there can be extensive fibrosis (Andoh *et al.* 1993; Daniels and Fox 1992; Fox and Kang, 1992; Fox and Speight, 1996). In this classical model, this loss of apparently normal secretory epithelia, presumably by apoptosis, results in the decrease of saliva or tear production (reviewed in Dawson *et al.* 2006; Fox and Speight 1996; Garcia-Carrasco *et al.* 2006; Manganelli et al 1997; Manganelli and Fietta 1997; Ramos-Casals and Font, 2005). More recently, the role of acinar cell death in loss of secretory function has come into question. First, there is discordance between the amount of lymphocytic infiltration, loss of acinar tissue and reduction of fluid production (Bloch *et al.* 1965; Dawson *et al.* 2000, 2005, 2006; Fox and Kang, 1992; Fox and Maruyama 1997; Greenspan *et al.* 1974; Jonsson *et al.* 1993; Manganelli et al 1997). Most individuals with secretory hypofunction and significant infiltration still retain relatively large amounts of normal-appearing acini, while other individuals may have marked loss of salivary function despite relatively low infiltration and loss of acini. Second, there is a 'normal' age-related decline in the acinar cell volume that does not typically produce SS-like dryness (Kikuchi *et al.* 2004). Third, labial gland acinar cells from SS patients can still secrete, but they show a marked decrease in sensitivity to acetylcholine stimulation, suggesting the residual acinar tissue is dysfunctional (Dawson *et al.* 2001).

In addition to these observations, the relationship between apoptosis and loss of secretion has become less clear. Several studies have reported an elevation in apoptosis of epithelial cells in SS salivary glands, in contrast to minimal apoptosis in normal glands (e.g., Polihronis *et al.* 1998, reviewed in Manganelli and Fietta, 2003). However, the range in acinar apoptotic frequencies reported in these studies (from "a few" to 37%) is very high, and even higher for ductal epithelium (Ohlsson *et al.* 2001). Two candidate mechanisms of induction of apoptotic cell death in acinar cells are binding of FasL (produced by T lymphocytes or epithelial cells) to Fas, and release of perforin and granzyme B by cytotoxic T lymphocytes. Consistent with a role for apoptosis in SS, a number of studies have reported dysregulation of expression of several apoptotis-related molecules, including Fas/FasL, in salivary glands of SS patients (reviewed in Ramos-Casals and Font, 2005; Manganelli and Fietta, 2003). Further, perforin-expressing cytotoxic $CD4^+$ T cells are present in SS labial glands (Xanthou *et al.* 1999). However, a study by Ohlsson *et al.* (2001) of apoptosis in labial gland biopsies of SS patients found minimal levels of apoptosis in acinar and ductal epithelium, and they suggested that the high levels of apotosis observed in other studies could, in part, be due to technical issues with the terminal deoxynucleotidyl transferase mediated dUTP-digoxygenin nick end labeling (TUNEL) method used. In addition, they raised the possibility that the observed increased levels of Fas and FasL in SS epithelial tissue might in fact be due to infiltrating T cells that are hard to distinguish based solely on morphology.

The Non-Obese Diabetic (NOD) Mouse Model for SS

Further insight into the pathophysiology of SS has come from animal models, particularly the NOD mouse, which is considered to be one of the best models for the human disease (Cha *et al.* 2002; Jonsson *et al.* 2007; van Blokland and Versnel 2002). Generation of congenic strains of mice carrying various alleles from the NOD background has allowed various aspects of the glandular exocrinopathy to be dissected. Focal lymphocytic infiltrations that resemble those of human SS occur in the submandibular gland at about 8 weeks of age. As in humans, there is a dysregulation of expression of apoptosis-related molecules, but an uncertain role for apoptosis in the pathogenesis of the exocrinopathy (Kong *et al.* 1998; Masago *et al.* 2001; Qi *et al.* 2007; van Blokland *et al.* 2003). Significantly, there is also a severe impairment of secretory function that does not correlate with the more modest degree of acinar cell loss or degree of inflammation (Jonsson *et al.* 2006; Rosignoli *et al.* 2005). Importantly, NOD.*scid* mice that lack a functional immune system still show characteristic abnormalities in their salivary protein profile, and loss of acinar cells in the submandibular gland despite the absence of a lymphocytic infiltrate (Robinson *et al.* 1996; Humphreys-Beher and Peck, 1999). NOD.Igμ^{null} mice that lack functional B lymphocytes still develop submandibular T-cell infiltrates, but fail to develop a loss of secretory function (Robinson *et al.* 1998). Further, infusion of purified IgG from NOD mice or human primary SS patients can partially block stimulated secretion, likely through interaction with muscarinic receptors. These observations are consistent with a two-stage model in which an initial genetically determined lymphocyte-independent abnormality in the homeostasis of the exocrine tissue, associated with apoptosis (Kong *et al.* 1998), triggers a subsequent self-sustaining immune response, and autoantibodies suppress the functionality of seemingly intact acinar cells (Kong *et al.* 1998; Humphreys-Beher and Peck, 1999; Humphreys-Beher *et al.* 1998; 1999a,b).

The Non-Apoptotic Model for SS

Observations in SS patients and animal models have led to a 'non-apoptotic' model for SS, in which glandular hypofunction occurs as a result of immune-mediated inhibition of acinar cell function, and glandular atrophy is a consequence, rather than a cause, of loss of function (Dawson *et al.* 2006; Humphreys-Beyer *et al.* 1999a,b; Ramos-Casals and Font 2005). In this model, environmental factors, such as a viral infection, act in conjunction with a predisposing genetic background to initiate the disease by expression of proinflammatory cytokines and autoantigens, perhaps due to aberrant processing or accumulation on the surface of apoptotic cells (reviewed in Delaleu *et al.* 2005; Fox and Speight 1996; Fox 2005; Garcia-Carrasco *et al.* 2006; Ramos-Casals and Font 2005; Todaro *et al.* 2004). In parallel, changes in the cytokine profile and upregulation of adhesion molecules in the glandular vascular endothelium lead to recruitment of lymphocytes and dendritic cells into the gland (Fox and Speight 1996). Within the glands, T and B lymphocytes are activated by interaction with HLA-DR-restricted antigen presenting cells, possibly including the glandular epithelial cells themselves (Tapinos et al, 1999; Delaleu *et al.* 2005), leading to local production of autoantibodies. The profiles of cytokines and chemokines released by the lymphocytes and epithelial cells sustains the inflammatory response. Cytokines and aberrantly expressed matrix metalloproteinases could also contribute to salivary hypofunction (Fox 2005). Significantly, autoantibodies have been identified is SS patients and the NOD mouse that inhibit muscarinic receptors that are essential to the secretory function of acinar cells (Dawson *et al.* 2005; Cha *et al.* 2002). Chronic inhibition of secretion could contribute to gland atrophy (e.g., Teymoortash *et al.* 2007).

Emerging Data on the Effects of Green Tea Polyphenols on Exocrinopathy in NOD Mice

At present, treatment of SS is generally symptomatic (Kassan and Moutsopoulos 2004), and there is an urgent need for agents that can prevent or block the progression of SS. GTPs may provide one such agent. GTPs have potent anti-inflammatory, antioxidant and anti-apoptotic effects, and epidemiological evidence is consistent with a beneficial effect from GTP consumption (reviewed in Hsu and Dickinson, 2006). Expression of autoantigens (including SS-A/Ro and SS-B-La) by normal human primary epidermal keratinocytes and an immortalized human salivary acinar cell line was reduced by treatment with (-)-epigallocatechin-3-gallate (EGCG), the most abundant and potent green tea polyphenol (Hsu *et al.* 2005). GTPs (as a complex natural extract of various compounds) have been shown to reduce the severity of some autoimmune disorders in animal models, including Sjogren's-like symptoms in the NOD mouse, and psoriasiform lesions in the flaky skin mouse model (Hsu et al. 2007a,b; reviewed in Hsu and Dickinson, 2006).

(i) Effects of Dietary EGCG on Autoimmune Disease in NOD Mice

We hypothesized initially that GTPs could influence the progression of SS-like disease in the NOD mouse by reducing the rate of lymphocytic infiltration and apoptosis in the glandular acinar cells. Recently, we reported that administration of GTPs in the diet of NOD mice reduced the autoimmune-induced lymphocytic infiltration of the submandibular gland

and reduced serum total autoantibody levels in mice that had progressed to development of diabetes (Hsu *et al.* 2007b). However, since these studies used a complex mixture of GTPs, it was important to examine the effects of dietary EGCG. Lymphocytic infiltration of the submandibular gland can be detected from about 8 weeks of age, and a significant decrease in salivary flow rate occurs between 14 and 24 weeks of age (Jonsson *et al.* 2006, 2007; Rosignoli et al., 2005; van Blokland and Versnel, 2002). Therefore, as an initial test of this hypothesis, we administered EGCG in the diet to NOD mice for 19 weeks, and examined the effects on the Sjogren's-like pathology at 22 weeks of age, when disease progression is well established. At 22 weeks of age, 3 of the 12 animals in the water-fed group were negative for urine glucose, while 7 of the 12 EGCG-fed animals were negative. However, this difference was not statistically significant due to the relatively small number of animals used (χ^2 =0.213). Similarly, there was no significant difference in body weight average between the groups, and in each group 2 animals showed significant decline in body weight (Table 1). As expected, dietary EGCG was tolerated well.

Table 1. Disease status and body weight of NOD mice fed with either water only or water-EGCG. NOD/ShiLtJ (001976) mice were purchased at the age of 3 weeks from Jackson Laboratory, MN. The animal were housed at 5 mice/cage, fed ad libitum, and maintained in a pathogen-free environment. All animal protocols in this study were approved by the Institutional Animal Care and Use Committee. The mice were fed with either EGCG (>95%, Sigma-Aldrich, St. Louis, MO). or water (12 animals per treatment group). EGCG exposure (0.1% w/v) was initiated at 4 weeks of age, and the concentration increased to 0.2% at the age of 8 weeks, when the animals reached reproductive age. Water bottles for each cage were filled daily with freshly prepared EGCG-water. The autoimmune disease condition was determined by a test of urinary glucose using glucotest strips (Glucotest, Boehringer Mannheim, Mannheim, Germany). The body weight of each mouse was monitored and recorded. C, water-fed; T, EGCG-fed

Animal#	Weight (g)	Diabetes	Animal#	Weight (g)	Diabetes
C25	25.5	P	T25	25.8	N
C26	23.7	P	T26	27.8	N
C27	28.1	N	T27	25.2	N
C36	23.9	P	T28	26.7	N
C34	25.5	P	T29	22.1	P
C32	17.4	P	T35	26.1	P
C33	21.3	P	T36	23.7	N
C35	22.8	N	T32	18.5	P
C28	21.0	P	T33	26.4	N

C29	16.6	P	T30	15.1	P
C30	29.8	N	T31	24.0	P
C31	25.0	P	T34	24.5	N

The total serum autoantibody levels were significantly increased ($p<0.05$) in the water-fed group (0.424 ± 0.09), in comparison to the EGCG-fed group (0.318 ± 0.038) (unpublished data, manuscript in preparation). This is consistent with our observation that EGCG can reduce the expression of autoantigens by epithelial cells *in vitro* (Hsu *et al.* 2005). At this age, there is a significant lymphocytic infiltration of the NOD submandibular glands (e.g. Figure 1). The average area of lymphocytic infiltration between the two treatment groups (water-fed 60599.66 ± 40230.24 vs. EGCG-fed 51442.32 ± 31730.66, p = 0.599, unpublished data) was not statistically different. Previously, we reported that three weeks after urinary glucose detection the average area of lymphocytic infiltration in the salivary glands of NOD mice was significantly reduced by GTP consumption (Hsu *et al.* 2007b). NOD mice start to show positive urinary glucose as early as 12 weeks old. A similar reduction at 16 weeks of age was seen in EGCG fed NOD mice (data not shown). Thus, it appears that EGCG or GTP intervention can inhibit lymphocytic infiltration at earlier stages, but not at late (22 weeks old) stages.

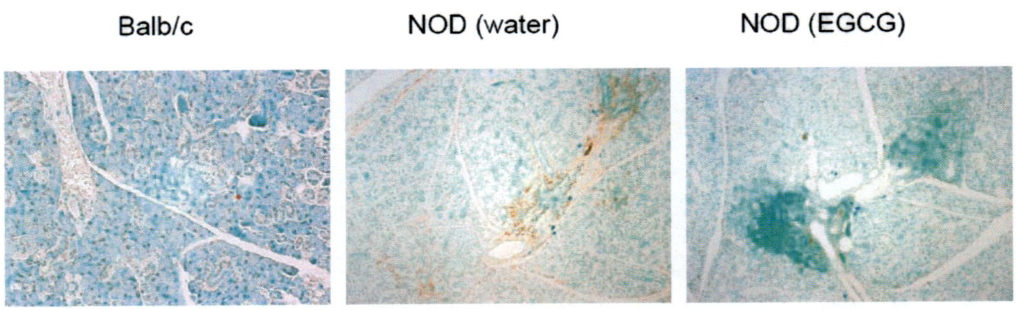

Figure 1. Submandibular gland apoptosis analysis (TUNEL assay) results. At the end of week 22, animals (including BALB/c mice) were euthanized by CO_2 inhalation followed by thoracotomy. The submandibular glands were surgically collected, weighed, fixed in 10% neutral-buffered formalin, and paraffin-embedded for pathological and immunohistochemistry analysis. Five micron-thick (5 μm) serial sections were prepared, and cells with nuclear DNA fragmentation were visualized by the TUNEL method using the ApopTag Plus Peroxidase in situ apoptosis detection kit (Chemicon International, CA, U.S.A.) according to the manufacturer's directions. Methyl green was used for counterstaining. TUNEL indices (TI) were defined as the ratio of TUNEL-positive cells/total number of cells counted (at least 1000 cells per sample). A one-way ANOVA and two-tailed Student's *t* tests were used to analyze statistical significant. Differences were considered statistically significant at $p<0.05$.

(ii) Effect of EGCG on Apoptosis in NOD Submandibular Glands

The apoptotic activity in the NOD submandibular glands fed either EGCG or water was determined by TUNEL staining. In 22 week old NOD mice fed with water alone, there was a modest level of apoptosis in the non-infiltrated glandular epithelium (0.35±0.11%) that was slightly higher than that observed in the BALB/c control mice (0.1)(Table 2, Figure 1). EGCG had no significant effect on the level of apoptosis in the non-infiltrated glandular epithelium (p=0.23). In contrast, there was a significant increase in the apoptotic index in lymphocyte-infiltrated areas in water fed mice. Dietary EGCG reduced this level of apoptosis to about 2-fold higher than that of the non-infiltrated epithelium (Table 2).

Table 2. Summary and statistical analysis of TUNEL, PCNA and Ki-67 results

DC surface Marker	Supernatant from NKT cell cultures stimulated three days with Mitomycin C-treated CD11c^{+} cells and the following glycolipids.		
	Vehicle	aGal.Cer	C20:2
CD40	12% ± 3	36% ± 8	39% ± 13
MHCII	8% ± 2	51% ± 11	50% ± 19
CD86	7% ± 2	42% ± 13	37% ± 12
CD8	11% ± 4	1% ± 1	2% ± 1
DC stimulation	pg/ml of IL-10 in DC supernatants		
Medium	<10	<10	<10
CpG	523 ± 39	1287 ± 123	1098 ± 251
	pg/ml of IL-12 in DC supernatants		
Medium	<10	<10	<10
CpG	1312 ± 437	153 ± 59	287 ± 73

As seen in studies of apoptosis in human SS glands, there is some discordance in the reported values for apoptotic indices in the NOD mouse. For example, van Blokland *et al.* (2003) observed a modest level of apoptosis in NOD submandibular glands, and no change in the level between 5 and 20 weeks. In addition, the levels of apoptosis were not significantly different from those seen in control C57BL/10 mice. They concluded that it was unlikely that apoptosis had a role in either the initiation of NOD sialadenitis or the subsequent immune-mediated effector phase. Cha *et al.* (2004) observed about a 3-fold higher level of apotosis in

20 week old NOD mice (6 cells per 8 mm^2, calculated from their Table 2) than observed by van Blokland *et al.* (2003)(about 2 cells per 7.5 mm^2, estimated from their Figure 2).

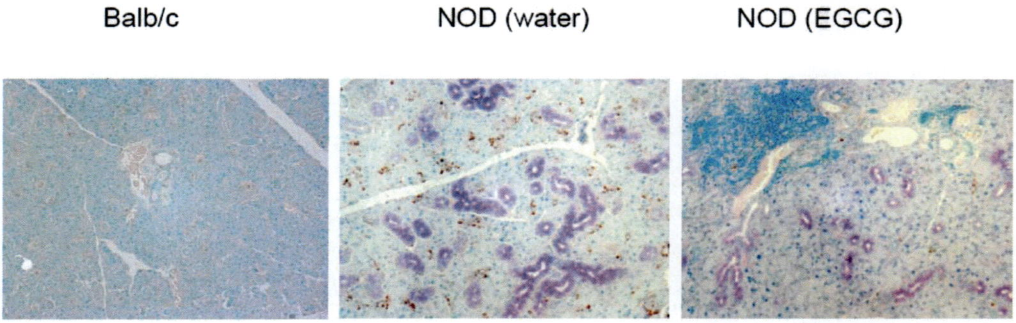

Figure 2. Nuclear protein PCNA expression in the submandibular glands of NOD mice. Immunohistochemical staining was performed using a standard protocol with Histo-plus Kits (ZYMED Laboratories, CA, U.S.A.) according to the manufacturer's directions. Deparaffinized sections were immersed in methanol containing 3% hydrogen peroxide for 20 min. The sections were incubated with anti-PCNA polyclonal antibody (FL-261; Santa Cruz Biotechnology, CA, U.S.A., diluted 1:100) overnight at 4°C. The sections were then incubated with the biotinylated secondary antibody for 10 min and HRP-streptavidin for 10 min. Peroxidase staining was performed for 3~7 min using a solution of DAB chromogen. The sections were counterstained with 0.5% methyl green. At least 1000 cells were counted per animal, and the percentage of cells showing positive nuclear staining was designated as the PCNA index. A one-way ANOVA and two-tailed Student's *t* tests were used to analyze statistical significant. Differences were considered statistically significant at $p<0.05$.

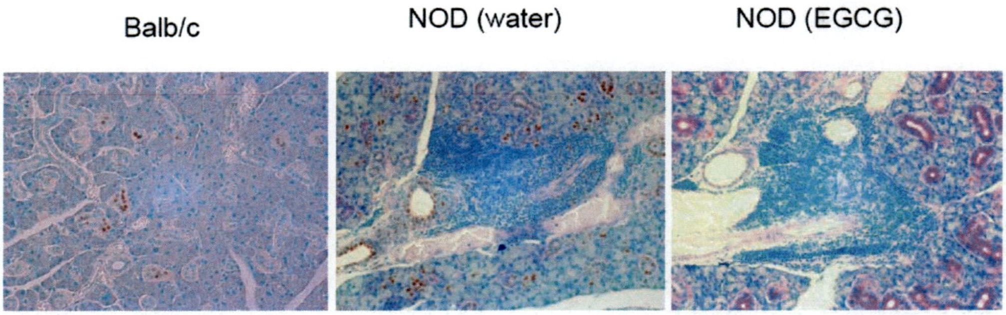

Figure 3. Nuclear protein Ki-67 expression in the submandibular glands of NOD mice. Immunohistochemical staining was performed using a standard protocol with Histo-plus Kits (ZYMED Laboratories, CA, U.S.A.) according to the manufacturer's directions. Sections of samples were incubated with anti-Ki-67 polyclonal antibody (Abcam Inc, MA, U.S.A. diluted 1:1500) for 1 hour at room temperature, followed by the procedures described in Figure 2.

In contrast, Qi *et al.* (2007) observed a 2.5-fold increase in apoptosis in the NOD mouse between 5 and 20 weeks, to levels 3-fold higher than seen in control BALB/c mice. Kong et al. (1998) observed a similar increase between 8 and 18 weeks, to levels nearly 6-fold higher than in BALB/c. Our observations of modest levels of apoptosis in 22 week old NOD mice and BALB/c controls, with moderately higher levels in areas of lymphocytic infiltration, are generally consistent with these reports, although the levels of apoptosis we observed in NOD and BALB/c non-infiltrated epithelium (0.35% and 0.1%; Table 2) were much lower than those seen by Kong *et al.* (1998)(11.2 and 2.0% respectively at 18 weeks). EGCG reduced the level of apoptosis in infiltrated, but not in non-infiltrated, areas. We cannot at this time know if it is the lymphocytes, epithelial cells or both undergoing apoptosis. However, SS lymphocytes are resistant to apoptosis (Garcia-Garasco *et al.* 2006; Ramos-Casals and Font 2005), raising the possibility that it is the acinar cells undergoing apoptosis in association with proximity to the lymphocytes. This could be examined using a combination of cell-specific immunostaining and the TUNEL assay. The dysregulation of apoptosis control pathways in the NOD mouse is an early event (Masago *et al.* 2001; Qi *et al.* 2007; van Blokland *et al.* 2003), consistent with (although not proving) some role for apoptosis in initiation of the autoimmune response (Humphreys-Beher *et al.* 1999b). An interesting possibility raised by our observations of the effects of EGCG is that some of the range in apoptotic indices observed for SS patients might be due to dietary factors.

(iii) Effect of EGCG on Epithelial Cell Proliferation

Homeostasis in the normal gland requires a balance of cell death and proliferation. In contrast to epithelial cell death in SS, epithelial cell division has received relatively little attention. However, the various cell populations of normal salivary glands in humans and rodents do show a low-modest level of cell proliferation (Dardick *et al.* 1990; Denny *et al.* 1997; Ihrler *et al.* 2004). Interestingly, in the parotid gland of SS patients, there is typically a hyperplasia of the salivary ductal epithelium, and numerous Ki67-positive proliferating epithelial cells (Daniels and Fox 1992; Ihrler *et al.* 1999). A hyperplasia of airway secretory cells in SS has also been reported (Andoh *et al.* 1993).

Immunostaining was used to assess the expression of two cell proliferation markers; PCNA (an autoantigen) and Ki67 (Figs. 2 and 3). BALB/c control mice showed a modest level of proliferation in the non-infiltrated glandular epithelium. In contrast, 22 week old water-fed NOD mice showed a considerably higher proliferation index with both markers 14.6$\pm$8.83% PCNA; 3.71$\pm$1.96% Ki67; Table 2). Remarkably, treatment with dietary EGCG reduced the glandular epithelial proliferation indices to BALB/c control levels. In comparison to the non-infiltrated glandular epithelium of water-fed NOD mice, regions of infiltration had near-control proliferation indices with PCNA and Ki67. These levels were further reduced by EGCG treatment (Table 2).

This preliminary data demonstrates a remarkably high level of cell proliferation (as measured by PCNA and Ki67 positive cells) in the epithelial cells of 22 week old NOD mouse submandibular glands in comparison to cells of BALB/c control mice. To our knowledge, cell proliferation in the submandibular gland of NOD mice has not been examined before. Importantly, dietary EGCG reduces the level of proliferation to near normal levels. These results are similar to those we obtained in the flaky skin mouse model for psoriasis. This disease involves hyperproliferation and aberrant differentiation of epidermal keratinocytes. Although it is associated with inflammation, the development of psoriasiform lesions may be independent of T and B-cells (Zenz *et al.* 2005). Application of GTPs to the lesions that develop in the flaky skin mouse reduced the symptoms of epidermal pathology, increased processing of caspase 14 (a marker of terminal differentiation) and reduced the number of PCNA-positive cells (Hsu et al., 2007a).

In chronic sialadenitis of the human parotid gland, there is a significant increase in the proliferation of acinar cells (Ihrler *et al.* 2004), suggesting a reparative response to injury. In the rat ductal ligation model for parotid sialadenitis, the majority of acinar cells are lost. However, 14 days after duct release, the parotid glands appear essentially normal (Burgess and Dardick 1998). These data indicate that under certain circumstances there is considerable regenerative potential in the glands following loss of acinar cells. Viewed in this light, the proliferation of epithelial cells in the NOD mouse suggests a chronically activated proliferative, reparative response. Consistent with this, trefoil factor family 1 (TFF1, pS2) peptide, a protein important in maintaining the surface integrity of secretory epithelia (Giraud *et al.* 2007), is expressed by a significant percentage of acinar and ductal cells in the minor glands of SS patients (Polihronis *et al.* 1998; reviewed in Ramos-Casals and Font, 2005).

An abnormal proliferative response associated with tissue dysfunction in this animal model for SS has similarities to other diseases of unknown etiology such as idiopathic pulmonary fibrosis (IPF) and chronic obstructive pulmonary disease (COPD). IPF is a progressive, generally fatal lung disease characterized by extracellular matrix remodeling associated with fibroblast proliferation and irreversible distortion of the tissue architecture. Like SS, it was originally thought to be the result of a chronic inflammatory process, in this case leading to fibrotic scarring; however, there is a poor correlation between inflammation and the fibrotic response (reviewed in Selman *et al.* 2001). More recently, it has been suggested that IPF is the result of cycles of epithelial cell injury, perhaps triggered by a viral infection, followed by abnormal wound healing resulting from defects in epithelial cell migration, proliferation and differentiation associated with hyperplasia of type II alveolar epithelial progenitor cells, and apoptosis of alveolar epithelial cells (Selman *et al.* 2001, Selman and Pardo, 2006). These defects are associated with disruption of the basement membrane, possibly due in part to upregulation of MMP activity (Bove *et al.* 2007; Pardo and Selman 2006). Similarly, in COPD, an airway injury, perhaps due to bacterial infection, leads to abnormal remodeling and repair associated with basal and mucus cell hyperplasia (Puchelle *et al.* 2006).

(iv) Proteomic Profiling of SMG Proteins in NOD Mice Treated with EGCG

Abnormal proliferation of differentiated tissue can be accompanied by the loss of differentiated cell protein synthesis and function (Morley and Hodes 1988). Alternatively, dysregulation of glandular homeostasis might lead to the expression of novel proteins. Proteomic technology has been applied recently in an effort to use whole saliva as a diagnostic tool for SS (e.g., Baldani *et al.* 2008; Hu *et al.* 2007). These studies have provided evidence for dysfunction of acinar cells, e.g., reduction in levels of amylase, cystatins and proline-rich proteins (glandular secreted proteins), but have not yet yielded information related to the mechanisms underlying the pathology of SS.

We have begun to explore the use of laser capture microdissection in conjunction with proteomic analysis to identify protein differences between NOD and BALB/c mice whose expression in the NOD mouse can be modulated and normalized by EGCG. Proteomic profiling of submandibular gland acinar cells from 22 week old BALB/c, NOD (with diabetes), and NOD (with or without diabetes) mice fed EGCG identified 11 proteins with >10-fold changes in expression levels. Among these, 3 proteins were differentially expressed in BALB/c and NOD mice regardless of disease status or EGCG treatment. The expression of 3 other differentially expressed proteins in NOD mice was regulated to BALB/c levels by dietary EGCG. The other 5 proteins were regulated in association with frank diabetes or a combination of diabetes and dietary EGCG. These proteins are excellent candidates for proteins that have a role in the abnormality of the acinar cells that preceeds the inflammatory infiltrate, especially if they are dysregulated in young NOD and NOD.*scid* mice. Further investigation is currentlty is underway.

Conclusion

Collectively, our observations are consistent with a model for development of SS-like pathology in the NOD mouse in which developmental abnormalities created a defect in the normal glandular homeostasis. Differentiation, proliferation and apoptosis are alternative fates for cells that are normally tightly regulated and integrated with ECM directed signaling (Chen *et al.* 1997). For example, in the mammary gland, differentiation and survival of exocrine cells requires a specific 3-dimensional interaction of cells with the extracellular matrix (ECM)(Katz and Streuli 2007). A balance between these alternative fates is essential to tissue homeostasis. Abberations in the submandibular gland ECM, likely created in part by elevated expression of MMPs (Goicovich *et al.* 2003; Konttinen *et al.* 2006; Laine et al. 2004; Perez *et al.* 2000, 2005; Yamachika *et al.* 1998), could lead to failure of the acini to fully differentiate due to inappropriate intracellular signaling. MMP9 has a key role in epithelial regeneration (Mohan *et al.* 2002), but overexpression is associated with defective re-epithelialization (Fini *et al.* 1996). Consistent with a role in the exocrinopathy seen in the NOD mouse, MMP9 is upregulated in the submandibular glands (Cha *et al.* 2001).

These events would likely lead to conflicting signals: while glandular epithelial cells would normally differentiate as a terminal fate, the aberrant signaling may be interpreted as a need for a reparative, proliferative response. Although some submandibular acinar cells might respond by dividing, other may undergo apoptosis as a common safety default response to signaling leading to conflicting fates. Dysregulation of cellular function, perhaps in conjunction with apoptosis, would then lead to autoantigen presentation (Todaro *et al.* 2004). Proinflammatory cytokine and chemokine expression could also result from the attempt to establish a reparative response. GTPs such as EGCG are known to modulate intracellular signaling (reviewed in Hsu and Dickinson 2006). A plausible explanation for the beneficial effects of EGCG in the NOD mouse model, consistent with its established pro-differentiation and anti-apoptotic effects, is that the effects on signaling pathways in acinar cells mimic the normal signaling of an appropriate ECM environment and over-ride the genetic abnormalities. In effect, the behavior of the acinar cells would be normalized. This effect would be consistent with the partial return of the SMG protein expression profile of NOD mice to that of the parental BALB/c strain after EGCG treatment, and with the suppression of the proliferative reparative and apoptotic responses. In various models, EGCG reduces expression of autoantigens by epithelial cells, and proinflamatory cytokine expression. This would be consistent with the reduction in the inflammatory infiltrates seen here after EGCG treatment.

If this testable hypothesis is correct, and applies to SS patients, it raises the possibility that complementary and alternative approaches to SS treatment, such as green tea polyphenols, could protect secretory glands from autoimmune-induced tissue destruction. In addition, and early detection of autoimmune risk for disease might be possible by examination of protein markers in saliva and serum that result from abnormalities in acinar cell differentiation that preceed significant lymphocytic infiltration and loss of glandular function.

References

Andoh Y, Shimura S, Sawai T, Sasaki H, Takishima T, Shirato K. Morphometric analysis of airways in Sjögren's syndrome. *Am. Rev. Respir. Dis.* (1993) 148:1358-1362.

Baldini C, Giusti L, Bazzichi L, Lucacchini A, Bombardieri S. Proteomic analysis of the saliva: a clue for understanding primary from secondary Sjögren's syndrome? *Autoimmun. Rev.* (2008) 7:185-191.

Bloch KJ, Buchanan WW, Wohl MJ, Bunim JJ. Sjögren's syndrome. A clinical, pathological, and serological study of sixty-two cases. *Medicine (Baltimore).* (1965) 44:187-231.

Bove PF, Wesley UV, Greul AK, Hristova M, Dostmann WR, van der Vliet A. Nitric oxide promotes airway epithelial wound repair through enhanced activation of MMP-9. *Am. J. Respir. Cell Mol. Biol.* (2007) 36:138-146.

Burgess KL, Dardick I. Cell population changes during atrophy and regeneration of rat parotid gland. *Oral Surg. Oral Med. Oral Pathol. Oral Radiol.Endod.* (1998) 85:699-706.

Cha S, van Blockland SC, Versnel MA, Homo-Delarche F, Nagashima H, Brayer J, Peck AB, Humphreys-Beher MG. Abnormal organogenesis in salivary gland development may initiate adult onset of autoimmune exocrinopathy. *Exp. Clin. Immunogenet.* (2001) 18:143-160.

Cha S, Peck AB, Humphreys-Beher MG. Progress in understanding autoimmune exocrinopathy using the non-obese diabetic mouse: an update. *Crit. Rev Oral Biol. Med.* (2002) 13:5-16.

Cha S, Brayer J, Gao J, Brown V, Killedar S, Yasunari U, Peck AB. A dual role for interferon-gamma in the pathogenesis of Sjogren's syndrome-like autoimmune exocrinopathy in the nonobese diabetic mouse. *Scand. J. Immunol.* (2004) 60:552-565.

Chen CS, Mrksich M, Huang S, Whitesides GM, Ingber DE. Geometric control of cell life and death. *Science.* (1997) 276:1425-1428.

Daniels TE, Fox PC. Salivary and oral components of Sjögren's syndrome. *Rheum. Dis. Clin. North Am*. (1992) 18:571-589.

Dardick I, Byard RW, Carnegie JA. A review of the proliferative capacity of major salivary glands and the relationship to current concepts of neoplasia in salivary glands. *Oral Surg. Oral Med. Oral Pathol*. (1990) 69:53-67.

Dawson LJ, Smith PM, Moots RJ, Field EA. Sjögren's syndrome-time for a new approach. *Rheumatology* (Oxford). (2000) 39:234-237.

Dawson LJ, Field EA, Harmer AR, Smith PM. Acetylcholine-evoked calcium mobilization and ion channel activation in human labial gland acinar cells from patients with primary Sjögren's syndrome. *Clin. Exp. Immunol*. (2001) 124:480-485.

Dawson L, Tobin A, Smith P, Gordon T. Antimuscarinic antibodies in Sjögren's syndrome: where are we, and where are we going? *Arthritis Rheum*. (2005) 52:2984-2995.

Dawson LJ, Fox PC, Smith PM. Sjogrens syndrome--the non-apoptotic model of glandular hypofunction. *Rheumatology* (Oxford). (2006) 45:792-798.

Delaleu N, Jonsson R, Koller MM. Sjögren's syndrome. *Eur. J. Oral Sci*. (2005) 113:101-113.

Denny PC, Ball WD, Redman RS. Salivary glands: a paradigm for diversity of gland development. *Crit. Rev. Oral Biol. Med*. (1997) 8:51-75.

Fini ME, Parks WC, Rinehart WB, Girard MT, Matsubara M, Cook JR, West-Mays JA, Sadow PM, Burgeson RE, Jeffrey JJ, Raizman MB, Krueger RR, Zieske JD. Role of matrix metalloproteinases in failure to re-epithelialize after corneal injury. *Am. J. Pathol*. (1996) 149:1287-1302.

Fox PC, Speight PM. Current concepts of autoimmune exocrinopathy: immunologic mechanisms in the salivary pathology of Sjögren's syndrome. *Crit. Rev. Oral Biol. Med*. (1996) 7:144-158.

Fox PC. Autoimmune diseases and Sjögren's syndrome: an autoimmune exocrinopathy. *Ann. NY Acad. Sci*. (2007) 1098:15-21.

Fox RI, Kang HI. Pathogenesis of Sjögren's syndrome. Rheum Dis Clin North Am. (1992) 18:517-538.

Fox RI, Maruyama T. Pathogenesis and treatment of Sjögren's syndrome. *Curr. Opin. Rheumatol*. (1997) 9:393-399.

Fox RI. Sjögren's syndrome. *Lancet*. (2005) 366:321-331.

Gao J, Cha S, Jonsson R, Opalko J, Peck AB. Detection of anti-type 3 muscarinic acetylcholine receptor autoantibodies in the sera of Sjögren's syndrome patients by use of a transfected cell line assay. *Arthritis Rheum*. (2004) 50:2615-2621.

García-Carrasco M, Fuentes-Alexandro S, Escárcega RO, Salgado G, Riebeling C, Cervera R. Pathophysiology of Sjögren's syndrome. *Arch. Med. Res*. (2006) 37:921-932.

Giraud AS, Jackson C, Menheniott TR, Judd LM. Differentiation of the Gastric Mucosa IV. Role of trefoil peptides and IL-6 cytokine family signaling in gastric homeostasis. *Am. J. Physiol. Gastrointest. Liver Physiol*. (2007) 292:G1-5.

Goicovich E, Molina C, Pérez P, Aguilera S, Fernández J, Olea N, Alliende C, Leyton C, Romo R, Leyton L, González M. Enhanced degradation of proteins of the basal lamina and stroma by matrix metalloproteinases from the salivary glands of Sjögren's syndrome patients: correlation with reduced structural integrity of acini and ducts. *Arthritis Rheum.* (2003) 48:2573-2584.

Greenspan JS, Daniels TE, Talal N, Sylvester RA. The histopathology of Sjögren's syndrome in labial salivary gland biopsies. *Oral Surg. Oral Med. Oral Pathol.* (1974) 37:217-229.

Hsu S, Dickinson DP, Qin H, Lapp C, Lapp D, Borke J, Walsh DS, Bollag WB, Stöppler H, Yamamoto T, Osaki T, Schuster G. Inhibition of autoantigen expression by (-)-epigallocatechin-3-gallate (the major constituent of green tea) in normal human cells. *J. Pharmacol. Exp. Ther.* (2005) 315:805-811.

Hsu S, Dickinson D. A new approach to managing oral manifestations of Sjogren's syndrome and skin manifestations of lupus. *J. Biochem. Mol. Biol.* (2006) 39:229-239.

Hsu S, Dickinson D, Borke J, Walsh DS, Wood J, Qin H, Winger J, Pearl H, Schuster G, Bollag WB. Green tea polyphenol induces caspase 14 in epidermal keratinocytes via MAPK pathways and reduces psoriasiform lesions in the flaky skin mouse model. *Exp. Dermatol.* (2007a) 16:678-684.

Hsu SD, Dickinson DP, Qin H, Borke J, Ogbureke KU, Winger JN, Camba AM, Bollag WB, Stöppler HJ, Sharawy MM, Schuster GS. Green tea polyphenols reduce autoimmune symptoms in a murine model for human Sjogren's syndrome and protect human salivary acinar cells from TNF-alpha-induced cytotoxicity. *Autoimmunity.* (2007b) 40:138-147.

Hu S, Wang J, Meijer J, Ieong S, Xie Y, Yu T, Zhou H, Henry S, Vissink A, Pijpe J, Kallenberg C, Elashoff D, Loo JA, Wong DT. Salivary proteomic and genomic biomarkers for primary Sjögren's syndrome. *Arthritis Rheum.* (2007) 56:3588-3600.

Humphreys-Beher MG, Peck AB. New concepts for the development of autoimmune exocrinopathy derived from studies with the NOD mouse model. *Arch. Oral Biol.* (1999) 44 Suppl 1:S21-25.

Humphreys-Beher MG, Brayer J, Yamachika S, Yamamoto H, Maeda N, Nakagawa Y, Peck AB, Robinson CP. Salivary gland changes in the NOD mouse model for Sjögren's syndrome: is there a non-immune genetic trigger? *Eur. J. Morphol.* (1998) 36, Suppl:247-251.

Humphreys-Beher MG, Brayer J, Yamachika S, Peck AB, Jonsson R. An alternative perspective to the immune response in autoimmune exocrinopathy: induction of functional quiescence rather than destructive autoaggression. *Scand. J. Immunol.* (1999a) 49:7-10.

Humphreys-Beher MG, Peck AB, Dang H, Talal N. The role of apoptosis in the initiation of the autoimmune response in Sjögren's syndrome. *Clin. Exp. Immunol.* (1999b) 116:383-387.

Ihrler S, Zietz C, Sendelhofert A, Riederer A, Löhrs U. Lymphoepithelial duct lesions in Sjögren-type sialadenitis. *Virchows Arch.* (1999) 434:315-323.

Ihrler S, Blasenbreu-Vogt S, Sendelhofert A, Rössle M, Harrison JD, Löhrs U. Regeneration in chronic sialadenitis: an analysis of proliferation and apoptosis based on double immunohistochemical labeling. *Virchows Arch.* (2004) 444:356-361.

Jonsson R, Kroneld U, Bäckman K, Magnusson B, Tarkowski A. Progression of sialadenitis in Sjögren's syndrome. *Br. J. Rheumatol.* (1993) 32:578-581.

Jonsson MV, Delaleu N, Brokstad KA, Berggreen E, Skarstein K. Impaired salivary gland function in NOD mice: association with changes in cytokine profile but not with histopathologic changes in the salivary gland. *Arthritis Rheum*. (2006) 54:2300-2305.

Jonsson MV, Delaleu N, Jonsson R. Animal models of Sjögren's syndrome. *Clin. Rev. Allergy Immunol*. (2007) 32:215-224.

Kassan SS, Moutsopoulos HM. Clinical manifestations and early diagnosis of Sjögren syndrome. *Arch. Intern. Med*. (2004) 164:1275-1284

Katz E, Streuli CH. The extracellular matrix as an adhesion checkpoint for mammary epithelial function. *Int. J. Biochem. Cell Biol*. (2007) 39:715-726.

Kikuchi M, Inagaki T, Ogawa K, Banno S, Matsumoto Y, Ueda R, Hanaki H. Histopathological investigation of salivary glands in the asymptomatic elderly. *Arch. Gerontol. Geriatr*. (2004) 38:131-138.

Kong L, Robinson CP, Peck AB, Vela-Roch N, Sakata KM, Dang H, Talal N, Humphreys-Beher MG. Inappropriate apoptosis of salivary and lacrimal gland epithelium of immunodeficient NOD-scid mice. *Clin. Exp. Rheumatol*. (1998) 16:675-681.

Konttinen YT, Porola P, Konttinen L, Laine M, Poduval P. Immunohistopathology of Sjögren's syndrome. *Autoimmun. Rev*. (2006) 6:16-20.

Laine M, Virtanen I, Salo T, Konttinen YT. Segment-specific but pathologic laminin isoform profiles in human labial salivary glands of patients with Sjogren's syndrome. *Arthritis Rheum*. (2004) 50:3968-3973.

Manganelli P, Quaini F, Andreoli AM, Lagrasta C, Pilato FP, Zuccarelli A, Monteverdi R, D'Aversa C, Olivetti G. Quantitative analysis of apoptosis and bcl-2 in Sjögren's syndrome. *J. Rheumatol*. (1997) 24:1552-1557.

Manganelli P, Fietta P. Apoptosis and Sjögren syndrome. *Semin. Arthritis Rheum*. (2003) 33:49-65.

Masago R, Aiba-Masago S, Talal N, Zuluaga FJ, Al-Hashimi I, Moody M, Lau CA, Peck AB, Brayer J, Humphreys-Beher MG, Dang H. Elevated proapoptotic Bax and caspase 3 activation in the NOD.scid model of Sjögren's syndrome. *Arthritis Rheum*. (2001) 44:693-702.

Mohan R, Chintala SK, Jung JC, Villar WV, McCabe F, Russo LA, Lee Y, McCarthy BE, Wollenberg KR, Jester JV, Wang M, Welgus HG, Shipley JM, Senior RM, Fini ME. Matrix metalloproteinase gelatinase B (MMP-9) coordinates and effects epithelial regeneration. *J. Biol. Chem*. (2002) 277:2065-2072.

Morley D, Hodes M. Amylase expression in human parotid neoplasms: evidence by in situ hybridization for a lack of transcription of the amylase gene. *J. Histochem. Cytochem*. (1988) 36:487-491.

Ohlsson M, Skarstein K, Bolstad AI, Johannessen AC, Jonsson R. Fas-induced apoptosis is a rare event in Sjögren's syndrome. *Lab. Invest*. (2001) 81:95-105.

Pardo A, Selman M. Matrix metalloproteases in aberrant fibrotic tissue remodeling. *Proc. Am. Thorac. Soc*. (2006) 3:383-388.

Pérez P, Goicovich E, Alliende C, Aguilera S, Leyton C, Molina C, Pinto R, Romo R, Martinez B, González MJ. Differential expression of matrix metalloproteinases in labial salivary glands of patients with primary Sjögren's syndrome. *Arthritis Rheum*. (2000) 43:2807-2817.

Pérez P, Kwon YJ, Alliende C, Leyton L, Aguilera S, Molina C, Labra C, Julio M, Leyton C, González MJ. Increased acinar damage of salivary glands of patients with Sjögren's syndrome is paralleled by simultaneous imbalance of matrix metalloproteinase 3/tissue inhibitor of metalloproteinases 1 and matrix metalloproteinase 9/tissue inhibitor of metalloproteinases 1 ratios. *Arthritis Rheum.* (2005) 52:2751-2760.

Polihronis M, Tapinos NI, Theocharis SE, Economou A, Kittas C, Moutsopoulos HM. Modes of epithelial cell death and repair in Sjögren's syndrome (SS). *Clin. Exp. Immunol.* (1998) 114:485-90.

Puchelle E, Zahm JM, Tournier JM, Coraux C. Airway epithelial repair, regeneration, and remodeling after injury in chronic obstructive pulmonary disease. *Proc. Am. Thorac. Soc.* (2006) 3:726-733.

Qi G, Hua H, Gao Y, Lin Q, Yu GY. Sialoadenitis progression in nonobese diabetic mice and its correlation with expression of apoptosis-associated proteins in salivary glands and serum IgG levels. *Chin. Med. J.* (Engl). (2007) 120:1426-1431.

Ramos-Casals M, Font J. Primary Sjögren's syndrome: current and emergent aetiopathogenic concepts. *Rheumatology* (Oxford). (2005) 44:1354-1367.

Robinson CP, Yamamoto H, Peck AB, Humphreys-Beher MG. Genetically programmed development of salivary gland abnormalities in the NOD (nonobese diabetic)-scid mouse in the absence of detectable lymphocytic infiltration: a potential trigger for sialoadenitis of NOD mice. *Clin. Immunol. Immunopathol.* (1996) 79:50-59.

Robinson CP, Brayer J, Yamachika S, Esch TR, Peck AB, Stewart CA, Peen E, Jonsson R, Humphreys-Beher MG. Transfer of human serum IgG to nonobese diabetic Igmu null mice reveals a role for autoantibodies in the loss of secretory function of exocrine tissues in Sjögren's syndrome. *Proc. Natl. Acad. Sci. USA.* (1998) 95:7538-7543.

Rosignoli F, Roca V, Meiss R, Leceta J, Gomariz RP, Pérez Leirós C. Defective signalling in salivary glands precedes the autoimmune response in the non-obese diabetic mouse model of sialadenitis. *Clin. Exp. Immunol.* (2005) 142:411-418.

Selman M, Pardo A. Role of epithelial cells in idiopathic pulmonary fibrosis: from innocent targets to serial killers. *Proc. Am. Thorac. Soc.* (2006) 3:364-372.

Selman M, King TE, Pardo A. Idiopathic pulmonary fibrosis: prevailing and evolving hypotheses about its pathogenesis and implications for therapy. *Ann. Intern. Med.* (2001) 134:136-151.

Tapinos NI, Polihronis M, Tzioufas AG, Moutsopoulos HM. Sjögren's syndrome. Autoimmune epithelitis. *Adv. Exp. Med. Biol.* (1999) 455:127-134.

Teymoortash A, Sommer F, Mandic R, Schulz S, Bette M, Aumüller G, Werner JA. Intraglandular application of botulinum toxin leads to structural and functional changes in rat acinar cells. Br. *J. Pharmacol.* (2007) 152:161-167.

Todaro M, Zeuner A, Stassi G. Role of apoptosis in autoimmunity. *J. Clin. Immunol.* (2004) 24:1-11.

van Blokland SC, Versnel MA. Pathogenesis of Sjögren's syndrome: characteristics of different mouse models for autoimmune exocrinopathy. *Clin. Immunol.* (2002) 103:111-124.

Van Blokland SC, Van Helden-Meeuwsen CG, Wierenga-Wolf AF, Tielemans D, Drexhage HA, Van De Merwe JP, Homo-Delarche F, Versnel MA. Apoptosis and apoptosis-related molecules in the submandibular gland of the nonobese diabetic mouse model for Sjögren's syndrome: limited role for apoptosis in the development of sialoadenitis. *Lab. Invest.* (2003) 83:3-11.

Xanthou G, Tapinos NI, Polihronis M, Nezis IP, Margaritis LH, Moutsopoulos HM. CD4 cytotoxic and dendritic cells in the immunopathologic lesion of Sjögren's syndrome. *Clin. Exp. Immunol.* (1999) 118:154-163.

Yamachika S, Nanni JM, Nguyen KH, Garces L, Lowry JM, Robinson CP, Brayer J, Oxford GE, da Silveira A, Kerr M, Peck AB, Humphreys-Beher MG. Excessive synthesis of matrix metalloproteinases in exocrine tissues of NOD mouse models for Sjögren's syndrome. *J. Rheumatol.* (1998) 25:2371-2380.

Zenz R, Eferl R, Kenner L, Florin L, Hummerich L, Mehic D, Scheuch H, Angel P, Tschachler E, Wagner EF. Psoriasis-like skin disease and arthritis caused by inducible epidermal deletion of Jun proteins. *Nature*. (2005) 437:369-375.

In: Autoimmunity: Role, Regulation and Disorders
Editor: Fynn L. Vogel and L. F. Zimmermann
ISBN 978-1-60456-833-2

Chapter 7

Coxsackievirus B3 Induced Autoimmune Heart Disease: Role of the Innate Immune Response in Controlling Autoimmunity

S. A. Huber and Jessica Schwartz
Department of Pathology, University of Vermont, Colchester VT 05446

Abstract

Virus infections can initiate autoimmunity to self molecules, but not all infections have this effect. A deciding factor in whether infection induces autoimmunity is the nature of the innate immune response initiated by the pathogen. The innate immune system is the initial response to infection and not only helps control microbial growth but modulates the type and intensity of the developing adaptive (antigen-specific) immune response to the microbe. One type of cell affected by the innate immune system is the T regulatory cell. T regulatory cells are a special population of lymphocytes which can inhibit inflammation and autoimmunity. Control of T regulatory cell activation and/or function often determines whether autoimmunity will occur, and many factors, including the role of antigen-presenting cells, signaling through Toll-Like Receptors (TLRs), and innate effectors including natural killer cells and T cells expressing the gamma-delta (γδ) T cell receptor, affect T regulatory cell generation. This review discusses how virus infection, and the innate immune response it generates, determines whether T regulatory cells are activated.

Coxsackievirus B3 Biology

Coxsackieviruses are members of the Picornavirus family of small (~30 nm in diameter), non-enveloped icosahedral viruses containing a single strand RNA genome of between 7200 and 8450 nucleotides [1, 2]. These viruses are distinguished by their physical properties (pH stability and buoyant density), clinical syndromes, and RNA sequence. The family is composed of nine genera: aphthovirus, cardiovirus, enterovirus, erbovirus, hepatovirus, kobuvirus, parechovirus, rhinovirus, and teschovirus [3]. The Enterovirus genus includes polioviruses (3 serotypes), coxsackieviruses (23 serotypes), echoviruses (28 serotypes), human enteroviruses (4 serotypes), and many other nonhuman enteric viruses. Infection is initiated by attachment of the virus to specific membrane proteins (virus receptors). Coxsackievirus B3 (CVB3) uses two known receptors. Coxsackievirus-adenovirus receptor (CAR) is a 46 kDa glycoprotein which is a junction associated molecule (JAM) located in tight junctions [4-6]. JAMs are required for the structural formation and stabilization of tight junctions, primarily in epithelial and endothelial cells, and also promote leukocyte transmigration through epithelial or endothelial barriers. Different JAMs promote transmigration of distinct leukocyte populations. CAR binds immunoglobulin and most likely is required for transmigration of B lymphocytes [5, 7]. All six coxsackievirus B serotypes use CAR as a virus receptor [8] and the extracellular domain of the molecule is adequate to promote virus entry [9]. Decay-acceleration factor (DAF) or CD55, is a 70-kDa glycosylphosphotidylinositol (GPI)- anchored glycoprotein which is primarily involved in inactivation of C3 [10]. Both DAF and CAR are widely expressed throughout the body. In polarized epithelial cells, virus attaches to DAF on the apical which activates Abl kinase and induces Rac-dependent actin rearrangements leading to the virus movement into the epithelial tight junction where the virus binds CAR [6] in the canyon regions of the virus capsid [11]. Both virus binding to CAR and DAF will activate Fyn kinases and phosphorylation of caveolin-1 that will allow virus entry in caveolin coated vesicles. Receptor binding also leads to conformational changes in the capsid, and release of VP4 which inserts into the cell membrane where it forms pores that allow RNA entry into the cytoplasm. Some coxsackieviruses apparently fail to bind DAF [12]. Conceptually, one might wonder how virus can bind CAR hidden in tight junctions without DAF. However, exposing cells to TNFα and IFNγ causes relocation of JAMs outside of tight junctions which improves accessibility of leukocytes to these molecules for transmigration but also improves accessibility to viruses [13].

The genome is divided into 5' and 3' non-translated regions and a central open reading frame [14]. Picornaviruses are positive sense viruses, which means that the viral genome acts like a messenger RNA (mRNA) and is directly translated in the infected cell to produce viral proteins. A small protein (VPg; ~2400 MW) is covalently linked to the 5' terminus of the viral RNA. This protein acts as a primer in the initiation of translation along with the secondary structure of the 5' and 3' NTRs and an internal ribosome entry site (IRES). The open reading frame is translated into a single polyprotein which is processed by viral proteases into at least 11 proteins. Total shutdown of host cell RNA and protein synthesis is complete by 6-8 hours after infection, and molecules produced by infected cells after this point are almost exclusively of viral origin making the infected cell a viral factory. The 2A viral protease degrades the host eukaryotic initiation factor 4G (eIF-4G) which disrupts the cellular p220 protein cap-dependent binding complex and results in the shutdown of cap-dependent host protein synthesis [15, 16]. It also degrades the poly(A)-binding protein [17]. Although picornavirus infections are usually considered lysogenic, many cells can be infected and replicate virus without showing cytopathic effects. These viruses can produce a persistent infection [18-20]. Induction of viral persistence may depend upon the cell cycle at the time of infection since these viruses replicate in cells during G1 and G1/S but not in cells during G0 or G2/M [18]. However, cells infected during non-permissive cell cycle phases retain the viral genome and should these cells enter cycle may begin an active viral replication. Once the initial viral polyproteins are produced and processed, replication of the viral genome occurs using the RNA-dependent-RNA polymerase (3D). The VPg primer and the 3D polymerase bind to the poly-A tail on the 3' NTR to initiate negative-strand synthesis which is a complementary copy of the viral genome. The negative strand is then used as the template for further positive strand RNA synthesis; these positive strand RNAs are used for additional viral protein translation and as new viral genomes. During RNA synthesis, double stranded RNA replicative intermediates (RI) are formed. Virus assembly occurs in the cytoplasm by coalescing of the viral capsid proteins into a procapsid. Entry of the new virus genome into the procapsid causes structural rearrangement of the procapsid sealing in the genome and maturation of the progeny virion. Cellular RNAs are not packaged into progeny virus and trans encaspidation of unrelated viral RNA is rare. Evidence suggests that only newly synthesized viral RNAs can be encapsidated and suggest direct physical interactions between the RNA replication complex and the forming procapsid [21].

Autoimmunity

Autoimmunity is the immune response to self antigens, and three factors must exist for development of an autoimmune disease. These are: 1) the presence of a repertoire of autoreactive lymphocytes; 2) activation of the autoreactive cells; and 3) absence of the normal immunoregulatory mechanisms which suppress autoimmunity [22]. T lymphocytes are better targets for tolerance than B cells. T cells are the central players in the immune response, both directly mediating inflammation through release of chemokines and cytokines, and by cell mediated cytotoxicity of target tissues; and providing B cell help for IgG, IgA, and IgE responses. Tolerance is induced either centrally or peripherally. Central tolerance occurs in the thymus during T cell ontogeny. Self-reactive prothymocytes enter the thymus where high affinity interactions between the T cell receptors on the developing T cells and thymic epithelium major histocompatibility complex (MHC) antigen presenting self antigens cause clonal deletion through apoptosis of these autoreactive T cells. Often, infections with viruses (HIV, rabies), bacteria (*F. turalenesis*), parasites (*T. cruzi, P. chaubi, S.mansoni, T. spiralis*) and fungi (*H. capsulatum, P. brasiliensis*) produce significant thymic atrophy partly due to increased levels of glucorticoid hormone levels (reviewed in [23]). This results in activation of caspases 3 and 8 leading to T cell apoptosis. However, intrathymic T cell migration is also altered during infections resulting in increased immature T cell migration into the periphery. The immature T cells contain increased numbers of self-reactive cells indicating that infection can abort depletion of these autoreactive cells in the thymus [23].

Generally, thymic deletion of self-reactive T cell clones should be restricted to widely expressed self antigens. Autoreactive T cells recognizing tissue-restricted antigens which would not be present in the thymus should escape the thymus and populate the peripheral lymphoid organs. Peripheral tolerance can result in either deletion of self-reactive T cells by exposure of these cells to high levels of self-antigen, or anergy of the cells by inappropriate antigen presentation [24, 25]. Initiation of a primary immune response requires a stable interaction between the antigen presenting cell and naïve T cell for 20 hours [26]. Thus, usually only "professional" antigen presenting cells (dendritic cells) can activate naïve T cells [27, 28]. However, once T cells have been activated, re-stimulation of memory or effector T cells requires significantly less stringent T cell-APC-antigen interaction [29]. Although many cells can be induced to express MHC molecules through exposure to cytokines such as interferon-gamma [30], antigen presentation by these cells places the naïve T cell in a stable state of unresponsiveness (anergy). Anergized T cells show impaired tyrosine kinase phosphorylation of the T cell receptor and defects in downstream signal kinase (MAPK, ERK, JNK) pathways [31, 32]. Such anergized cells remain alive for extended periods, but are incapable of responding even when the appropriate antigen is presented by professional antigen presenting cells. Anergized T cells can be rescued either by inhibition of p38 MAPK, or by high levels of interleukin-2 [33, 34].

There are several mechanisms besides loss of tolerance by which infections might trigger autoimmunity. The earliest mechanism hypothesized is antigenic mimicry in microbial and self-molecules share sufficient similarity to induce cross-reactive immunity [35-37]. Cross-reactive T cells or antibodies between microbes and self antigens are found in various autoimmune diseases. Several of these include: ankylosing spondylitis between HLA B27 and *Krebsiella pneumoniae* [38, 39]; myasthenia gravis between the acetylcholine receptor and herpes simplex virus [40]; type I diabetes between glutamic acid decarboxylase and human cytomegalovirus [41]; rheumatic heart disease between the M protein of group A streptococcus and cardiac myosin [42]; multiple sclerosis between myelin basic protein and Epstein Barr Virus DNA polymerase [43]; and Sjogren's syndrome between the Ro60 kD autoantigen in salivary gland and hepatitis C virus [44]. When cross-reactive antibodies but not T cells are observed [41, 45], mimicry probably involves the tertiary conformation of the antigens. In contrast, cross-reactive T cell clones [41] must involve the primary amino acid sequence of the peptides since T cells recognize peptides of only 9 to 10 amino acids presented by MHC molecules. Only limited sequence homology between the microbial and self antigens is required for cross-reactivity[43, 46]. The ability of T cells to recognize epitopes with minimal amino acid homology should increase the probability of antigenic mimicry. There is evidence for antigenic mimicry between enteroviruses and self molecules in several autoimmune diseases. Numerous studies correlate enterovirus/coxsackievirus infections and Sjogren's syndrome [47-51] and have found cross-reactivity between coxsackievirus peptides and the Ro/SSA 60 kD autoantigen. It should be noted, however, that at least one study failed to find a correlation between coxsackieviruses and Sjogren's syndrome [52]. Enteroviruses have also been associated with type 1 diabetes [53] and cross-reactivity between coxsackievirus proteins and the glutamic acid decarboxylase (GAD65) autoantigen [45, 54, 55], although again other studies fail to find such antigenic mimicry [56-58]. Antigenic mimicry between cardiac myosin and coxsackieviruses has been shown in experimental myocarditis [59], but evidence of such mimicry occurring in patients is lacking. The probable conclusion to date is that while antigenic mimicry might explain at least some cases of autoimmune disease, the evidence is not conclusive. Presence of cross-reactive T cells or antibody does not necessitate that these are major pathogenic factors in the disease.

Another mechanism by which infections can initiate autoimmunity is production of cryptic epitopes. Cryptic epitopes are immunogenic peptides which are either not generated during normal antigen processing or generated at too low concentrations for effective T cell activation [60, 61]. Our current understanding is that the cryptic epitope is not produced during antigen processing most likely because the normal proteases in antigen presenting cells cleave within the epitope. However, there are situations where cryptic epitopes might be rescued and initiate pathogenic immune responses. Several mechanisms for induction of autoimmunity to cryptic epitopes have been proposed [61]. Increasing the amount of the self protein entering into the antigen processing compartment could result in enough cryptic epitope generation for T cell activation. Coxsackievirus downregulates cyclin D1 by increasing its degradation through the ubiquitin-proteosome pathway [62]. The ability of virus to increase cellular protein degradation could result in more cryptic epitope generation. Similarly, increasing expression of MHC and accessory molecules on cells would allow more efficient presentation of low concentrations of cryptic antigens and improve T cell sensitivity to stimulatory signals [61]. Alternatively, types of proteases can vary among distinct antigen presenting cells which might produce distinct peptide repertoires for T cell activation [63]. IFNγ and TNFα exposure alter protease expression in cells and may change the peptides produced [64]. Finally, protein-protein interactions can affect antigen processing. For example, internalization of HIV-CD4 complexes results cryptic epitope production of the CD4 molecule and autoreactivity [65, 66]. Similarly, antigen-antibody complexes may alter protease access to cleavage sites in antigens during antigen processing [67]. FcR up-take of immune complexes may deliver antigen to different compartments of the endosome pathway which may also alter antigen processing [68]. Another specific method for virus infections to cause cryptic epitopes is the viral proteases. As discussed above, coxsackievirus proteases not only cleave the viral polyprotein into individual viral proteins during viral replication, but these viral proteases also cleave cellular proteins such as eIF-4G. Another protein cleaved by coxsackievirus protease 2A is dystrophin, a contractile protein in myocytes [69]. Cleavage of dystrophin itself could result in cardiomyopathy [69], but it is also likely that the viral protease cleaves dystrophin differently than cellular proteases and this could result in cryptic epitope generation.

Innate Immunity and Autoimmunity

Innate immunity represents a constitutive or rapidly induced host response to infection which reacts broadly with many different microbial agents. This is in contrast to adaptive immunity which is highly antigen-specific. Innate immunity is usually less effective in controlling infection than the adaptive immune response and rarely is adequate to clear the invading microbe. However, innate immunity restrains microbial growth during the 7-10 days required for generation of the adaptive immune response which reduces tissue injury that might occur with uncontrolled infection. Innate effectors are generally concentrated in potential sites of microbe invasion (skin, gut, mucosa) but also are present in all tissues and the peripheral lymphoid organs. While innate immunity is important in the initial control of infection, it is now clear that innate immunity also influences the developing adaptive immune response and can determine whether autoimmunity arises or not.

Virus Receptor Signaling

As discussed above, virus cross-linking of cellular receptors is crucial for virus internalization and infection. However, virus-cellular receptor binding also initiates the host response to infection. Many virus receptors belong to the immunoglobulin, integrin, cytokine or chemokine receptor superfamilies of molecules which have important biological functions. The coxsackievirus capsid consists of 60 protomers each of which has a receptor binding site, and virus-receptor interactions have high avidity. Thus, the probability is that virus will cross-link and signal through the receptor at least as well as the receptor's natural ligand. There are several examples of virus signaling through receptor cross-linking. HIV uses CD4 and co-receptors CCR5 and CXCR4, and can activate various kinase pathways leading to increased cytokine and MMP9 induction [70-73]. Epstein-Barr virus gp350 cross-links CD21 and results in B cell proliferation and cytokine induction [74-76]. Herpesvirus uses herpesvirus entry mediator protein, a member of the TNF receptor superfamily, as its receptor and can suppress T cell proliferation and activation [77]. Coxsackieviruses employ DAF which induces calcium flux [78], activates p56lck and p59fyn and promotes T cell proliferation and cytokine induction [79, 80]. Increasing evidence indicates that signaling through DAF is immunosuppressive to CD8+ cell responses since mice lacking DAF generate aggravated T cell responses [81, 82].

Antigen-independent polyclonal T cell activation is an important host defense to infection as it rapidly induces production of pro-inflammatory cytokines without requiring activation of antigen-specific cells. These pro-inflammatory cytokines can improve antigen presentation by initiating maturation of dendritic cells and up-regulation of MHC and accessory molecules. However, this process may also predispose to autoimmunity [83, 84]. Studies demonstrate that persistent up-regulation of accessory molecules such as CD40L in the epidermis causes systemic autoimmunity, possibly through breaking of immune tolerance. Picornavirus infections induce high expression levels of IL-2 and IL-2 mRNA [85-87] and as discussed above, high IL-2 concentrations can break anergy leading to activation of autoreactive T cells.

Toll-Like Receptors

Pattern recognition receptors (PRR) are cellular molecules which recognize pathogen-associated molecular patterns (PAMPs). PAMPs are conserved microbial molecules which are found in broad ranges of infectious agents. These molecules are usually important in either microbial infection of replication, which means that they can't be readily mutated without inhibiting microbial infection [88]. Host response to PAMPs allows very rapid cytokine responses. The most recognized PPR are Toll-Like Receptors (TLR). TLR likely play an important role in infection induced autoimmunity. Certainly, experimental models of autoimmune disease inject self antigen in complete Freund's adjuvant containing LPS which would activate TLR4[89-91]. There are 12 toll-like receptors (TLR) in humans and mice which react to different molecular species[88, 92-96]. TLR are type I integral membrane glycoproteins that have an extracellular domains with variable numbers of leucine-rich repeat (LRR) motifs and conserved intracellular domains with a homologous Toll/interleukin (IL)-1 response domain [88, 97]. TLR4 recognizes the lipopolysaccharide of gram-negative bacteria while TLR2 recognizes peptidoglycan of gram-positive bacteria. Also most TLR are expressed on the plasma membrane, TLRs 3,7, 8, and 9 are expressed in the endosomal membrane [98]. TLR3 recognizes double stranded RNA. TLRs 7 and 8 recognize single stranded RNA and TLR9 recognizes CpG DNA motifs. Other TLR and their ligands are: TLR1, triacyl lipopeptides; TLR5, flagellin; TLR6, peptidoglycan; and TLR11, profiling-like molecule. Other TLR ligands are unknown. All tissues express at least one TLR, and several cells/tissues express multiple TLRs [99]. Besides expressing individual TLR, additional complexity of PAMP recognition is provided by the formation of heterodimers between different TLR, such as between TLR1/TLR6, TLR1/TLR2 or TLR2/TLR6 [100]. Different lymphoid cell populations express distinct sets of TLR. CD8+ cells express high levels of TLR3 but very low levels of TLR2 and TLR4. B cells express high levels of TLR9 and TLR10. Thus, some immune effectors may respond to some microbes but not others (reviewed in [101] and [102]). This may be especially important when considering different dendritic cells. There are two major types of dendritic cells in lymphoid tissue. These are myeloid and lymphoid/pasmacytoid dendritic cells. In the resting stage, plasmacytoid dendritic cells express TLR7 and TLR9 but not TLR3 while monocyte-derived dendritic cells express TLR3 but not TLRs7 and 9 suggesting that the different dendritic cell subsets might have distinct responses to pathogens. Generally, TLRs 3, 4, 5 and 9 are considered to preferentially activate Th1 responses while TLR2 preferentially induces Th2 immunity [102]. In addition to the type of TLR, the intensity of signaling through TLR can determine Th response. Low dose LPS stimulation of TLR4 promotes Th2 response while higher doses of ligand promote Th1 responses. Interestingly, naïve CD4+ cells may express TLR2 and TLR4 mRNA and intracellular protein but not cell-surface protein, but after activation, CD4+ cells rapidly express cell-surface TLR2 and TLR4 [103]. Only the TLR2 may be functional in these cells since TLR2 stimulation of activated CD4+ cells with bacterial lipoprotein increases IFNγ, IL-2 and TNFα expression but LPS stimulation of TLR4 has little effect.

The TLR intracellular domain contains toll-interleukin (IL)-1 response (TIR) domains which are homologous to IL-1/IL-18 receptors [88, 104]. Basically, there are two signal transduction pathways: MyD88-dependent and MyD88-independent. MyD88 is an adaptor molecule which binds to the cytoplasmic domain of TLRs 1, 2, 4, 5, 7, and 9. MyD88 recruits interleukin receptor-associated kinases (IRAK1 and IRAK4) which subsequently activates TNFR-associated factor 6 (TRAF6), and ultimately activates IKK which phosphorylates IkB. Release of IkB allows nuclear translocation of NFkB and production of pro-inflammatory cytokines (IL-1β, TNFα, and IL-6) as well as inducible nitric oxide synthetase [105, 106]. Nitric oxide has important anti-microbial activity and has been shown to inactivate coxsackievirus B3 [107]. Other molecules upregulated through MyD88 signaling are CD80 and CD86 which bind CD28 on T lymphocytes during antigen presentation [108]. MyD88-independent signaling usually uses another adaptor molecule, Toll-IL-1 receptor domain-containing adaptor-inducing interferon-beta (TRIF) and TRIF-related adaptor molecule (TRAM). TRIF binds to TLR3 and TLR4 [93, 104]. TRAM interacts with TRIF, but only in TLR4 signal pathways. The TRIF/TRAM pathways activate interferon response factors (IRF3 and IRF7) resulting in expression of type I interferons, RANTES and IP-10. MyD88 also can activate type 1 interferon gene expression through IRF5 and IRF7 [96, 104]. Only TLR4 signals through both MyD88 dependent and independent mechanisms.

In coxsackievirus infections, mice deficient in MyD88 have reduced production of pro-inflammatory cytokines; type I interferon expression is increased; and virus titers are reduced [109-111]. Cardiocytes express minimal amounts of TLR1-8 before infection, but TLR7 and TLR8 increase after infection [112]. Signaling through TLR8 activates NFkB and pro-inflammatory cytokine expression. Another TLR important in coxsackievirus infections is TLR4 which one would not expect to be activated by viruses [113]. However, IFNγ up-regulates and IL-4 down-regulates both TLR4 and TLR3 expression [114], and coxsackievirus B3 infections induce strong IFNγ responses [115].

Recently, a growing literature has arisen relative to TLR influence on immune regulation, specifically on Th17 and T regulatory cells. CD4+ cells stimulated by antigen presenting cells in the presence of TGFβ have the potential to differentiate into either Th17 or T regulatory cells Th17 cells (see [116]). In the additional presence of IL-6 and possibly IL-23, CD4+ cells differentiate into Th17 cells while in the absence of these two cytokines, differentiation is into T regulatory cells. IL-23 may not be required for the differentiation of Th17 cells but may be necessary for Th17 cell survival [96]. Th17 cells express retinoic acid orphan receptor-γt transcription factor while most Tregulatory cells express FoxP3. Th17 cells increase expression of IL-1, IL-6 and G-CSF and enhance autoimmunity in both humans and animals. Diseases associated with Th17 include rheumatoid arthritis and multiple sclerosis. While Th17 cells promote autoimmunity, Tregulatory cells suppress it. Tregulatory cells are characterized as natural or adaptive. Natural T regulatory cells are CD4+CD25+FoxP3+ and are directly generated in the thymus as a consequence of T cell ontogeny. In contrast, adaptive Tregulatory cells arise in the periphery upon antigen stimulation. These cells are also CD4+CD25+ but may or may not express FoxP3 [117]. While natural Tregulatory cells can suppress through direct cell-cell contact, the adaptive Tregulatory cells, Tr1 and Th3, primarily inhibit immunity through Il-10 and TGFβ, respectively. Various TLR affect Tregulatory cell activity. TLR8-MyD88 signaling suppresses Tregulatory cell function[118], while TLR2, and TLR5 both increase Tregulatory cell numbers and activity [119, 120]. Most studies indicate that TLR affect Tregulatory response via alterations in dendritic cell cytokine or accessory molecule expression [121]. Mice lacking CD80, CD86 and CD40 have fewer Tregulatory cells than wild-type mice [122]. IL-2, IL-4 and IL-7 stregnthen the Tregulatory response [123, 124]. However, T regulatory cells also express TLR and can be directly modulated without dendritic cell involvement [125]. Human Tregulatory cells express TLR4, 5 and 8 and do not express TLR7. Other TLR have not been determined. Mouse Tregulatory cells express TLR1, 2, 4, 5, 6, 7, and 8 but not TLR3 or 9.

TLR are not the only PRR active in microbial infections. Retinoic acid inducible protein (RIG-1) and melanoma differentiation associated gene 5 (MDA5) are two DEXD/H box RNA helicases which directly bind cytosolic viral dsRNA. These helicases contain two caspase recruiting domains (CARDs) in the N terminal portion of the molecule and activate IRF-3 resulting in type 1 interferon expression [126-128]. RIG-1 and MDA5 have different virus specificities. RIG-1 is more important in controlling Japanese Encephalitis Virus, Vesticular Stomatitis Virus and NewCastle Disease virus than picornaviruses while MDA5 has better antiviral actitivy to picornaviruses [129]. Nucleotide-binding oligomerization domain (NOD)-like receptors are also cytoplasmic PRR which recognize peptidoglycans. NOD2 recognizes both gram positive and negative bacteria but NOD1 recognizes only gram negative bacteria [130]. NOD signaling activates the MAP kinases and NFkB signal pathways.

Natural Killer T cells and γδ+ T Cells

Innate immunity is either constituitive or rapidly induced subsequent to infection and has broad reactivity to multiple microbial agents. Innate effectors include natural killer, natural killer T, and γδ+ T cells. Natural killer (NK) cells are non-T cells and lack a T cell receptor and CD3 [131]. NK cell cytotoxicity is mediated through perforin and is enhanced by type 1 interferons. The purpose for killing infected cells is to abort virus replication before mamimum progeny virus has been produced. The earlier cell killing occurs, the less virus produced and the better for the host. Killing can occur within 30-60 minutes of cell infection. NK cells express receptors which can either increase or suppress their cytotoxic activities. Killer Immunoglobulin-like (KIR) receptors recognize MHC molecules and suppress NK cytotoxicity. The ability to recognize MHC molecules provides one mechanism for distinguishing between infected/transformed and normal cells as transformation or virus infection causes down-regulation of MHC molecules [132, 133]. In opposition to the KIRs are natural cytotoxic receptors (NCR). Signaling through these receptors activate NK cells making them more cytolytic [133]. Ox40L expressed on NK cells interacts with OX40 on dendritic cells and activated T cells causing increased immune response [134].

A second population of innate lymphoid effectors are the semi-invariant natural killer T cells (iNKT cells). These effectors express a T cell receptor comprised of an invariant alpha chain (Vα14-Jα18 mice; Vα24-Jα18 humans) and one of several different beta chains (Vβ2, Vβ7 and Vβ8.2) [135]. NKT cells can either be CD4+ or CD4-. NKT cells are cytolytic, but also are potent producers of cytokines, either Th1 or Th2, which modulate the developing adaptive immune responses. iNKT cells recognize CD1 molecules, a family of non-classical MHC class I antigens. CD1 is comprised of two groups of molecules, CD1 group I and group II. Group I consists of CD1a, CD1b, CD1c and CD1e while Group II consists of CD1d [136, 137]. Most species, except mice, express both group I and II CD1 molecules, but mice express only CD1d. CD1d presents self and microbial glycolipid antigens [138, 139]. iNKT cells are not the only innate effectors responding to CD1. T cells expressing the Vγ4 T cell receptor are also CD1d restricted [140].

Innate effectors often accumulate at inflammatory sites [141-148], and can have either beneficial or detrimental effects [144, 146, 147, 149, 150]. iNKT cells promote tolerance in various autoimmune diseases and allograft transplantation [151, 152]. It is hypothesized that the success of type 1 interferon therapy in multiple sclerosis is due to the cytokine's effect on dendritic cells resulting in increased CD1, CD80 and CD40 expression, activation of iNKT cells and bias of the immune response toward a Th2 phenotype (IL-4 and IL-5) which suppresses the pathogenic Th1 response implicated in this disease [152]. However, iNKT cells might also interact with Tregulatory cells in autoimmunity suppression. iNKT cells inhibit the development of type 1 diabetes in NOD mice and nickel hypersensitivity [153, 154]. Various studies demonstrate that iNKT cells are required for the generation of T regulatory cells [154, 155]. Once generated, the T regulatory cells act independently of the iNKT cells. In the diabetes model, suppression by iNKT cells requires functional CD4+CD25+ T regulatory cells, but in this case, the iNKT cells are not required for T regulatory cell generation. Rather, the T regulatory cells are important in production of the inhibitory iNKT cell population. γδ+ T cells also have important immunosuppressive activities [156]. TLR8 and MyD88 signaling in the γδ+ T cells effectively reversed their immunosuppressive activity. As with iNKT cells, at least some studies indicate that γδ+ T cells may be necessary for induction of T regulatory cells and the maintenance of self-tolerance [157].

Conclusion

Infections are often implicated in the induction of autoimmune diseases [37, 158]. The mechanisms how infection impacts autoimmunity are less clear. Although the concept of antigenic mimicry has been around for decade, the definitive evidence that this plays a decisive role in autoimmune diseases is still lacking. Recent studies provide stronger evidence that infection alters immunoregulation. The probable pathways predominantly involve PRR and the recognition of microbial PAMPs. Thus, as reviewed by Rose [158], infection may act more as an adjuvant in promoting autoreactivity. Signaling through TLR activates NFkB up-regulates over 100 genes, many of these involved in inflammatory responses, such as accessory molecules and cytokines. Production of high levels of IL-2 by itself could reverse T cell anergy and restore functional activity to autoreactive T cells. TLR signaling directly on T regulatory cells or indirectly on dendritic cells can abrogate immunosuppression and promote both non-autoimmune and autoimmune responses. Similarly, innate effectors including iNKT and γδ+ T cells can modulate T regulatory responses so that infections which either induce or suppress the innate effectors could alter self-tolerance. In addition to PRRs, however, it is important to remember that direct interactions of microbes with cells they infect can dramatically alter immunoregulation. Virus cross-linking of cellular receptors can be a potent inducer of cytokines which may affect the balance between Th17 and T regulatory cell generation. The IL-6 and IL-1β induced in certain virus infections by virus receptor signaling should bias toward a Th17 cell response and therefore increased autoimmunity and away from the protective T regulatory cell response.

References

[1] Rueckert, R., Picronaviruses, in 3rd Ed. ed. *Fundamental Virology*, D.M.K. B.N. Fields, P.M. Howley, Editor. 1996, Lippincott-Raven: Philadelphia, PA. p. 477-522.

[2] Muckelbauer, J.K., et al., The structure of coxsackievirus B3 at 3.5 A resolution. *Structure*, 1995. 3(7): p. 653-67.

[3] Racaniello, V.R., Picornaviridae: The Viruses and Their Replication, in *Fields Virology*, D.M. Knipe, Editor. 2007, Lippincott Williams and Wilkins: Philadelphia. p. 796-838.

[4] Huber, S., T cells in coxsackievirus-induced myocarditis. *Viral Immunol.*, 2004. 17(2): p. 152-64.

[5] Carson, S.D., Receptor for the group B coxsackieviruses and adenoviruses: CAR. *Rev. Med. Virol.*, 2001. 11(4): p. 219-26.

[6] Coyne, C.B. and J.M. Bergelson, Virus-induced Abl and Fyn kinase signals permit coxsackievirus entry through epithelial tight junctions. *Cell*, 2006. 124(1): p. 119-31.

[7] Carson, S.D. and N.M. Chapman, Coxsackievirus and adenovirus receptor (CAR) binds immunoglobulins. *Biochemistry*, 2001. 40(48): p. 14324-9.

[8] Martino, T.A., et al., The coxsackie-adenovirus receptor (CAR) is used by reference strains and clinical isolates representing all six serotypes of coxsackievirus group B and by swine vesicular disease virus. *Virology*, 2000. 271(1): p. 99-108.

[9] Wang, X. and J.M. Bergelson, Coxsackievirus and adenovirus receptor cytoplasmic and transmembrane domains are not essential for coxsackievirus and adenovirus infection. *J. Virol.,* 1999. 73(3): p. 2559-62.

[10] Bergelson, J.M., et al., Coxsackievirus B3 adapted to growth in RD cells binds to decay-accelerating factor (CD55). J Virol, 1995. 69(3): p. 1903-6.

[11] Hafenstein, S., et al., Interaction of decay-accelerating factor with coxsackievirus B3. *J. Virol.*, 2007. 81(23): p. 12927-35.

[12] Spiller, O.B., et al., Coxsackie B viruses that use human DAF as a receptor infect pig cells via pig CAR and do not use pig DAF. *J. Gen. Virol.*, 2002. 83(Pt 1): p. 45-52.

[13] Ozaki, H., et al., Cutting edge: combined treatment of TNF-alpha and IFN-gamma causes redistribution of junctional adhesion molecule in human endothelial cells. *J. Immunol.*, 1999. 163(2): p. 553-7.

[14] Gauntt, C. and S. Huber, Coxsackievirus experimental heart diseases. *Front Biosci.*, 2003. 8: p. E23-35.

[15] Cornell, C.T., J.E. Brunner, and B.L. Semler, Differential rescue of poliovirus RNA replication functions by genetically modified RNA polymerase precursors. *J. Virol.,* 2004. 78(23): p. 13007-18.

[16] Rueckert, R., Picronaviruses. 3rd Ed. ed. *Fundamental Virology*, ed. B.N. Fields, D.M. Knipe, and P.M. Howley. 1996, Philadelphia, PA: Lippincott-Raven. 477-522.

[17] Kerekatte, V., et al., Cleavage of Poly(A)-binding protein by coxsackievirus 2A protease in vitro and in vivo: another mechanism for host protein synthesis shutoff? *J. Virol.*, 1999. 73(1): p. 709-17.

[18] Feuer, R., et al., Cell cycle status affects coxsackievirus replication, persistence, and reactivation in vitro. *J. Virol.*, 2002. 76(9): p. 4430-40.

[19] Feuer, R., et al., Coxsackievirus replication and the cell cycle: a potential regulatory mechanism for viral persistence/latency. *Med. Microbiol. Immunol.* (Berl), 2003.

[20] Kandolf, R., et al., Mechanisms and consequences of enterovirus persistence in cardiac myocytes and cells of the immune system. *Virus Res.*, 1999. 62(2): p. 149-58.

[21] Nugent, C.I., et al., Functional coupling between replication and packaging of poliovirus replicon RNA. *J. Virol.*, 1999. 73(1): p. 427-35.

[22] Horwitz, M. and N. Sarvetnick, Viruses, host responses, and autoimmunity. *Immunol. Rev.*, 1999. 169: p. 241-253.

[23] Savino, W., The thymus is a common target organ in infectious diseases. *PLoS Pathog.*, 2006. 2(6): p. e62.

[24] Theofilopoulos, A., The basis for autoimmunity: Part I, mechanisms of aberrant self-recognition. *Immunol. Today*, 1995. 16: p. 90-98.

[25] Pugliese, A., Central and peripheral autoantigen presentation in immune tolerance. *Immunology*, 2004. 111(2): p. 138-46.

[26] Iezzi, G., K. Karjalainen, and A. Lanzavecchia, The duration of antigenic stimulation determines the fate of naive and effector T cells. *Immunity,* 1998. 8(1): p. 89-95.

[27] Steinman, R.M., The dendritic cell system and its role in immunogenicity. *Annu. Rev. Immunol.*, 1991. 9: p. 271-96.

[28] Eriksson, U., et al., Dendritic cell-induced autoimmune heart failure requires cooperation between adaptive and innate immunity. *Nat. Med.*, 2003. 9(12): p. 1484-90.

[29] Flynn, K. and A. Mullbacher, The generation of memory antigen-specific cytotoxic T cell responses by CD28/CD80 interactions in the absence of antigen. *Eur. J. Immunol.*, 1997. 27(2): p. 456-62.

[30] Romieu-Mourez, R., et al., Regulation of MHC class II expression and antigen processing in murine and human mesenchymal stromal cells by IFN-gamma, TGF-beta, and cell density. *J. Immunol.*, 2007. 179(3): p. 1549-58.

[31] Li, W., et al., Blocked signal transduction to the ERK and JNK protein kinases in anergic CD4+ T cells. *Science,* 1996. 271(5253): p. 1272-6.

[32] Sloan-Lancaster, J., et al., Partial T cell signaling: altered phospho-zeta and lack of zap70 recruitment in APL-induced T cell anergy. *Cell,* 1994. 79(5): p. 913-22.

[33] Bendiksen, S. and O.P. Rekvig, Interleukin-2, but not interleukin-15, is required to terminate experimentally induced clonal T-cell anergy. *Scand. J. Immunol.*, 2004. 60(1-2): p. 64-73.

[34] Ohkusu-Tsukada, K., et al., Regulation of the maintenance of peripheral T-cell anergy by TAB1-mediated p38 alpha activation. *Mol. Cell Biol.*, 2004. 24(16): p. 6957-66.

[35] Fujinami, R.S. and M.B. Oldstone, Amino acid homology between the encephalitogenic site of myelin basic protein and virus: mechanism for autoimmunity. *Science*, 1985. 230(4729): p. 1043-5.

[36] Fujinami, R.S. and M.B. Oldstone, Molecular mimicry as a mechanism for virus-induced autoimmunity. *Immunol. Res.*, 1989. 8(1): p. 3-15.

[37] Rose, N.R. and I.R. Mackay, Molecular mimicry: a critical look at exemplary instances in human diseases. *Cell Mol. Life Sci.*, 2000. 57(4): p. 542-51.

[38] Schwimmbeck, P.L. and M.B. Oldstone, Molecular mimicry between human leukocyte antigen B27 and Klebsiella. Consequences for spondyloarthropathies. *Am. J. Med.,* 1988. 85(6A): p. 51-3.

[39] Schwimmbeck, P.L. and M.B. Oldstone, Klebsiella pneumoniae and HLA B27-associated diseases of Reiter's syndrome and ankylosing spondylitis. *Curr. Top Microbiol. Immunol,* 1989. 145: p. 45-56.

[40] Schwimmbeck, P.L., et al., Molecular mimicry and myasthenia gravis. An autoantigenic site of the acetylcholine receptor alpha-subunit that has biologic activity and reacts immunochemically with herpes simplex virus. *J. Clin. Invest*, 1989. 84(4): p. 1174-80.

[41] Hiemstra, H.S., et al., Cytomegalovirus in autoimmunity: T cell crossreactivity to viral antigen and autoantigen glutamic acid decarboxylase. *Proc. Natl. Acad. Sci. USA,* 2001. 98(7): p. 3988-91.

[42] Cunningham, M., et al., A study of anti-group A streptococcal monoclonal antibodies crossreactive with myosin. *J. Immunol.*, 1986. 136: p. 293.

[43] Wucherpfennig, K. and J. Strominger, Molecular mimicry in T cell-mediated autoimmunity: Viral peptides activate human T cell clones specific for myelin basic protein. *Cell,* 1995. 80: p. 695-705.

[44] Ramos-Casals, M., S. De Vita, and A.G. Tzioufas, Hepatitis C virus, Sjogren's syndrome and B-cell lymphoma: linking infection, autoimmunity and cancer. *Autoimmun. Rev.*, 2005. 4(1): p. 8-15.

[45] Vreugdenhil, G.R., et al., Analysis of antibody responses against coxsackie virus B4 protein 2C and the diabetes autoantigen GAD(65). *J. Med. Virol.*, 1999. 59(2): p. 256-61.

[46] Evavold, B., et al., Specific T cell recognition of minimally homologous peptides: evidence for multiple endogenous ligands. *Immunity,* 1995. 2: p. 655.

[47] Benoist, C. and D. Mathis, Autoimmunity provoked by infection: how good is the case for T cell epitope mimicry? Nat Immunol, 2001. 2(9): p. 797-801.

[48] Stathopoulou, E.A., et al., Cross-reaction between antibodies to the major epitope of Ro60 kD autoantigen and a homologous peptide of Coxsackie virus 2B protein. *Clin. Exp. Immunol.*, 2005. 141(1): p. 148-54.

[49] Triantafyllopoulou, A. and H.M. Moutsopoulos, Autoimmunity and coxsackievirus infection in primary Sjogren's syndrome. *Ann NY Acad. Sci.*, 2005. 1050: p. 389-96.

[50] Triantafyllopoulou, A., N. Tapinos, and H.M. Moutsopoulos, Evidence for coxsackievirus infection in primary Sjogren's syndrome. *Arthritis Rheum.*, 2004. 50(9): p. 2897-902.

[51] Youinou, P., et al., Viruses contribute to the development of Sjogren's syndrome. *Clin. Exp. Immunol.,* 2005. 141(1): p. 19-20.

[52] Gottenberg, J.E., et al., Failure to confirm coxsackievirus infection in primary Sjogren's syndrome. *Arthritis Rheum,* 2006. 54(6): p. 2026-8.

[53] Elfaitouri, A., et al., Recent enterovirus infection in type 1 diabetes: evidence with a novel IgM method. *J. Med. Virol.*, 2007. 79(12): p. 1861-7.

[54] Lonnrot, M., et al., Antibody cross-reactivity induced by the homologous regions in glutamic acid decarboxylase (GAD65) and 2C protein of coxsackievirus B4. Childhood Diabetes in Finland Study Group. *Clin. Exp. Immunol.,* 1996. 104(3): p. 398-405.

[55] Maclaren, N.K. and M.A. Alkinson, Insulin-dependent diabetes mellitus: the hypothesis of molecular mimicry between islet cell antigens and microorganisms. *Mol. Med. Today*, 1997. 3(2): p. 76-83.

[56] Marttila, J., et al., Responses of coxsackievirus B4-specific T-cell lines to 2C protein-characterization of epitopes with special reference to the GAD65 homology region. *Virology,* 2001. 284(1): p. 131-41.

[57] Ou, D., et al., Cross-reactive rubella virus and glutamic acid decarboxylase (65 and 67) protein determinants recognised by T cells of patients with type I diabetes mellitus. *Diabetologia,* 2000. 43(6): p. 750-62.

[58] Vreugdenhil, G.R., et al., Acute onset of type I diabetes mellitus after severe echovirus 9 infection: putative pathogenic pathways. *Clin. Infect. Dis*., 2000. 31(4): p. 1025-31.

[59] Cunningham, M.W., T cell mimicry in inflammatory heart disease. *Mol. Immunol.* 2004. 40(14-15): p. 1121-7.

[60] Sercarz, E., et al., Dominance and crypticity of T cell antigenic determinants. *Ann. Rev. Immunol,* 1993. 11: p. 729-766.

[61] Lanzavecchia, A., How can cryptic epitopes trigger autoimmunity? *J. Exp. Med*., 1995. 181(6): p. 1945-8.

[62] Luo, H., et al., Ubiquitin-dependent proteolysis of cyclin D1 is associated with coxsackievirus-induced cell growth arrest. *J. Virol*., 2003. 77(1): p. 1-9.

[63] Vidard, L., K.L. Rock, and B. Benacerraf, Heterogeneity in antigen processing by different types of antigen-presenting cells. Effect of cell culture on antigen processing ability. *J. Immunol*., 1992. 149(6): p. 1905-11.

[64] Gresser, O., et al., Immunocompetent astrocytes and microglia display major differences in the processing of the invariant chain and in the expression of active cathepsin L and cathepsin S. *Eur. J. Immunol.* 2001. 31(6): p. 1813-24.

[65] Caporossi, A.P., et al., Autoimmune T-cell response to the CD4 molecule in HIV-infected patients. *Viral Immunol*., 1998. 11(1): p. 9-17.

[66] Salemi, S., et al., HIVgp120 activates autoreactive CD4-specific T cell responses by unveiling of hidden CD4 peptides during processing. *J. Exp. Med*., 1995. 181(6): p. 2253-7.

[67] Simitsek, P.D., et al., Modulation of antigen processing by bound antibodies can boost or suppress class II major histocompatibility complex presentation of different T cell determinants. *J. Exp. Med*., 1995. 181(6): p. 1957-63.

[68] Driessen, C., A.M. Lennon-Dumenil, and H.L. Ploegh, Individual cathepsins degrade immune complexes internalized by antigen-presenting cells via Fcgamma receptors. *Eur. J. Immunol,* 2001. 31(5): p. 1592-601.

[69] Badorff, C., et al., Enteroviral protease 2A cleaves dystrophin: evidence of cytoskeletal disruption in an acquired cardiomyopathy. *Nat. Med*., 1999. 5(3): p. 320-6.

[70] Collman, R.G., et al., Chemokine signaling and HIV-1 fusion mediated by macrophage CXCR4: implications for target cell tropism. *J. Leukoc. Biol*., 2000. 68(3): p. 318-23.

[71] Del Corno, M., et al., HIV-1 gp120 and chemokine activation of Pyk2 and mitogen-activated protein kinases in primary macrophages mediated by calcium-dependent, pertussis toxin-insensitive chemokine receptor signaling. *Blood*, 2001. 98(10): p. 2909-16.

[72] Liu, Q.H., et al., HIV-1 gp120 and chemokines activate ion channels in primary macrophages through CCR5 and CXCR4 stimulation. *Proc. Natl. Acad. Sci. USA*, 2000. 97(9): p. 4832-7.

[73] Misse, D., et al., HIV-1 glycoprotein 120 induces the MMP-9 cytopathogenic factor production that is abolished by inhibition of the p38 mitogen-activated protein kinase signaling pathway. *Blood,* 2001. 98(3): p. 541-7.

[74] D'Addario, M., et al., Epstein-Barr Virus and its glycoprotein-350 upregulate IL-6 in human B-lymphocytes via CD21, involving activation of NF-kappaB and different signaling pathways. *J. Mol. Biol.*, 2001. 308(3): p. 501-14.

[75] D'Addario, M., et al., Binding of the Epstein-Barr virus major envelope glycoprotein gp350 results in the upregulation of the TNF-alpha gene expression in monocytic cells via NF-kappaB involving PKC, PI3-K and tyrosine kinases. *J. Mol. Biol.*, 2000. 298(5): p. 765-78.

[76] D'Addario, M., et al., Epstein-Barr virus envelope glycoprotein gp350 induces NF-kappaB activation and IL-1beta synthesis in human monocytes-macrophages involving PKC and PI3-K. *Faseb J.,* 1999. 13(15): p. 2203-13.

[77] Cheung, T.C., et al., Evolutionarily divergent herpesviruses modulate T cell activation by targeting the herpesvirus entry mediator cosignaling pathway. *Proc. Natl. Acad. Sci. USA,* 2005. 102(37): p. 13218-23.

[78] Peiffer, I., A.L. Servin, and M.F. Bernet-Camard, Piracy of decay-accelerating factor (CD55) signal transduction by the diffusely adhering strain Escherichia coli C1845 promotes cytoskeletal F-actin rearrangements in cultured human intestinal INT407 cells. *Infect. Immun.*, 1998. 66(9): p. 4036-42.

[79] Shenoy-Scaria, A.M., et al., Signal transduction through decay-accelerating factor. Interaction of glycosyl-phosphatidylinositol anchor and protein tyrosine kinases p56lck and p59fyn 1. *J. Immunol.*, 1992. 149(11): p. 3535-41.

[80] Davis, L.S., et al., Decay-accelerating factor functions as a signal transducing molecule for human T cells. *J. Immunol.*, 1988. 141(7): p. 2246-52.

[81] Liu, J., et al., The complement inhibitory protein DAF (CD55) suppresses T cell immunity in vivo. *J. Exp. Med.*, 2005. 201(4): p. 567-77.

[82] Heeger, P.S., et al., Decay-accelerating factor modulates induction of T cell immunity. *J. Exp. Med.*, 2005. 201(10): p. 1523-30.

[83] Smith, H.R., et al., Induction of autoimmunity in normal mice by thymectomy and administration of polyclonal B cell activators: association with contrasuppressor function. *Clin. Exp. Immunol.*, 1983. 51(3): p. 579-86.

[84] Mehling, A., et al., Overexpression of CD40 ligand in murine epidermis results in chronic skin inflammation and systemic autoimmunity. *J. Exp. Med.*, 2001. 194(5): p. 615-28.

[85] Chang, J.R., et al., Differential expression of TGF-beta, IL-2, and other cytokines in the CNS of Theiler's murine encephalomyelitis virus-infected susceptible and resistant strains of mice. *Virology*, 2000. 278(2): p. 346-60.

[86] Vreugdenhil, G.R., et al., Enterovirus-induced production of pro-inflammatory and T-helper cytokines by human leukocytes. *Cytokine*, 2000. 12(12): p. 1793-6.

[87] Seko, Y., et al., Expression of cytokine mRNAs in murine hearts with acute myocarditis caused by coxsackievirus B3. *J. Pathol.*, 1997. 183: p. 105-108.

[88] Abreu, M.T. and M. Arditi, Innate immunity and toll-like receptors: clinical implications of basic science research. *J. Pediatr.*, 2004. 144(4): p. 421-9.

[89] Kaya, Z., et al., Cutting edge: a critical role for IL-10 in induction of nasal tolerance in experimental autoimmune myocarditis. *J. Immunol.,* 2002. 168(4): p. 1552-6.

[90] Bebo, B.F., Jr., et al., Low-dose estrogen therapy ameliorates experimental autoimmune encephalomyelitis in two different inbred mouse strains. *J. Immunol.*, 2001. 166(3): p. 2080-9.

[91] Pelegri, C., et al., Depletion of gamma delta T cells does not prevent or ameliorate, but rather aggravates rat adjuvant arthritis. *Arthritis Rheum*. 1996. 38: p. 204-215.

[92] Netea, M.G., J.W. Van der Meer, and B.J. Kullberg, Toll-like receptors as an escape mechanism from the host defense. *Trends Microbiol.*, 2004. 12(11): p. 484-8.

[93] O'Neill, L.A., TLRs: Professor Mechnikov, sit on your hat. *Trends Immunol.*, 2004. 25(12): p. 687-93.

[94] Lauw, F.N., D.R. Caffrey, and D.T. Golenbock, Of mice and man: TLR11 (finally) finds profilin. *Trends Immunol.*, 2005. 26(10): p. 509-11.

[95] Hasan, U., et al., Human TLR10 is a functional receptor, expressed by B cells and plasmacytoid dendritic cells, which activates gene transcription through MyD88. *J. Immunol.*, 2005. 174(5): p. 2942-50.

[96] Wang, R.F., Y. Miyahara, and H.Y. Wang, Toll-like receptors and immune regulation: implications for cancer therapy. *Oncogene*, 2008. 27(2): p. 181-9.

[97] Means, T.K., D.T. Golenbock, and M.J. Fenton, The biology of Toll-like receptors. *Cytokine Growth Factor* Rev., 2000. 11(3): p. 219-32.

[98] Akira, S. and K. Takeda, Toll-like receptor signalling. *Nat. Rev. Immunol.*, 2004. 4(7): p. 499-511.

[99] Zarember, K.A. and P.J. Godowski, Tissue expression of human Toll-like receptors and differential regulation of Toll-like receptor mRNAs in leukocytes in response to microbes, their products, and cytokines. *J. Immunol.*, 2002. 168(2): p. 554-61.

[100] Schroder, N.W., et al., Heterozygous Arg753Gln polymorphism of human TLR-2 impairs immune activation by Borrelia burgdorferi and protects from late stage Lyme disease. *J. Immunol.*, 2005. 175(4): p. 2534-40.

[101] Pulendran, B., Variegation of the immune response with dendritic cells and pathogen recognition receptors. *J. Immunol.*, 2005. 174(5): p. 2457-65.

[102] Netea, M.G., et al., From the Th1/Th2 paradigm towards a Toll-like receptor/T-helper bias. *Antimicrob Agents Chemother,* 2005. 49(10): p. 3991-6.

[103] Liew, F.Y., M. Komai-Koma, and D. Xu, A toll for T cell costimulation. *Ann. Rheum. Dis.*, 2004. 63 Suppl 2: p. ii76-ii78.

[104] Vogel, S.N., K.A. Fitzgerald, and M.J. Fenton, TLRs: differential adapter utilization by toll-like receptors mediates TLR-specific patterns of gene expression. *Mol. Interv.*, 2003. 3(8): p. 466-77.

[105] Michelsen, K.S., et al., TLR signaling: an emerging bridge from innate immunity to atherogenesis. *J. Immunol.*, 2004. 173(10): p. 5901-7.

[106] Hosoi, T., et al., Bacterial DNA induced iNOS expression through MyD88-p38 MAP kinase in mouse primary cultured glial cells. *Brain Res. Mol. Brain Res.*, 2004. 124(2): p. 159-64.

[107] Lowenstein, C., et al., Nitric oxide inhibits viral replication in murine myocarditis. *J. Clin. Invest,* 1996. 97: p. 1837-1843.

[108] Horng, T., et al., The adaptor molecule TIRAP provides signalling specificity for Toll-like receptors. *Nature*, 2002. 420(6913): p. 329-33.

[109] Fuse, K., et al., Myeloid differentiation factor-88 plays a crucial role in the pathogenesis of Coxsackievirus B3-induced myocarditis and influences type I interferon production. *Circulation*, 2005. 112(15): p. 2276-85.

[110] Liu, P., et al., The tyrosine kinase p56lck is essential in coxsackievirus B3-mediated heart disease. *Nat. Med.,* 2000. 6(4): p. 429-34.

[111] Lutton, C. and C. Gauntt, Ameliorating effect of IFN-B and anti-IFN-B on coxsackievirus B3-induced myocarditis in mice. *J. Interferon Res.*, 1985. 5: p. 137-146.

[112] Triantafilou, K., et al., Human cardiac inflammatory responses triggered by Coxsackie B viruses are mainly Toll-like receptor (TLR) 8-dependent. *Cell Microbiol.*, 2005. 7(8): p. 1117-26.

[113] Fairweather, D., S. Frisancho-Kiss, and N.R. Rose, Viruses as adjuvants for autoimmunity: evidence from Coxsackievirus-induced myocarditis. *Rev. Med. Virol.*, 2005. 15(1): p. 17-27.

[114] Mueller, T., et al., Th2 cytokines down-regulate TLR expression and function in human intestinal epithelial cells. *J. Immunol.*, 2006. 176(10): p. 5805-14.

[115] Huber, S., A. Mortensen, and G. Moulton, Modulation of cytokine expression by CD4+ T cells during coxsackievirus B3 infections of BALB/c mice initiated by cells expressing the gamma-delta+ T cell receptor. *J. Virol.*, 1996. 70: p. 3039-3045.

[116] Gutcher, I. and B. Becher, APC-derived cytokines and T cell polarization in autoimmune inflammation. *J. Clin. Invest*, 2007. 117(5): p. 1119-27.

[117] Curiel, T.J., Tregs and rethinking cancer immunotherapy. *J. Clin. Invest,* 2007. 117(5): p. 1167-74.

[118] Peng, G., et al., Toll-like receptor 8-mediated reversal of CD4+ regulatory T cell function. *Science,* 2005. 309(5739): p. 1380-4.

[119] Crellin, N.K., et al., Human CD4+ T cells express TLR5 and its ligand flagellin enhances the suppressive capacity and expression of FOXP3 in CD4+CD25+ T regulatory cells. *J. Immunol.*, 2005. 175(12): p. 8051-9.

[120] Netea, M.G., et al., Toll-like receptor 2 suppresses immunity against Candida albicans through induction of IL-10 and regulatory T cells. *J. Immunol,* 2004. 172(6): p. 3712-8.

[121] Lehner, T., Special regulatory T cell review: The resurgence of the concept of contrasuppression in immunoregulation. *Immunology*, 2008. 123(1): p. 40-4.

[122] Sakaguchi, S., et al., Naturally arising Foxp3-expressing CD25+CD4+ regulatory T cells in self-tolerance and autoimmune disease. *Curr. Top Microbiol. Immunol.*, 2006. 305: p. 51-66.

[123] Thornton, A.M., C.A. Piccirillo, and E.M. Shevach, Activation requirements for the induction of CD4+CD25+ T cell suppressor function. *Eur. J. Immunol*, 2004. 34(2): p. 366-76.

[124] Harnaha, J., et al., Interleukin-7 is a survival factor for CD4+ CD25+ T-cells and is expressed by diabetes-suppressive dendritic cells. *Diabetes*, 2006. 55(1): p. 158-70.

[125] Sutmuller, R.P., et al., Toll-like receptors on regulatory T cells: expanding immune regulation. *Trends Immunol.*, 2006. 27(8): p. 387-93.

[126] Yoneyama, M., et al., The RNA helicase RIG-I has an essential function in double-stranded RNA-induced innate antiviral responses. *Nat. Immunol.*, 2004. 5(7): p. 730-7.

[127] Yoneyama, M., et al., Direct triggering of the type I interferon system by virus infection: activation of a transcription factor complex containing IRF-3 and CBP/p300. *Embo J.,* 1998. 17(4): p. 1087-95.

[128] Andrejeva, J., et al., The V proteins of paramyxoviruses bind the IFN-inducible RNA helicase, mda-5, and inhibit its activation of the IFN-beta promoter. *Proc. Natl. Acad. Sci. USA*, 2004. 101(49): p. 17264-9.

[129] Kato, H., et al., Differential roles of MDA5 and RIG-I helicases in the recognition of RNA viruses. *Nature*, 2006. 441(7089): p. 101-5.

[130] Strober, W., et al., Signalling pathways and molecular interactions of NOD1 and NOD2. *Nat. Rev. Immunol.*, 2006. 6(1): p. 9-20.

[131] Biron, C.A., et al., Natural killer cells in antiviral defense: function and regulation by innate cytokines. *Annu. Rev. Immunol.*, 1999. 17: p. 189-220.

[132] Vossen, M.T., et al., Viral immune evasion: a masterpiece of evolution. I*mmunogenetics*, 2002. 54(8): p. 527-42.

[133] Moretta, L. and A. Moretta, Unravelling natural killer cell function: triggering and inhibitory human NK receptors. *Embo J.*, 2004. 23(2): p. 255-9.

[134] Zingoni, A., et al., NK cell regulation of T cell-mediated responses. *Mol. Immunol.*, 2005. 42(4): p. 451-4.

[135] Godfrey, D.I. and M. Kronenberg, Going both ways: immune regulation via CD1d-dependent NKT cells. *J. Clin. Invest*, 2004. 114(10): p. 1379-88.

[136] Stanic, A.K., J.J. Park, and S. Joyce, Innate self recognition by an invariant, rearranged T-cell receptor and its immune consequences. *Immunology*, 2003. 109(2): p. 171-84.

[137] Maitre, B., et al., Control of the Intracellular Pathway of CD1e. Traffic, 2008.

[138] Bendelac, A., et al., Mouse CD1-specific NK1 T cells: development, specificity, and function. *Annu. Rev. Immunol.*, 1997. 15: p. 535-62.

[139] Burdin, N. and M. Kronenberg, CD1-mediated immune responses to glycolipids. *Curr. Opin. Immunol.*, 1999. 11: p. 326-331.

[140] Huber, S., D. Sartini, and M. Exley, Role of CD1d in coxsackievirus B3-induced myocarditis. *J. Immunol*, 2003. 170(6): p. 3147-53.

[141] Carding, S.R., A role for gamma/delta T cells in the primary immune response to influenza virus. *Res. Immunol.*, 1990. 141(7): p. 603-6.

[142] Carding, S.R., et al., Late dominance of the inflammatory process in murine influenza by gamma/delta + T cells. *J. Exp. Med.*, 1990. 172(4): p. 1225-31.

[143] Carding, S.R. and P.J. Egan, The importance of gamma delta T cells in the resolution of pathogen-induced inflammatory immune responses. *Immunol. Rev.*, 2000. 173: p. 98-108.

[144] Sandor, M., et al., Two waves of gamma delta T cells expressing different V delta genes are recruited into schistosome-induced liver granulomas. *J. Immunol.,* 1995. 155: p. 275.

[145] O'Brien, R., et al., Stimulation of a major subset of lymphocytes expressing T cell receptor gamma/delta by an antigen derived from Myocbacterium tuberculosis. *Cell,* 1989. 57: p. 667.

[146] Mukasa, A., et al., Evidence that the same gamma delta T cells respond during infection-induced and autoimmune inflammation. *J. Immunol.*, 1997. 159: p. 5787-5794.

[147] Olive, C., Gamma delta T cell receptor variable region usage during the development of experimental allergic encephalomyelitis. *J. Neuroimmunol.*, 1995. 62: p. 1.

[148] Peterman, G.M., et al., Role of gamma delta T cells in murine collagen-induced arthritis. *J. Immunol.,* 1993. 151(11): p. 6546-58.

[149] Roark, C., et al., Response of a gamma delta+ T cell receptor invariant subset during bacterial infection. *J. Immunol.*, 1996. 156: p. 2214-2220.

[150] Mukasa, A., et al., Gamma delta T cells in infection-induced and autoimmune-induced testicular inflammation. *Immunol,* 1998. 95: p. 395-401.

[151] Morita, M., et al., Spontaneous tolerance involving natural killer T cells after hepatic grafting in mice. *Transpl. Immunol.*, 2007. 18(2): p. 142-5.

[152] Gigli, G., et al., Innate immunity modulates autoimmunity: type 1 interferon-beta treatment in multiple sclerosis promotes growth and function of regulatory invariant natural killer T cells through dendritic cell maturation. *Immunology*, 2007. 122(3): p. 409-17.

[153] Ly, D., et al., Protection from type 1 diabetes by invariant NK T cells requires the activity of CD4+CD25+ regulatory T cells. *J. Immunol.*, 2006. 177(6): p. 3695-704.

[154] Roelofs-Haarhuis, K., X. Wu, and E. Gleichmann, Oral tolerance to nickel requires CD4+ invariant NKT cells for the infectious spread of tolerance and the induction of specific regulatory T cells. *J. Immunol.*, 2004. 173(2): p. 1043-50.

[155] Nakamura, T., et al., CD4+ NKT cells, but not conventional CD4+ T cells, are required to generate efferent CD8+ T regulatory cells following antigen inoculation in an immune-privileged site. *J. Immunol.*, 2003. 171(3): p. 1266-71.

[156] Peng, G., et al., Tumor-infiltrating gammadelta T cells suppress T and dendritic cell function via mechanisms controlled by a unique toll-like receptor signaling pathway. *Immunity*, 2007. 27(2): p. 334-48.

[157] Locke, N.R., et al., TCR gamma delta intraepithelial lymphocytes are required for self-tolerance. *J. Immunol.*, 2006. 176(11): p. 6553-9.

[158] Rose, N.R., The Adjuvant Effect in Infection and Autoimmunity. *Clin. Rev. Allergy Immunol.*, 2008.

In: Autoimmunity: Role, Regulation and Disorders
Editor: Fynn L. Vogel and L. F. Zimmermann
ISBN 978-1-60456-833-2

Chapter 8

Innate Autoimmunity: Basic Mechanisms and Clinical Association

Maria Ramos and Ming Zhang*
Department of Anesthesiology,
State University of New York (SUNY)-Downstate Medical Center,
Brooklyn, NY 11204, USA

Abstract

Innate autoimmunity refers to that innate immune system recognizes self targets and initiate inflammatory response in a similar way as with pathogens. One novel example of this innate autoimmunity is ischemia-reperfusion (I/R) injury. Recent advance in this field reveals a general mechanism of I/R injury by which ischemic stress leads to expose a highly conserved self-antigen on the cell surface, and such antigen is recognized by the innate immune system resulting in acute inflammation. Studies of different I/R models showed that reperfusion of ischemic tissues elicits an acute inflammatory response involving serum complement system which is activated by natural IgM. A monoclonal natural IgM that initiates I/R injury has been identified. This led to the subsequent identification of nonmuscle myosin heavy chain type II A and C as the self-targets in two different tissues. In addition, studies of the downstream pathway of this innate response found that IgM binds initially to ischemic antigen providing a binding site for mannan binding lectin (MBL), which subsequently leads to activation of complement and results in tissue injury. The discovery of natural IgM mediated innate autoimmunity opens up a new area of biomedical research and may lead to the development of potential interventions for I/R injury.

* Corresponding Author: Ming Zhang, M.D., Ph.D. Department of Anesthesiology, SUNY-Downstate Medical Center. 450 Clarkson Avenue, Brooklyn, NY 11203. Tel: 718-270-1413. Fax: 718-270-3928. E-mail: ming.zhang@downstate.edu

Introduction

The innate immune system provides immediately available defense mechanisms against antigens without requiring prior exposure. This system of pathogen recognition is ubiquitous in multicellular organisms from plants to humans [4]. Natural antibody, CRP, mannan-binding lectin and toll-like receptor 4 are three preformed innate immune receptors that recognize pathogenic molecular patterns and consequently activate multiple inflammatory pathways, such as complement, capable of attacking and eliminating a wide variety offending pathogens in a coordinated fashion. In addition this innate response may activate and orientate an adaptive immune response that will be aimed against persistent microorganisms [1, 3, 5]. Even though the immune system is capable of recognizing self from non-self [2], cross-reactivity may inevitably happen when such conserved patterns exist on host antigens. An example of this is that under certain circumstances, heat shock protein 70 is able to present pathogen-associated molecular patterns for toll-like receptors (TLR) and this con initiate a sterile inflammatory response [6]. Besides toll-like receptors, natural antibodies are recently demonstrated to be able to induce inflammatory response against self-antigens [6-8, 73]. This type of response is coined as “innate autoimmunity”, as the initial event is triggered by the innate recognition of self-molecules [7].

Innate Autoimmunity and the Ischemia / Reperfusion Injury

Innate autoimmunity is now known to be an important contributor to the severity of injury following an ischemic event. Ischemia/Reperfusion (I/R) injury has been implicated in many pathological entities such as myocardial infarction (MI), cerebral ischemic events, intestinal ischemia, vascular surgery, transplantation, trauma [9] and most recently its been shown to exacerbate burn wound depth [10]. The incidence of ischemic assaults in heart and brain are the highest among all diseases in the United States. About every 26 seconds, an American will have a coronary event. Coronary heart disease caused 1 of every 5 deaths in the United States in a recent survey. Each year, about 780,000 people experience a new or recurrent stroke [11]. Every year approximately 2 million people seek medical attention due to burns; about 7,000 will die due to complications [12]. Although intestinal ischemia is not as common as MI or stroke it has proven to be lethal with a mortality rate of 70-90% [13]. Given the ample spectrum of pathologies in which I/R injury have been implicated and the high morbidity and mortality caused, there have been many efforts to try to elucidate its pathogenesis and design specific interventions.

Eukaryotic cells are very sensitive to changes in oxygen supply. If hypoxic conditions ensue the cell will undergo disruptions in intracellular process that may lead to cell death if hypoxic conditions are sustained. Some of the intracellular alterations include mitochondrial dysfunction [14-16], production of reactive oxygen species (ROS) [17-20], Calcium and other ion imbalances [21], activation of kinases, proteases and lipases [22-25], damage to membrane proteins and lipids [26-37], NF-kB signaling [28-33], and activation of poly (ADP-ribose) polymerase (PARP) [34-35]. If a period of hypoxia is followed by reperfusion a phenomenon described as I/R injury will develop. Many studies confirm the mounting of an inflammatory response including, neutrophils [36-42], mast cells [43-46] and cytokines [57-50] described as the extrinsic response to I/R. An early hypothesis was that hypoxic cells activated neutrophils which by producing ROS caused the vascular reperfusion injury. However, this hypothesis was not supported by the observation of I/R injury in situations with limited number of inflammatory cells [45, 63-65] which pointed scientist toward alternative mechanisms of injury. The current view of the pathogenesis of I/R injury is illustrated in Figure 1 and explained as following [73]: For the duration of an interruption of blood flow, cells are exposed to hypoxic conditions which initiate several changes, such as these previously mentioned, that can lead to cell death through the apoptotic and the necrotic pathways. During this period there are morphological changes in the cell membrane, such as the presentation of neo-epitopes, which are recognized by natural IgM as pathological. Subsequently, complement is activated perpetuating the injury beyond that caused by the intracellular processes alone. The evidence leading to these conclusions will be further discussed.

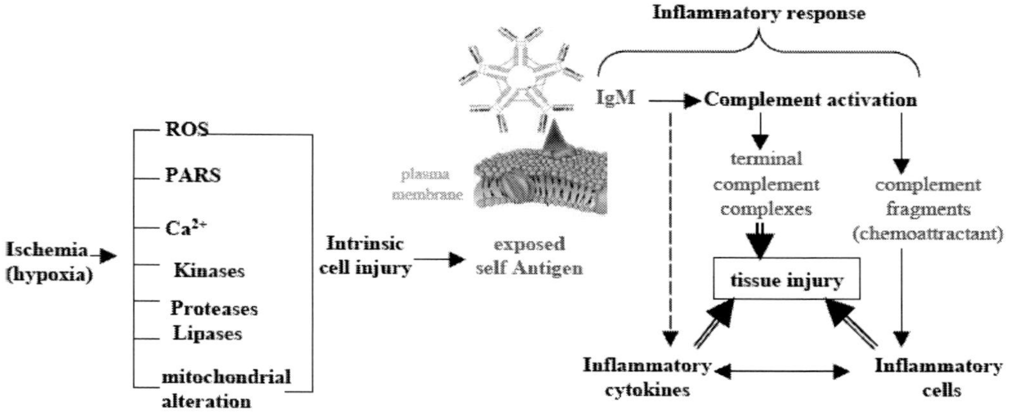

Figure 1 A model for the initiation of the inflammatory response in I/R injury [73]. Single lines indicate a pathway, double lines indicate an effector-target relationship. PARP, poly(ADP-ribose) polymerase.

Natural IgM and Complement Activation

In 1990 Weisman et al., demonstrated that pretreatment with a soluble inhibitor of complement C3b (i.e., sCR1) significantly reduced I/R injury in a heart model [66]. These findings were reproducible in other I/R models, such as the intestinal [56] and skeletal muscle model [67]. Complement can be activated by different pathways such as the classical pathway which requires antigen-antibody complexes to be activated starting at C1, alternate pathway which do not require antibody to commence C3 hydrolysis and mannan binding lectin (MBL) pathway which cleaves C2 and C4 and subsequently activates C3 convertase. In an earlier study of skeletal muscle I/R injury it was suggested that an intact classical pathway of complement was required to produce injury [70]. More recent studies using genetically modified animals demonstrated that C2 and MBL, but not C1q, are necessary for gut injury after Gastrointestinal I/R [68,72], which pointes towards the lectin pathway as the pathway for complement activation in I/R injury. MBL has been shown binding to immunoglobulins [73]. This interaction provides a route of clearance of immune complexes from the serum, and a mechanism of complement activation to Ig-coated cells [69]. Mice deficient in immunoglobulin (RAG-1$^{-/-}$) showed protection against I/R injury in the skeletal [70] and intestinal model [71]. In the same studies reconstitution of RAG-1 $^{-/-}$ mice with IgM from wild-type (WT) mouse sera restored injury. These observations led to a hypothesis that I/R injury is initiated by recognition and binding of pre-existing or natural IgM to neo-epitopes expressed by hypoxic cells (Figure 2) [70]. IgM- self antigen complex thus provides an attachment site for MBL and subsequent complement activation. Cleavage products of complement can also act as chemoattractants for inflammatory cells which will further perpetuate the injury.

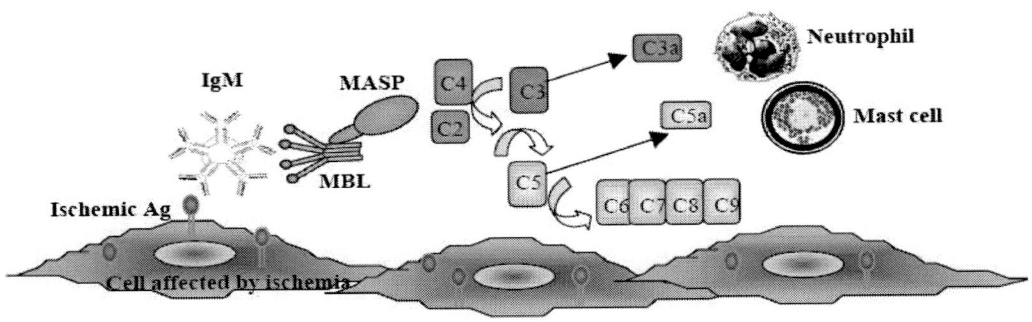

Figure 2. A model illustrating the activation of the lectin pathway by natural IgM in ischemia/reperfusion injury [73]. IgM binds to the neo-epitope in self-antigen and activates the lectin pathway of complement. The downstream events include the releasing of proinflammatory factors C3a and C5a, deposition of the membrane attack complex C5-C9, recruitment of inflammatory cells, and resulting in direct cell damage.

Specific IgM Leads the Way to the Identification of Its Self-Antigen

To identify the specific I/R IgM producing cells, a panel of hybridomas was generated from an enriched fraction of B-1 cell and their IgM products were screened in vivo for reconstitution of injury in RAG-1 $^{-/-}$ mice [74]. A single pathogenic IgM, named CM22, was identified. This was supported by the observation of deposition of IgM, C4 and C3 within reperfused intestinal tissue of antibody-deficient mice reconstituted with IgM from clone 22 but not from other hybridomas [74].

The identification of the specific IgM was crucial for the identification of the self-antigen targets (neo-epitope). IgM-antigen from RAG-1 $^{-/-}$ mice reconstituted with CM22 were isolated and separated on SDS-PAGE. A unique band was identified in ischemia treated mice. This band was analyzed by tandem mass-spectrometry. The self-antigen was identified as non-muscle myosin heavy chain II (NMHC-II) [75]. Such myosins constitute part of a superfamily of several classes of proteins expressed in almost all eukaryotic cell types. NMHC II is a molecular motor which is an important component of the cytoskeleton and plays a major role in cell motility and chemotaxis [76]. Five lines of evidence support a role for NMHC-II as the critical self-ligand in I/R injury: (1) protein sequence analysis of natural IgM-bound NMHC-II isolated from lysates of I/R injury (2)binding of NMHC-II by pathogenic CM22 in an ELISA assay (3) initiation if intestinal I/R injury in RAG-1$^{-/-}$ mice with an anti-myosin antibody (4) sequence homology with a synthetic peptide isolated from phage display library that binds pathogenic CM22 and blocks intestinal I/R injury in WT mice (5) a synthetic peptide representing a conserved region of NMHC-II binds CM22 in vitro and blocks I/R in WT mice in two distinct tissues [73].

Therapeutic Applications

Taking all this evidence into consideration a general mechanism of action can be suggested in which NMHC-II, a highly conserved self-antigen, is mobilized to the cell surface by hypoxia-related events and it is recognized by natural IgM which sets off an acute inflammatory reaction. The fact that RAG-1$^{-/-}$ mice showed decreased tissue injury after an ischemic insult [70] leads to the possibility that NMHC-II is exposed as a result of hypoxia but not necessarily cell death. This could be translated as the possibility that hypoxic cell injury may be reversible at least to the extent of the hypoxic conditions created in current experiments. It is expected that if hypoxic conditions are sustained cell death will be certain independently of the innate immune system. Inhibiting the innate immune system provides a new perspective to the development of effective therapeutic drugs that will increase survival and decrease morbidity following I/R injury.

To identify the ligand of pathogenic IgM CM-22 an M13 phage library of random 12-mer amino acid sequence was screened for potential inhibitors of the specific IgM. After four rounds of positive selection with IgM CM-22 and two rounds of negative selection with control IgM (CM-75) 10 phage clones were isolated and the nucleotide sequence of the relevant M13 gene was analyzed. All 10 clones bore a codon sequence rich in asparagines, and this also matches a conserved region in NMHC-II [75]. Clone P8 bound to IgM CM-22 with the highest efficiency, for which reason a 12-amino acid peptide was synthesized based on the phage sequence and tested in the intestinal I/R model [75]. Pretreatment of wild type mice with P8 peptide 5 min prior to reperfusion showed protective effects against I/R injury. Similar results were found in the skeletal muscle model [77].

Following the same reasoning another peptide with sequence homology to NMHC-II was synthesized. Figure 3 shows how this peptide successfully diminished I/R injury in the skeletal and intestinal models [75] [77]. More recently this peptide has proven useful in reducing inflammation in a burn model [10]. N2 peptide showed significant protection at concentrations of 32- and 40-μM, meanwhile P8 is protective at lower concentrations (10μM). This can be explained by the higher affinity of P8 relative to N2.

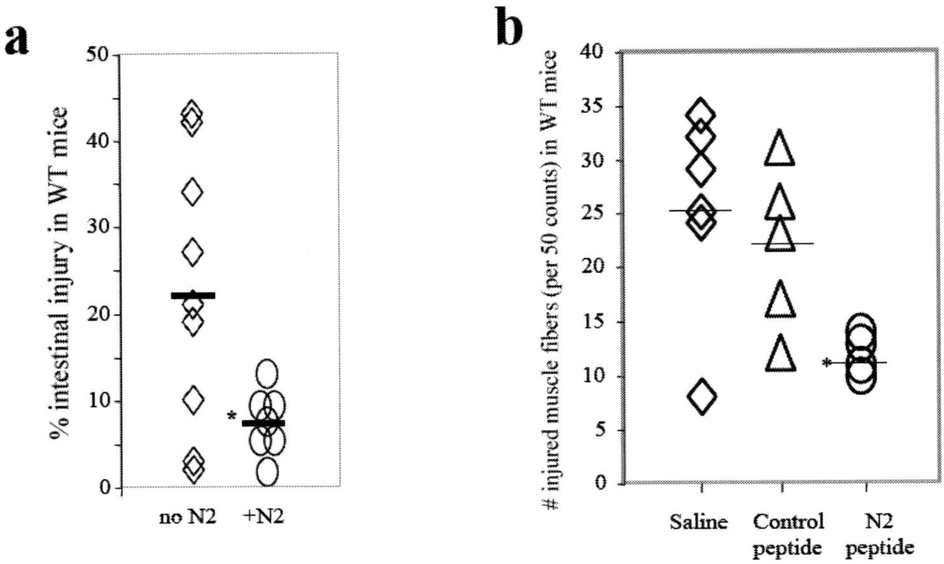

Figure 3. Treatment of mice with NMHC-II N2 peptide blocks I/R injury. (a) WT mice were treated for intestinal I/R and injected i.v. with either saline or 40 μM N2 peptide 5 min before reperfusion. Scatter plot shows injury scores of each treatment group. (b) WT mice were treated in the hindlimb model of I/R and administered either saline, control, or N2 peptide before reperfusion. Samples were stained with Masson's Trichrome for histology. Injury score based on the percentage of injured fibers per 50 counted.

Conclusion

Recent advances in this field revealed a general mechanism of I/R injury by which the ischemic cells expose a highly conserved self-antigen on the cell surface, and such antigen is recognized by natural IgM. This IgM provides a binding site for mannan binding lectin (MBL), which subsequently activates complement and results in tissue injury. The self-antigen has been characterized as non muscle myosin heavy chain type IIA and C in two different tissues. Short peptides generated from the genomic search i.e, P8 and N2 peptides may provide a new therapeutic approach to ameliorate I/R injury.

Bibliography

[1] Fearon DT, Locksley RM: The instructive role of innate immunity in the aquired immune response. *Science* (1996) 272:50-53.

[2] Janeway CA Jr: The immune system evolved to discriminate infectious nonself from noninfectious self. *Immunol. Today* (1992) 13:11-16.

[3] Medzhitov R, Janeway CA Jr: Innate immunity: the virtues of a nonclonal system of recognition. *Cell* (1997) 91:295-298.

[4] Dixon MS, Golstein C, Thomas M, van Der Biezen EA, Jones JD: Genetic complexity of pathogen perception by plants: the example of Rcr3, a tomato gene required sepecifically by Cf-2. *Proc. Natl. Acad. Sci. USA* (2000) 97:8807-8814.

[5] Vasselon T, Demeters P: Toll Receptors: a central element in innate immune responses. *Infection and Immunity* (2002) 70:1033-1041.

[6] Quintana FJ, Cohen IR: Heat shock proteins as endogenous adjuvants in sterile and septic inflammation. *J. Immunol.* (2005) 175: 2777-2782.

[7] Carroll MC, Holers VM: Innate autoimmunity. *Adv. Immunol.* (2005) 86:137-157.

[8] Krieg AM, Vollmer J: Toll-like receptors 7,8,9: linking innate immunity to autoimmunity. *Immunol. Rev.* (2007) 220:251-69.

[9] Cotran RS: ischemic and hypoxic injury. In: *Robbins Pathologic Basis of Disease.* (1999) W.B. Saunders Company, St. Louis, MO, pp. 7-12.

[10] Suber F, Carroll MC, Moore FD Jr.: innate response to self-antigen significantly exacerbates burn wound depth. *Proc. Natl. Acad. Sci. USA* (2007) 104: 3973-3977.

[11] Wayne R, *et al.* : Heart disease and stroke statistics 2008 update: A report from the AHA statistics committee and stroke statistics subcommittee. *Circulation* (2008) 117: e25-e146.

[12] Alexander AS, Adzick NS: *The surgical review* (2001), eds Krupnick KD, Kaiser AS. Lippincot, Philadelphia, pp. 123-138.

[13] Brandt JL: Mesenteric vascular disease. In: Friedman SL (Ed.), *Current Diagnosis and Treatment in Gastroenterology*. The McGraw-Hill Companies Inc., New York, Section 1.9.

[14] Halestrap AP, Clarke SJ, Javadov SA: Mitochondrial permeability transition pore opening during myocardial reperfusion- a target for cardioprotection. *Cardiovasc. Res.* (2004) 61:372-385.

[15] Madesh M, Bhaskar L, Balasubramanian KA: Enterocyte viability and mitochondrial function after graded intestinal ischemia and reperfusion in rats.*Mol. Cell. Biochem.* (1997) 167:81-87.

[16] Wu b, Ootani A, Iwakiri R *et al.*: Ischemic preconditioning attenuates ischemia-reperfusion induced mucosal apoptosis by inhibiting the mitochondrial dependent pathway in rat small intestine. *Am. J. Physiol. Gastrointest. Liver Physiol.* (2004) 286:G580-G587.

[17] Becker LB: New concepts in reactive oxygen spicies and cardiovascular reperfusion physiology. *Cardiovasc. Res.* (2004) 61:461-470.

[18] Grisham MB, Hernandez LA, Granger DN: Xanthine oxidase and neutophil infiltration in intestinal ischemia. *Am. J. Phisiol.* (1986) 251:G567-G574.

[19] Li C, Jackson RM: Reactive species mechanisms of cellular hypoxia-reoxygenation injury. *Am. J. Phisiol. Cell Physiol.* (2002) 282:C227-c241.

[20] Watts JA, Kline JA: Bench to bedside: the role of mitochondrial medicine in the pathogenesis and treatment of cellular injury. *Acad. Emerg. Med.* (2003) 10:985-997.

[21] Piper HM, Abdallah Y, Schafer C: The first minutes of reperfusion: a window of opportunity for cardioprotection. *Cardiovasc. Res.* (2004) 61:365-371.

[22] Armstrong SC: Protein kinase activation and myocardial ischemia/reperfusion injury. *Cardiovasc. Res.* (2004) 61:427-436.

[23] Um JW, Matthews JB, song JC, Mun EC: Role of protein kinase C in intestinal ischemic preconditioning. *J. Surg. Res.* (2005) 125:289-296.

[24] Zheng SY, Fu XB, Xu JG *et al.*: Inhibition of p38 mitogen-activated protein kinase may decrease intestinal epithelial cell apoptosis and improve intestinal epithelial barrier function after ischemia-reperfusion injury. *World J. Gastroenterol.* (2005) 11:656-660.

[25] El-Assal ON, Berner GE: HB-EGF enhances restitution sfter intestinal ischemia-reperfusion via P13K/Akt and MEK/ERK1/2 activation. *Gastroenterol.* (2005) 129:609-625.

[26] Spitteler G: Enzymatic lipid peroxidation- a consequence of cell injury? *Free Radic. Biol. Med.* (1996) 21:1003-1009.

[27] Moore RM, Muir WW, Granger DN: Mechanism of gastrointestinal ischemia-reperfusion injury and potential therapeutic interventions: a review and its implications in the horse. *J. Vet. Intern. Med.* (1995) 9:115-132.

[28] Kawano S, Kubota T, Monden Y *et al.*: Blockade of NF-kB improves cardiac function and survival after myocardial infarction. *Am. J. Physiol. Heart Circ. Physiol.* (2006).

[29] Misra A., Haudek SB, Knuefermann P *et al.*: NF-kB protects the adult cardiac myocyte against ischemia-induced apoptosis in a murine model of acute myocardial infarction. *Circulation* (2003) 108: 3075-3078.

[30] Yeh KY, Yeh M, Glass J, Granger DN : Rapid activation of NF-kB and AP-1 and target gene expression in postischemic rat intestine. *Gastroenterology* (2000) 118:525-534.

[31] Zou L, Attuwayabi B, Kone BC: Effects of NF-kB inhibition on mesenteric ischemia-reperfusion injury. *Am. J. Phisiol. Gastrointest. Liver Physiol.* (2003) 284:G713-G721.

[32] Chen LW, Egan L, Li ZW *et al.*: The two faces of IKK and NF-kB inhibition: prevention of systemic inflammation but increased local injury following intestinal ischemia-reperfusion. *Nat. Med.* (2003) 9:575-581.

[33] Dawn B, Guo y, Rezazadeh A *et al.*: TNF-alpha does not modulate ischemia-reperfusion injury in naive myocardium but is essential for the development of late preconditining. *J. Mol. Cell Cardiol.* (2004) 37:51-61.

[34] Szabo g, Liaudet L, Hagl S, Szabo C: Ploy(ADP-ribose) polymerase activation in the reperfused myocardium. *Cardiovasc. Res.* (2004) 61:471-480.

[35] Liaudet L, Szabo A, Soriano FG *et al.*: Poly(ADP-ribose) synthetase mediates intestinal mucosal barrier dysfunction alter mesenteric ischemia. *Shock* (2000) 14:134-141.

[36] Vinten-Johansen J: Involvement of neutrophils in the pathogenesis of lethal myocardial reperfusion injury. *Cardiovasc. Res.* (2004) 61:481-497.

[37] Schmeling DJ, Catay MG, Oldham KT *et al.*: Evidence for neutophil-related acute lung ijury after intestinal ischemia-reperfusion. *Surgery* (1989) 106:195-201; discussion 201-192.

[38] Zimmerman BJ, Grisham MB, Granger DN: Role of oxidants in ischemia/reperfusion induced granulocyte infiltration. *Am. J. Phisiol.* (1990) 258:G185-G190.

[39] Arndt H, Kubes P., Granger DN: Involvement of neutophils in ischemia-reperfusion injury in the small intestine. *Klin. Wochenschr.* (1991) 69:1056-1060.

[40] Kurtel H, Tso P, Granger DN: Granulocyte accumulation in postischemic intestine: role of leukocyte adhesion glycoprotein CD11/CD 18. *Am. J. Phisiol.* (1992) 262:G878-G882.

[41] Sisley AC, Desai T, Harig JM, Gewertz BL: Neutophil depletion attenuates human intestinal reperfusion injury. *J. Surg. Res.* (1994) 57:192-196.

[42] Carmody IC, Meng I, Shen XD *et al.*: P-selectin knockout mice have improved outcomes with both warm ischemia and small bowel transplantation. *Transplantat. Proc.* (2004) 36:263-264.

[43] Frangogianninis NG, Perrard JL, Mendoza LH *et al.*: Stem cell factor induction is associated with mast cell accumulation after canice muocardial ischemia and reperfusion. *Circulation* (1998) 98:687-698.

[44] Abonia JP, Friend DS, Austen WG *et al.*: mast cell protease 5 mediates ischemia-reperfusion injury of mouse skeletal muscle. *J. Immunol.* (2005) 174:7285-7291.

[45] Szabo A, Boros M, Kaszaki J, Nagy S: The role of mast cells in mucosal permeability changes during ischemia-reperfusion injury in the small intestine. *Shock* (1997) 8:284-291.

[46] Kanwar S, Hickey MJ, Kubes P: Postischemic inflammation: a role for mast cells in the intestine but not in the skeletal muscle. *Am. J. Phisiol.* (1998) 275:G212-G218.

[47] Frangogianninis NG, Smith CW, Entman ML: The inflammatory response in myocardial infarction. *Cardiovasc. Res.* (2002) 53: 31-47.

[48] Sorkine P, setton A, Halpern P *et al.*: Soluble TNF receptors reduce bowel ischemia induced lung permeability and neutrophil sequestration. *Crit. Care Med.* (1995) 23: 1377-1381.

[49] Cuzzocreas S, Nocentini G, Di Paola R *et al.*: Glucocorticoid induced TNF receptor family gene (GITR) knockout mice exhibit a resistance to splachnic artery occlusion (SAO) shock. *J. Leuk. Biol.* (2004) 76:933-940.

[50] Mbachu EM, Klein LV, Rubin BB, Lindsay TF: A monoclonal antibody against cytokine induced neutrophil chemoattractant attenuates injury in the small intestine in a model of ruptured abdominal aortic aneurysm. *J. Vasc. Surg.* (2002) 39:1104-1111.

[51] Arumugam TV, shiels IA, Woodruff TM *et al.*: The role of the complement system in ischemia-reperfusion injury. *Shock* (2004) 21:401-409.

[52] Horstick G: C1-esterase inhibitor in ischemia-reperfusion. *Immunobiology* (2002) 205:552-562.

[53] Patel MR, Granger CB: Pexelizumab: a novel therapy for ischemia-reperfusion. *Drugs Today* (Barc.) (2005) 41:165-170.

[54] Lutz HU, Jelezarova E: Complement amplification reviewed. *Mol. Immunol.* (2006) 43:165-170.

[55] Carroll mc, Holers VM: Innate autoimmunity. *Adv. Immunol.* (2005) 86:137-157.

[56] Hill J, Lindsay TF, Ortiz F *et al.*: soluble complement receptor type 1 ameliorates the local and remote organ injury after intestinal ischemia-reperfusion in the rat. *J. Immunol.* (1992) 149:1723-1728.

[57] Hill JH, Ward PA: The phlogistic role of C3 leukotactic fragments in myocardial infarcts in rats. *J. Exp. Med.* (1971) 133:885-900.

[58] Atkinson C. Song H, Lu B *et al.*: Targeted complement inhibition by C3d recognition ameliorates tissue injury without apparent increase in susceptibility to infection. *J. Clin. Invest.* (2005) 115:24444-2453.

[59] Karpel-Massler G, Fleming SD, Krischifink M, Tsokos GC: Human c1 esterase inhibitor attenuates murine mesenteric ischemia/reperfusion induced local organ injury. *J. Surg. Res.* (2003) 115:247-256.

[60] Sun Z, Wang X, Deng X *et al.*: The influence of intestinal ischemia and reperfusion on bidirectional intestinal barrier permeability, cellular membrane integrity, proteinase inhibitors, and cell death in rats. *Shock* (1998) 10:203-212.

[61] Wada K. Montalto MC, Stahl GL: Inhibition of complement C5 reduces local and remote organ injury after intestinal ischemia/reperfusion in the rat. *Gastroenterology* (2001) 120:126-133.

[62] Eror AT, Stojadinovic A, Starnes BW *et al.*: Antiinflammatory effects of soluble complement receptor type 1 promote rapid recovery of ischemia/reperfusion injury in rat small intestine. *Clin. Immunol.* (1999) 90:266-275.

[63] Li C, Jackson RM: Reactive species mechanisms of cellular hypoxia-reoxigenation injury. *Am. J. Physiol. Cell Physiol.* (2002) 282:C227-C241.

[64] Koike K, Moore EE, Moore FA *et al.*: CD11b blockade prevents lung injury despite neutrophil priming after gut ischemia/reperfusion. *J. Trauma* (1995) 39:23-27; discussion 27-28.

[65] Simpson R, Alon R, Kobzik L *et al.*: Neutrophil and nonneutrophil-mediated injury in intestinal ischemia-reperfusion. *Ann. Surg.* (1993) 218:444-453.

[66] Weisman HF, Bartow T, Leppo MK *et al.*: Soluble human complement receptor type 1: *in vivo* inhibitor of complement suppressing post-ischemic myocardial inflammation and necrosis. *Science* (1990) 249:146-151.

[67] Lindsay TF, Hill J, Ortiz F *et al.*: Blockade of complement activation prevents local and pulmonary albumin leak after lower torso ischemia-reperfusion. *Ann. Surg.* (1992) 216:677-683.

[68] Hart ML, Ceonzo KA, Shaffer LA *et al.*: Gastrointestinal ischemia-reperfusion injury is lectin complement pathway dependent without involving C1q. *J. Immunol.* (2005) 174:6373-6380.

[69] Arnold JN, Dwek R, Rudd P, Sim R: Mannan binding lectin and its interactions with immunoglobulins in health and in disease. *Immunol. Letters* (2006) 106:103-110.

[70] Weiser MR, Williams JP, Moore FD *et al.*: Reperfusion injury of ischemic skeletal muscle is mediated by natural antibody and complement. *J. Exp. Med.* (1996) 183:2343-2348.

[71] Williams JP, Pechet TT, Weiser MR *et al.*: Intestinal reperfusion injury is mediated by IgM and complement. *J. Appl. Phisiol.* (1999) 86:938-942.

[72] Zhang M, Takahashi K, Alicot EM *et al.*: Activation of the lectin pathway by natural IgM in a model of ischemia/reperfusion injury. *J. Immunol.* (2006) 177:4727-4734.

[73] Zhang M, Carroll MC: natural antibody mediated innate immune response. *Mol. Immunol.* (2007) 44:103-110.

[74] Zhang M, Austen WG Jr., Chiu I *et al.*: Identification of a specific self-reactive IgM antibody that initiates intestinal ischemia/reperfusion injury. *Proc. Nattl. Acad. Sci.* USA (2004) 101:3886-3891.

[75] Zhang M, Alicot EM, Chiu I *et al.*: Identification of the target self-antigens in reperfusion injury. *J. Exp. Med.* (2006) 203:141-152.

[76] Even-Faitelson L, Rosenberg M, Ravid S: PAK 1 regulates Myosin II-B phosphorilation filament assembly, localization and cell chemotaxis. *Cell Signal* (2005) 17:1137-11348.

[77] Chan RK, Verna N, Afnan J *et al.* : Attenuation of skeletal muscle reperfusion injury with intravenous 12 amino acid peptides that bind to pathogenic IgM. *Surgery* (2006) 139:236-243.

In: Autoimmunity: Role, Regulation and Disorders
Editor: Fynn L. Vogel and L. F. Zimmermann
ISBN 978-1-60456-833-2

Chapter 9

MHC-Anti MHC-Receptor Interactions Regulate Autoimmune Reactivity

Bent Rubin
Institut de Sciences et Technologies du Médicament de Toulouse
UMR 2587 CNRS-Pierre Fabre
3, rue des Satellites, 31400 Toulouse, France

Abstract

Major histocompatibility complex class I or class II molecules (MHCI or MHCII) are cell surface proteins involved in cell-cell interactions in the immune system, and among other body-cells. Anti-MHC receptors may be germ line encoded like killer cell activating receptors (KAR) or killer cell inhibitory receptors (KIR) expressed in particular on NK and NKT cells but also on some T lymphocytes. Anti-MHC receptors on T lymphocytes are rearranged from V, D, J, and C gene segments encoding antigen T-cell receptors (TCR), which react with peptides associated with the MHCI or MHCII binding groves. Among the more than 10^{12} different possible TCR molecules, several bind self-peptide-MHC molecules with high avidity. Such T cells are deleted in the thymus by negative selection, and in principle only non-self reacting T cells emigrate from the thymus. However, thymus negative selections are not infallible, and self-reactive T cells do enter the periphery, and some aggressive, auto-reactive T cells induce autoimmune diseases. We will discuss four examples of auto-reactivity: 1) TCR anti-TCR reactivity in experimental autoimmune encephalomyelitis (EAE) and immunity against T-cell lymphomas, 2) auto-reactivity to self-proteins with modulated amino acids in rheumatoid arthritis, 3) the role of harmless autoimmune reactions in natural immunity, and 4) NKT cell – dendritic cell – NK cell interactions in autoimmune reactions against spontaneous tumors and in type I Diabetes. We will attempt to formulate a strong point for the important role of MHC anti-MHC reactions in the regulation of autoimmune reactivity.

Introduction

Communication between individuals of a given species as well as between cells within an individual takes place via emitters from one individual/cell releasing messenger molecules, which are received by receptors on other individuals/cells. Major histocompatibility complex class I or class II molecules (MHCI or MHCII) are cell surface proteins involved in cell-cell interactions in the immune system, and among other body-cells. The importance of these interactions can be seen from the finding that MHC molecules can be traced back in evolution to bony fish, and it appears that receptor molecules with reactivity to MHC molecules have co-evolved with MHC molecules in these species [1, 2]. Reversely, MHC proteins can serve as receptors for physiological hormones like insulin or glucagons [3]. However, a major function of MHC molecules is to present "antigenic fragments" to T lymphocytes, and thereby initiate cellular and humoral, adaptive immune responses. The anti-MHC receptors may be germ line encoded like killer cell activating receptors (KAR) or killer cell inhibitory receptors (KIR) expressed in particular on NK and NKT cells [4]. T lymphocytes have rearranged anti-MHC receptors encoded by V, D, J, and C gene segments. Most αβ T cell receptors (TCRαβ) react with peptides associated with the MHCI or MHCII binding groves [5]. However, the antigen-binding site on TCRαβ heterodimers reacts with peptide structures as well as other structures like haptens, or sugar-moieties (6]. A specialized subset of T cells, the NKT cells, reacts with glycolipid molecules associated with particular non-classical MHCI molecules, the CD1 proteins [7]. Yet another subset of T cells bearing TCRγδ heterodimers react with small molecular weight phospho- or amido-entities, which may or may not be associated with the MHC-binding grove [8]. These ligand-TCRγδ interactions may resemble the interactions between TCRαβ and super-antigens, where the super-antigens react with non-binding site structures on both TCR and MHC molecules [9].

The rearrangement process among TCR gene segments allow for an αβ or γδ TCR repertoire of the range 10^{12} – 10^{15} possible TCR:s [5]. Among all these TCR, several bind self-peptide-MHC molecules with high avidity. T cells bearing such receptors may destroy body tissue due to their potential as killer cells or cytokine producing cells. In an attempt to diminish or avoid anti-self reactivity, i.e. autoimmune reactions, precursor-T cells are selected in the thymus, and in principle only non-self reacting T cells emigrate from the thymus. However, thymus positive and negative selections are not infallible, and self-reactive T cells do enter the periphery [10]. Many of these cells do no harm to the body, and possible reasons for this will be discussed in our paper. In contrast, some aggressive, auto-reactive T cells (called driver T cells) may induce autoimmune diseases [11]. To counteract the activity of such T driver cells, a fourth type of T cells is involved in the regulation of immune responses, the regulator T cells expressing TCRαβ [12]. These T_{reg} cells dampen the activity of autoimmune, driver T cells.

αβ and γδ TCR heterodimers are composed by transmembrane polypeptide chains with a very high degree of variability but with very short cytoplasmic tails, meaning that they are unable to connect with the intracellular signaling machinery [13, 14]. Therefore αβ and γδ TCR is associated non-covalently with CD3γ, δ, ε and ζ molecules, which collectively constitute the signal transmission CD3 complex. The energy produced by the interaction between the variable region of the TCR and its ligand can be transmitted to the interior of the

T cells by a series of allosteric structural changes in the extracellular part of the TCRβ chain followed by structural changes in the cytoplasmic tail of the CD3ε chain [15]. These changes allow the CD3ε chain to connect to the adapter protein Nck and thereby to the signaling machinery [16]. Like KAR and KIR molecules, it appears that TCR-reactivity in some way is tuned to MHC reactivity, i.e. TCR molecules may have a biased reactivity to MHC molecules. Thus, both thymocytes and peripheral T cells have partially phosphorylated CD3ζ chains, implicating that they are partially or recently activated [17, 18]. Thymocytes learn to react with low-medium avidity to self-peptides associated with MHC molecules in the thymus. Such self-reactive T cells recognize foreign antigenic peptides by cross-reactivity [19]. The biased reactivity of TCR against MHC proteins and the selection processes leading to a T-cell repertoire which in principle do not react with self, were two major arguments behind the self non-self discrimination phenomenon [20]. In contrast, if a major function of T cells is to survey the health of the different cells in the body (whether the cells are senescent, damaged by physical means or undergoing apoptosis, or transformed into tumor cells), then the low-medium reactivity of T cells with self pMHC is a normal beneficial and necessary process [4, 5]. $CD4^+CD25^+$ T_{reg} cells that control thymus-escaped, self-reactive T cells, are also selected in the thymus. It appears that expression of AIRE on thymic stromal cells, and of FOXP3 by maturing T_{reg} cells play an important role in this process. Compared with the thymic selection of conventional T cells, the selection of T_{reg} cells requires agonistic interactions of higher avidity between T cell receptors in developing thymocytes and self-peptide/MHC on thymic stromal cells [21].

As discussed above, the TCR on normal T cells have been selected to have relatively low avidity reactions with their ligands. Therefore, a certain number of TCR molecules on T cells and of ligands on the antigen-presenting cells must be available in order to activate full T-cell reactivity [22-24]. Thus, T-cell responses pose two major problems: 1) How does a T cell with its clonal receptors react with a few antigenic peptides associated with MHC molecules presenting mostly peptides from self-proteins, and 2) how does low avidity TCRαβ heterodimers attain sufficient binding efficiency to initiate ligand-specific signal transduction [25]. One appealing hypothesis (among others) is that during the recognition event, specific TCR receptors aggregate and associate with other co-receptor molecules and integrins in specialized surface membrane areas [26, 27]. These, so-called micro-domains, are in contact with similar surface membrane structures on the antigen-presenting cell (APC), thereby concentrating MHC molecules with relevant peptides to the TCR. TCR-ligand interactions may also be enforced by the activity of co-receptors like 1) CD4/CD8 molecules, which react with MHCII and MHCI, respectively, and 2) CD28 molecules which react with CD80/86 ligands on APC [28]. The CD4 and CD8 co-receptors are associated with protein tyrosine kinases like Lck, and these initiators of phosphorylation cascades are concentrated to the immunological synapse. This molecular rearrangement creates an optimal "phosphorylation milieu", where tyrosine phosphatases, like CD45, are excluded [see 29].

Among APCs are B cells, macrophages and dendritic (DC) cells, and these cells are responsible for the processing and presentation of either sufficient amounts of antigenic peptides to induce immune responses of T cells, or insufficient amounts of peptides to maintain tolerance or ignorance. The phagocytic capacity of APCs is important for these functions, because pathogens or their products enter phagocytes as a first defense system.

However, phagocytosis also is a mean to get nutrition. Thus, this possibly original function of phagocytosis was designed to degrade and catalyze sugars, lipids and proteins to their simplest building blocks. Such processes would not leave antigenic peptides for interactions with MHC molecules. It is outside the scope of the present article to go into details with these processes. It suffices to say that these phagocytosis processes are regulated [in APCs in contrast to e.g. neutrophils] by activation of toll-like receptors (TLR) on APC, by different compartments within the APC and by the stimulation of ligand-receptor pairs on the APCs like CD40 (CD40L). The end result is to have exactly the right amount of peptide-MHC complexes on the APC-surface to induce reactivity or tolerance/ignorance [30-35].

The purpose of this chapter is to summarize recent work on immune regulation by different T-cell subsets, and their collaboration with cells of the innate immune system. These regulations are controlled by MHC anti-MHC interactions and mediated by cytokine-anti-cytokine receptor interactions. However, whereas such regulations should dampen autoimmune reactions against normal self-components, beneficial autoimmune reactions against molecular structures specific to developing tumor cells, should be maintained. Thus, the immune system is confronted with a delicate balance between beneficial autoimmune reactivity towards cancer cells, and harmful autoimmune reactions against normal, healthy self-constituents.

1. Collaboration between the Innate and Adaptive Immune Systems

Helper T (Th) cells trigger differentiation of precursor cells into CD8$^+$ cytotoxic T lymphocytes (CTL) or into antibody-producing B cells. So-called Th1 cells induce preferentially the production of IL-2 and IFNγ, and the differentiation of CTL, whereas Th2 cells induce mostly the production of IL-4, IL-5 and IL-13 and the differentiation of B cells into plasma cells producing different antibody isotypes [36]. In order to elicit such responses, the antigens had to be in the form of cells, particles or aggregates, or emulsified in adjuvants such as Freund's adjuvants or aluminium salt precipitates [37]. A unifying concept of these phenomena was proposed by the late Charlie Janeway [38]: The innate immune system, natural killer T cells (NKT), NK cells, dendritic cells (DC), macrophages, granulocytes interacts with pathogen-associated molecular patterns by means of TLR [39], and secretion of inflammatory cytokines induce priming of subpopulations of CD4$^+$ Th cells (Th1, Th2, Th17). Immediately after infection, NKT cells release preformed IFNγ and IL-4 directing Th1 and Th2 cell differentiation, respectively, and DC produces IL-12, which induces Th1 priming and NK cell production of IFNγ and cytotoxicity [40, 41], see Figure 1. In addition, DC differentiates from immature, phagocyting cells to mature, non-phagocyting cells with increased levels of co-stimulatory molecules such as MHCII, CD40, CD80 and CD86. It is interesting to note (in particular in the context of this book) that whereas stimulation of the innate immune system may greatly help the initiation of adaptive cellular and humoral immune responses, the activation of the innate immune system may be a great risk due to the fatal cytokine storm that may issue [42, 43]. Thus, viral infection or poly(I:C) treatment of T-cell deficient mice cause death within a week. Adaptive immune T cells of either CD4$^+$ Th,

$CD8^+$ CTL or $CD4^+CD25^+$ T_{reg} type can down-regulate the activity of the innate immune system by a cell-cell contact and MHCII dependent mechanism [43]. Below, several examples of interactions between the innate and adaptive immune system in the induction of autoimmunity will be discussed.

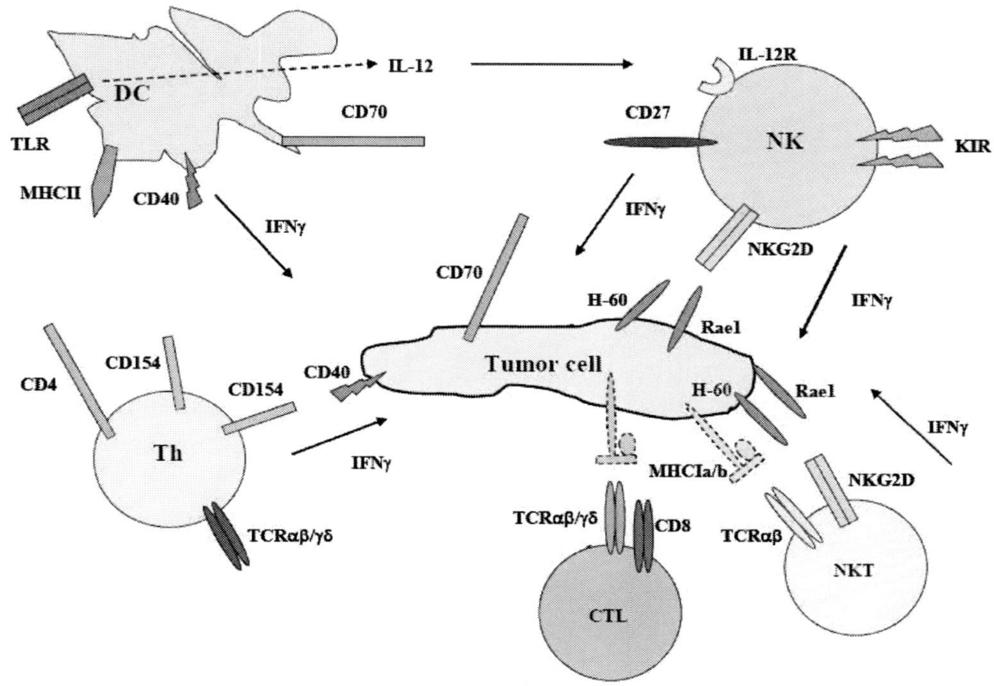

Figure 1. Interactions between the innate and the adaptive immune systems.

Cells from the innate immune system, DC, NK and NKT cells, initiate, cooperate and regulate the activity of adaptive immune cells like $CD4^+$ Th and $CD8^+$ CTL. The interactions between MHC or MHC-like proteins and anti-MHC receptors like CD4, CD8, KAR, KIR and TCR activate cellular crosstalk via release of cytokines like IFNγ.

2. Role of Natural Immunity on Autoimmune Reactions

Normal individuals express various amounts of immunoglobulins (Ig) in their body fluids [44]. These antibodies play an important role in induction of immune responses, and they have been thought of as a network of idiotypes and anti-idiotypes [45]. One example is that injection of purified, antigen-specific IgM antibodies (antigen-free, e.g. monoclonal antibodies) into naïve mice induces a specific antibody response with similar antigen-specificity whether against sheep red blood cells, dextran or trinitrophenol (TNP) hapten [40]. With the development of inbred mouse strains in specific pathogen-free (SPF) conditions, it became apparent e.g. that mice carrying transgenic TCRαβ genes encoding autoreactive αβTCR have a much higher frequency of autoimmune diseases, if raised in conventional compared to SPF conditions [47, 48]. Thus, natural immunity and/or cross-reactions between environmental antigens and the immune system may change the balance between beneficial and harmful autoimmune reactions.

We have observed two phenomema related to this issue during the last 15-20 years: 1) change in magnitudes of allogeneic T-cell responses, and 2) a much higher efficiency of protective immune responses against tumor cells in mice housed in conventional (conv.) compared to SPF conditions. We compared allogeneic T-cell responses in the two types of mice. As can be seen in Figure 2, it appears that T cells from conv. and SPF conditions respond equally well to allogeneic stimulator cells, whether the latter cells come from one or the other source. Thus, the repertoire of T-cell reactivities is not different in the two conditions. However, quantitatively allogeneic stimulator cells elicited much higher responses, when they derived from conv. mice. Furthermore, it seems to be DC:s and macrophages from conv. mice which are more potent stimulators, and the augmented stimulatory capacity was related to the increased expression by the stimulator cells of co-stimulatory molecules like MHCII, CD40, CD80 and CD86 (not shown). Thus, APC from mice raised under conv. conditions are probably activated via Toll-like receptors reacting against viral and bacterial "danger" ligands such as DNA, RNA, glycolipids, lipoproteins or proteins [39].

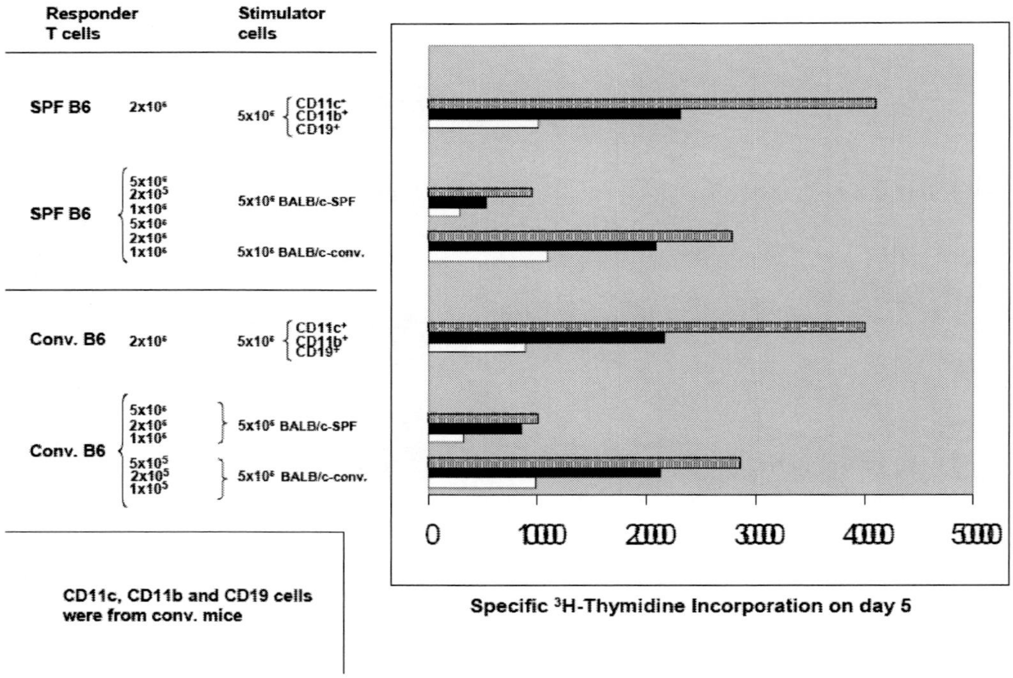

Figure 2. Allogeneic T-cell responses of conventional and SPF mice.

Responder T cells were purified using anti-MIg beads from spleens of mice raised under conventional or SPF conditions. They were analyzed in nthree different concentrations against Mitomycin-C treated stimulator cells from histoincompatible BALB/c mice from either conventional or SPF environment. Stimulator cells from conventional mice were purified using either anti-CD11c, anti-CD11b or anti-CD19 mAb beads.

We could find no reports on changed autoimmunity in conv. versus SPF mice (except in transgenic mice). Therefore, we investigated whether there were differences in frequency and/or activity of $CD4^+CD25^+$ T_{reg} cells in these mice; no differences were found (not shown). In order to analyze a functional autoimmune response against T lymphoma cells in the two types of mice, we immunized conv. or SPF mice with mitomycin C-treated L12R4 tumor cells. Normally, such an immunization induces long-lived protection against the tumor cells [49, 50]. As depicted in Figure 3, immunization of conv. mice protects against challenge with live tumor cells, thus confirming previous results. However, surprisingly immunization of SPF mice did only induce partial protection. The immune cells from conv., protected mice could transfer protection against the same L12R4 lymphoma cells (but not to other tumor cells; not shown), and the most efficient effector cells were $CD8^+$ T cells, NKT cells and DC:s. B cells and NK cells had no effect (not shown). Thus, it appears that immunization with mitomycin C-treated tumor cells induces a state of specific tumor protection, which looks quite similar to the spontaneous tumor protection described by Crui et al. [51, 52].

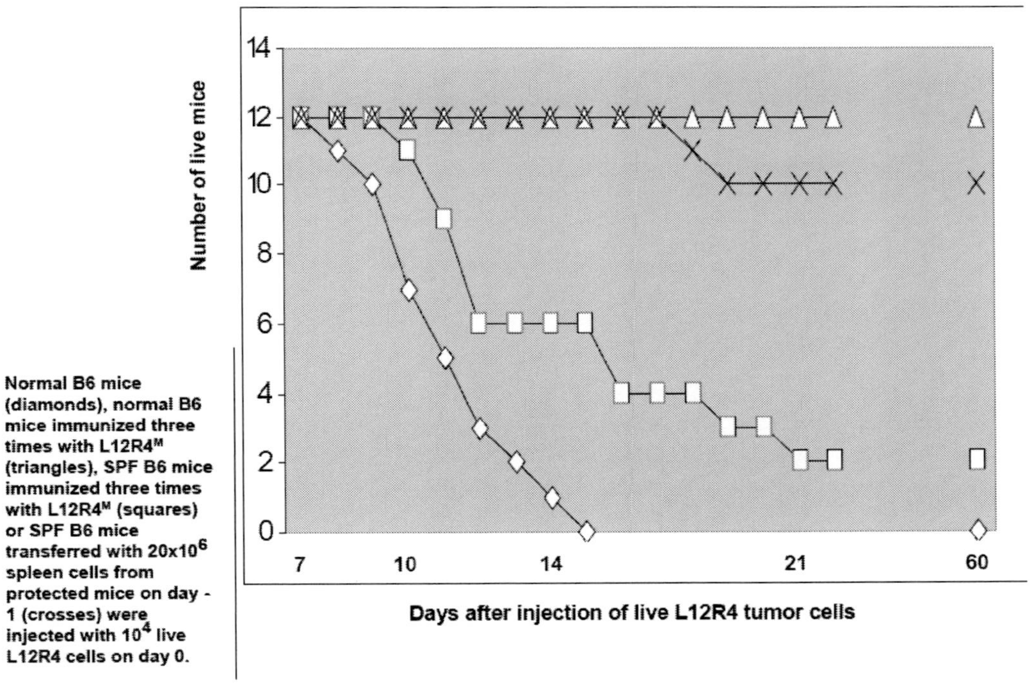

Figure 3. Natural Immunity augments protection against tumor cells.

Very interesting, induction of this tumor protection is dependent on the activation state of the animals. In conv. mice, the natural immunity is activated, and immunization with L12R4 lymphoma cells induces both specific and "non-specific" protection. Comparison of in vitro reactivity of immune cells from conv. and SPF mice show no difference in response to TCR-

Vβ12 peptide (p67-78, ref 50) (Figure 4a), whereas only immune cells from conv. mice protect against live L12R4 cells in vivo (Figure 4b).

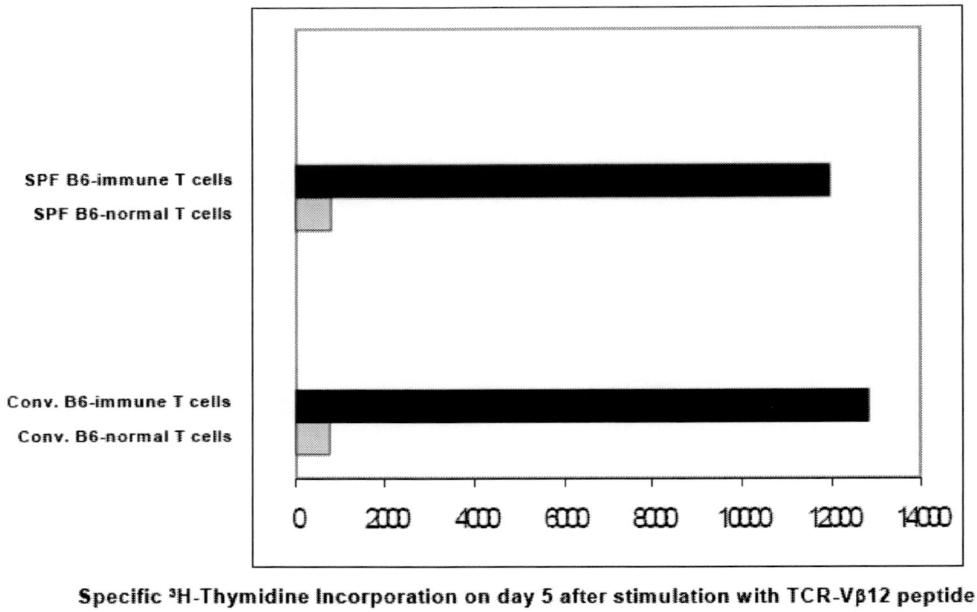

A

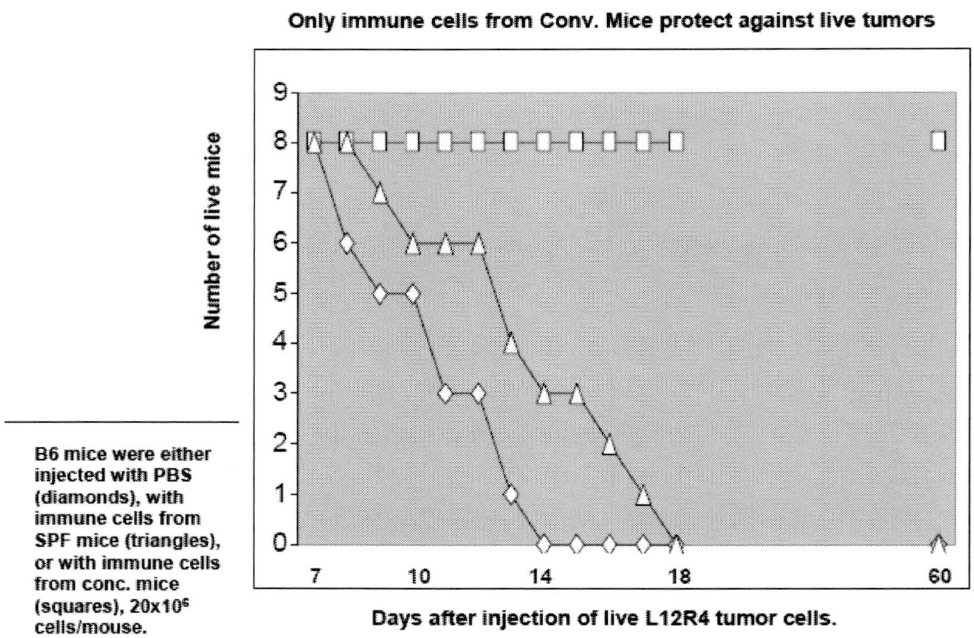

B

Figure 4. TCR-Vβ12 specific T-cell proliferation of cells from conv. or SPF mice.

Our explanation for these observations is that the innate immune system is much more activated in conv. mice compared to SPF mice. Such a hypothesis is supported by the finding that B6 mice carrying a transgenic TCR against a LCMV-epitope are only protected against B16 melanoma cells expressing the LCMV-epitope, if the mice were pre-immunized with live LCMV [53].

Natural immunity is defined as responses to naturally occurring virus, bacteria or parasites [54]. However, deliberate infections with different strains of mycobacteria, salmonella, streptococca, trypanosome, schistosoma mansoni parasites, and mouse hepatitis virus or gammaherpes virus [55, 56] may influence autoimmunity. Many of these microorganisms have glycolipids as cell-surface constituents, and such components may activate NKT cells when associated with CD1d molecules. Other products of microorganisms may activate Toll-like receptors, and thereby induce production of cytokines by DC:s and macrophages [39]. These cytokines may influence whether subsequent T-cell responses develop into Th1, Th2, Th17 (T_{reg}) subset manifestations. A recent example is that Flagellin from salmonella or Legionella bacteria is recognized by TLR5, which causes augmented production of IL-12 and decreased production of IL-10 and thus shaping the immune response of flagellated organisms towards Th1 type responses [57].

All together, it appears that an individual is much better protected by the positive and negative effects of the immune system, if they live in conventional environment and eat nutrients from none-sterilized, natural sources.

There are certain problems with these explanations, however. First of all, it has been shown that DCs can phagocytose apoptotic cells without being activated. This means that such DCs may present self-peptides to T cells in a non-immunogenic form [33]. If DCs take up foreign antigen and self-apoptotic cells at the same time, the antigen-specific T cells are not activated. In contrast, if the antigen is internalized together with TLR-ligand expressing bacteria, the adaptive immune system mounts a strong antigen-specific T-cell response. It seems that DCs may distinguish between non-TLR associated antigen inducing anergy/tolerance, and TLR-associated antigen, which is immunogenic [33].

In our vaccination model for induction of immunity and memory against tumor cells, the events do not exactly follow the logics of the above findings: 1) Immunization with mito-C treated L12R4 cells (apoptotic cells) induces an autoimmune CD8 T-cell response against the tumor cells; this response is performed by T cells that should have been eliminated in the thymus or controlled by specific T_{reg} cells, since the thymus has overwhelming amounts of APC that have phagocytized large amounts of TCR from negatively selected T cells. However, the amount of Vβ12-peptides presented in the thymus may be sufficient only to "eliminate" high avidity Vβ12-specific T cells. Thus, when immunizing with 20×10^6 L12R4 T-lymphoma cells, each expressing 10-50,000 Vβ12 TCR molecules at the cell-surface, the mouse is challenged with about 10^{12} Vβ12 TCR chains. This may be enough to activate medium-low avidity Vβ12-specific T cells. 2) If we immunize with live (or mito-C treated) L12R4 cells emulsified in complete Freund's adjuvant (CFA) and boost with L12R4 cells in incomplete Freund's adjuvant (IFA) 2 weeks later, no protective immunity is induced. This holds true for mice in both conv. or SPF conditions. In contrast, whereas the protective vaccination regime with mito-C treated tumor cells does not elicit L12R4-specific antibody production, the CFA vaccination scheme induces a strong antibody response. The anti-L12R4 antibodies are directed mostly against lymphoma cells in general (i.e. "non-specific") though there appears to be low amounts of anti-TCR clonotype antibodies produced. As expected, these hyperimmune antisera did not transfer protection against L12R4 cells; furthermore, sera from L12R4-protected mice do not transfer protection to naïve mice by themselves or together with immune cells [58]. CFA contains heat-killed mycobacteria, so immunization with L12R4 cells in CFA should have all the ingredients for a powerful vaccine. We did analyze whether spleen cells or draining popletal and inguinal lymph cells inhibited protection by L12R4-immune cells. However, no evidence of induction of regulatory T, B, or DC/macrophages was obtained. Rather it looks like the two vaccination regimes reflect the old dichonomy concerning induction of cellular immune responses by the i.v. or i.p. routes with live/inactivated cells, and induction of humoral immune responses by s.c. vaccination with adjuvant [37].

3. The Innate Immune System Regulates MHCI Expression on Tumor Cells

T lymphocytes, NK and NKT cells are involved in the protection against outgrowth of neoblastic cells. Spontaneous tumor cells are self-cells with abnormalities caused by structural changes in or altered levels of expression of house-hold proteins. These abnormalities may be due to irreversible genomic instability in the tumor cells, or to reversible pressure exerted on regulatory elements for genes encoding cell growth factors [59, 60]. Spontaneous tumor cells with either structurally changed membrane proteins or with changed expression levels of particular surface proteins have to be recognized by the immune system. Tumor-specific "antigens" have to activate the innate and adaptive immune system, the former by so-called danger signals, and the $CD4^+$ helper T cells by tumor-specific "antigens" presented by MHCII molecules. This may happen by endogenous MHCII molecules, if the tumor cells are MHCII positive, or by cross-presentation by MHCII positive, professional APC that have endocytozed dying tumor cells. Once the innate and adaptive immune systems are activated, effector cells (B cells, CTL or activated macrophages) and effector molecules (antibodies and cytokines) interact with and destroy the tumor cells by direct or antibody-mediated cytotoxicity [61-63]. The activating receptors (KAR and TCR) on NK and NKT cells interact with MHCI-like molecules presenting glycolipids or peptides (CD1, H60, Rae-1) [64]. Such MHCI-like molecules are often expressed in increased quantity on tumor cells. The activity of NK and NKT cells is strictly controlled as these cells are endowed with strong cytotoxic capacity, and they can release large quantities of cytokines upon stimulation. This activity is controlled by KIR, which are receptors linked to inhibitory signaling adaptor molecules [4]. NK and NKT cells (and $CD8^+$ CTL) express many different KIR molecules and the sum and activity of KIRs on the effector cells are related to the MHC haplotype of the cells [65]. Consequently, it is difficult to predict what level of MHCI molecules would be advantageous for the tumor cells. High levels of MHCI expression may suppress CTL responses due to the action of inhibitory receptors [4], intermediate levels of MHCI expression would favor CTL killing, and low levels of MHCI expression favors NK cell cytotoxicity [5, 66]. At the start of neoblastic cell development, it would be an advantage for the tumor cells to maintain high levels of MHCI expression as the frequency of tumor-specific CTL is very low, and the number of NKT and NK cells is high.

In order to cope with immune destruction, tumor cells have developed several escape strategies, many of which involve down-regulation of MHCI molecules or other molecules of the antigen-presenting machinery [59, 60, 67-70]. Consequently, tumor cells do not express tumor-specific antigens in an immunogenic way on the outer membrane, and thus they cannot be recognized by CTL. However, NK cells, NKT cells, polymorphonuclear leukocytes (PMN) and macrophages/DC may go into action against MHC^{low} tumor cells, as the former cells do not recognize tumor cells via peptide/MHCI ligands [51, 52, 71]. Other escape mechanisms used by tumor cells are e.g. release of inhibitory cytokines or expression of Fas.

So, how is the expression of MHC molecules controlled? MHCI antigens are expressed at various levels by all cells in the body from about day 12 of embryonic life with certain exceptions like brain, renal tubular cells or pancreatic acinar cells [72, 73]. Thus, MHCI expression is regulated and may change in response to the environment. It is not known whether regulation of MHCI expression is autonomous or induced by external factors such as type I interferons (α and β) or type II interferon γ, TNFα or others [72]. IFNγ is one of the major external regulators of MHCI expression, and it is produced mainly by T cells, NKT cells and NK cells but also to a lesser extent by macrophages and DC [74-76]. IFNγ exerts its function upon interaction with the IFNγ receptor (IFNγR) that is ubiquitously expressed on all cells [74].

Several tumor models use, as tumor antigens, peptides from proteins against which specific T-cell receptor (TCR) $\alpha\beta$ transgenic mice have been made [53, 77, 78]. These models systems have demonstrated that tumor cells may be killed directly by specific T cells or indirectly by released IFNγ. However, most systems showed that despite an overwhelming excess of tumor-specific T cells in the mice, the tumor cells will kill the hosts [53, 79]. The tumor cells used in these studies expressed rather low levels of MHCI at the cell surface. One possibility would be that the tumor-specific CTL had difficulties to recognize and kill the tumor cells due to their low expression of MHCI. Another possibility is that the innate and adaptive immune effector cells can not get sufficient contact with the tumor cells. In order to distinguish between these possibilities, we have used the P14 TCR-transgenic mouse model with the immunogenic LCMV-peptide gp33-41 expressed as a minigene in B16 melanoma [53, 79].

Normal B6 spleen cells (NSC) or spleen cells from P14 transgenic mice were mixed with the target cells at a 100:1 ratio. B16-C = parental B16.F10 melanoma cells; B16gp33 = B16 cells transfected with a LCMV minigene encoding the gp33-41 peptide; L12R4 = $H\text{-}2^b$ lymphoma cells; p33-41/L12R4 = L12R4 cells pulsed for three hours with gp33-41 peptide. % cytotoxicity waz determined as described [50].

As can be seen in Figure 5, NSC do kill very efficiently the MHC^{low} normal B16.F10 or gp33-transfected B16 cells due to their low MHCI expression (undetectable by anti-MHCI mAb in flow cytometry). NSC do not kill L12R4 lymphoma cells whether these were loaded with gp33 peptide or not. By contrast, spleen cells from P14 transgenic mice kill very efficiently B16gp33 cells and gp33 peptide loaded L12R4 cells but not normal B16 or L12R4 cells [80]. Thus, the majority of B16gp33 cells are killed by splenic NK cells, and the

B16gp33 cells express sufficient numbers of specific peptide-MHCI complexes on the cell surface to be recognized by P14-CTL.

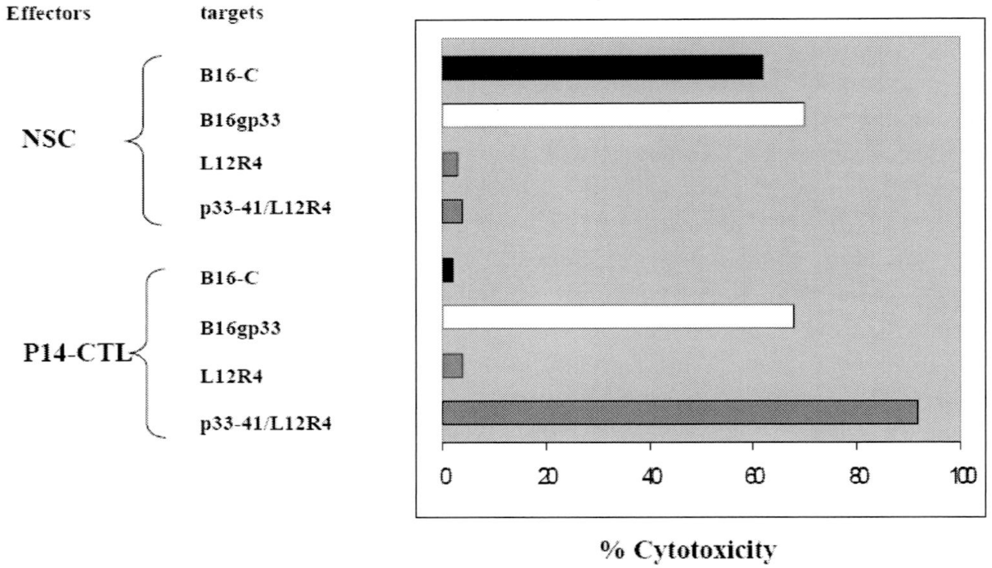

Figure 5. Cytotoxicity of NSC and P14 T cells against B16gp33 and gp33-peptide coated L12R4 cells.

Then, we tried to enrich the B16gp33 population for MHCI high expressing cells by co-culture with NSC. Our data showed that co-culture of MHCI^{low} tumor cells with NSC induced increased MHCI expression by a cell-cell contact dependent, IFNγ-mediated mechanism. The effector cells were found among the innate immune cells, and their frequency and/or activity was highest in spleen and lymph nodes, and lowest in bone marrow, thymus and peritoneum. IFNγ was the only effector molecules detected in the system and NSC from IFNγ$^{-/-}$ mice did not induce augmented MHCI expression in MHCI^{low} tumor cells. Cell fractionation experiments demonstrated that the major cell-subsets involved in the described phenomenon are CD4^{+}, CD1d-independent NKT cells, CD4^{+}, CD11c^{+} DC, and NK1.1^{+} NK cells. It seems that NKT, DC and NK cells function most efficiently together, e.g. 1) NSC from Rag$^{-/-}$ mice functions less well than NSC from wild type mice, 2) purified NK cells function less well than Rag$^{-/-}$ NSC and 3) both CD11c^{+} and CD11c^{-} sub-populations of CD4^{+}, CD8^{-}, Ig^{-} cells work suboptimally. Moreover, kinetic experiments have shown that the induction of augmented MHCI expression on MHCI^{low} tumor cells happens in two waves, an early peak around day 1 and a second, more important peak around day 2-3, with decreased synthesis of IFNγ from day 4-5 (not shown). Addition of mAb against IL-12 to cultures of NSC and MHCI^{low} tumor cells abolish the MHCI-inducing capacity of the effector cells. Therefore, it appears that the most probable scenario for our MHCI-inductive system is that NKT cells recognize the MHCI^{low} tumor cells, release stored IFNγ which induces DC to produce IL-12 that in turn activate NK cells [80].

A key-question is how the NKT cells recognize MHCI^{low} tumor cells and initiate the possible three-cell collaboration with DC and NK cells. The finding that the involved NKT cells were independent of CD1d appears to exclude the recognition of tumor-cell lipids, a process performed mostly by the $V\alpha14^+/V\beta8^+$, CD1d-restricted, classical iNKT cells [63, 81]. It follows that probable receptors were the activating (NKG2D or Ly-49D/H) or KIR on NKT or NK cells (purified NK-1.1$^+$ normal spleen cells) = triangles, and P14-CTL from day 5 in vitro cultures = squares, were analyzed for cytotoxicity against B16gp33 melanoma cells that were 1) stimulated overnight with different concentrations of IFNγ, and 2) quantitated for number of MHCI molecules expressed at the cell surface (flow cytometry) before the cytotoxicity assay [50, 80].

NK cells. However, none of the anti-KAR/KIR receptor mAb available to us influenced the capacity of NSC effector cells to induce MHCI expression on MHCI^{low} tumor cells, despite the fact that these mAb actively block NKT or NK cell cytotoxicity against YAC (MHCI^{low}) target cells. Therefore, we suggest that the recognition event under study may be carried out either 1) by an unknown receptor, 2) by ligand-receptor pairs not analyzed in our experiments, e.g. CD48-2B4 [82] or 3) by a combination of activating and inhibitory receptors [65]. The latter possibility is supported by the finding that B6 NSC is far more effective compared to (B6xCBA) F1 NSC [80], probably due to differences in expression of KAR and KIR among B6 and CBA strains [65].

Still, it is a mystery how tumor cells can resist the presence of high numbers of very active tumor-specific CTL in in vivo tumor models. IFNγ, produced early during recognition of MHCI^{low} tumor cells by the innate immune system, has 1) an up-regulatory function on MHCI expression rendering the MHCI^{low} tumor cells vulnerable to CTL, 2) a tumorocidal effect on the tumor cells [68, 83] and 3) an anti-angiogenetic effect on the tumor stroma cells [67]. The results depicted in Figure 6 show that NK cells and P14-CTL together kill very efficiently B16gp33 tumor cells whatever expression of MHCI they may have. Thus, it seems most reasonable to conclude that important components of the innate immune system do not get in contact with the tumor cells, and thus can not induce the necessary conditions for tumor cell killing [67].

It has been shown previously that MHC^{low} tumor cells maintained in naïve mice in vivo regain high MHCI expression [84]. The question arises whether it is the immune system that influences the tumor cells or whether tumor cell variants, insensitive to the immune system, are selected randomly. We cultured gp33-peptide loaded L12R4 cells with P14 CTL for prolonged periods of time, and analyzed whether this treatment selected MHC^{low} variant L12R4 cells. The data in Figures 5 and 7 clearly show that P14 CTLs kill almost all gp33 peptide-pulsed L12R4 cells. However, a few L12R4 cells survived such treatment. This could be due to insufficient loading of the L12R4 cells, or to lower expression of MHCI on the tumor cells. Then, these once-treated L12R4 cells were re-pulsed with gp33 peptide and P14 CTLs were added for 7 days. Again a few L12R4 cells survived, and as can be seen in Figure 7, the MHCI expression on these cells had decreased. Subsequent, similar treatments of L12R4 cells almost completely abolished MHCI expression, and these cells were very efficiently killed by splenic NK cells. However, all cloning experiments made to isolate stable MHCI^{low} L12R4 cells failed. As soon as the selective P14-CTL pressure was absent for a longer period (2-4 weeks), the MHCI expression regained normal levels (Figure 7). Thus, we may conclude that the immune system may induce reduced MHCI expression by an unknown reversible mechanism. However, it is not known how L12R4 cells manage to keep the MHCI expression so low as to avoid the cytotoxic activity of P14-CTLs for 7 days. As

MHCI expression is changing during the cell-cycle, the activity of factors regulating MHCI expression during the cell-cycle may be more active in the presence of highly active P14-CTLs.

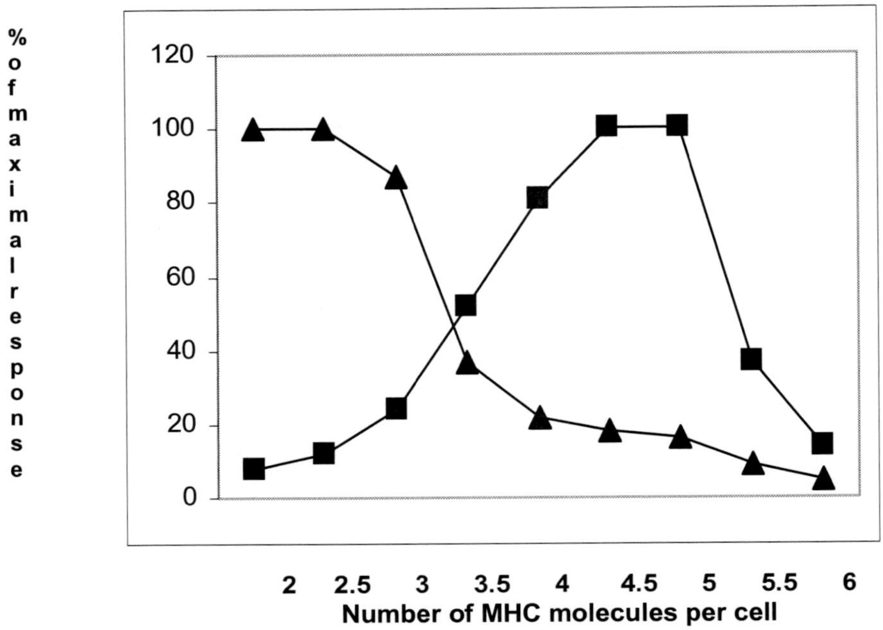

Figure 6. Response of NK cells and CTL to Melanoma cells with different expression of MHC class I antigen.

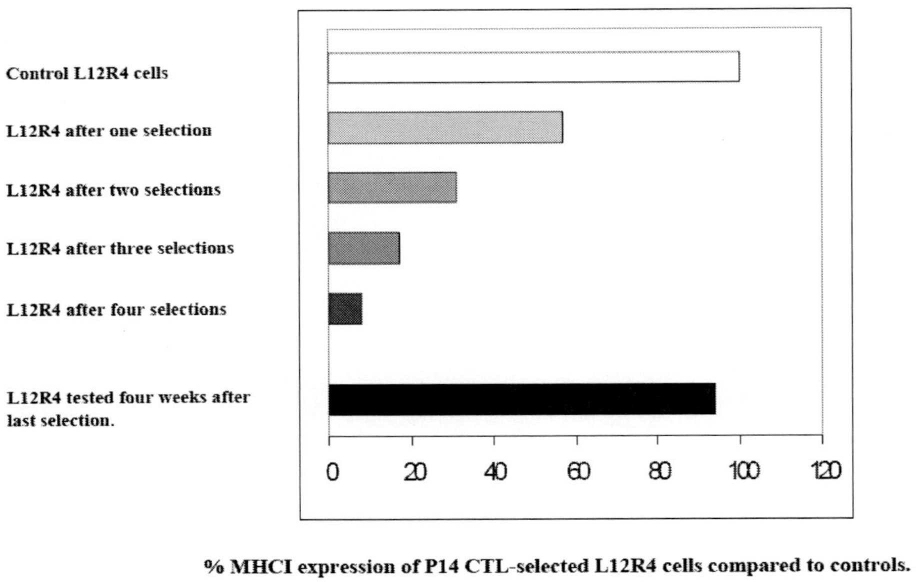

Figure 7. Down-regulation of MHCI in gp33-coated L12R4 cells by P14 CTL.

L12R4 lymphoma cells were pulsed for 3 hours with gp33-41 peptide before adding P14-CTL in a target to effector cell ration of 1:10. Seven days later, surviving L12R4 cells (< 1 %) were washed and expanded for 7 days (= one selection). Then, these cells were pulsed with gp33-41 peptide and added P14-CTL (= two selections) etc, etc. After four selections, the L12R4 cells expressed only ~8-10% MHCI molecules (compared to non-selected L12R4 cells cultured under the same conditions). When these 4x selected L12R4 MHC^{low} cells were cultured for four weeks without P14-CTL selection, they recovered almost full MHCI expression.

4. Chemical Modification of Protein/Peptides May Break Self-Tolerance and Induce Autoimmunity (Example, Rheumatoid Arthritis)

Immature DC and monocyte/macrophages are the first line of defense against microorganisms. In response to these interactions, DC/macrophages 1) process the "antigen" and present peptides or glycolipids to T cells and NKT cells, respectively, and 2) they produce cytokines. However, under certain conditions like local inflammations, proteins or glycolipids may be posttranslationally modified giving peptides with nitrated, phosphorylated or sulphonated tyrosines, oxidized tryptophans, arginines converted to citrulline and other modifications [85-87]. It seems that these processes occur mostly in DC and macrophages from different lymphoid organs; B cells seem not to express the enzymes relevant to the described modifications [88].

In the early days of T-B cell collaboration, we studied the immune responses to trinitrophenylated (TNP) mouse serum albumin (MSA) [89]. Three results emerged from these experiments: 1) T cells recognized TNP-MSA regardless of the level of trinitrophenylation, 2) B cells reacted against TNP structures and MSA epitopes altered by the hapten-coupling reaction, and 3) with increasing trinitrophenylation, B cells reacted only to the hapten, TNP. Thus, chemical modification of MSA resulted in a breakdown of T-cell tolerance. It was surprising that the immune response to TNP-MSA conjugates was so strong [89]. In contrast, immunization with hapten-coupled spleen cells induce hapten-specific tolerance [90], despite the fact that stimulation in vitro of naïve spleen cells with hapten-modified peptides induced strong, hapten-specific CTL responses [6]. Thus, it was clear early on that chemically modified proteins may play a role in autoimmune manifestations. Anti-Citrulline antibodies have been proposed as a diagnostic marker of Rheumatoid Arthritis (RA) [87, 91]. RA is a chronic inflammatory disease of the synovium characterized by synovial hyperplasia and inflammatory cell recruitment, intraarticular fibrin deposition, and, in its later stages, cartilage and bone destruction. Both autoreactive $CD4^+$ Th cells, autoantibodies, activated Fc receptor-bearing neutrophils and mast cells, and the alternative complement pathway may play active roles in the initiation and maintenance of RA [92].

We studied the immune response to normal or citrullinated, human or mouse fibrinogen (FBG) in different strains of mice [93]. The immune response to human fibrinogen in mice had been described as being independent on antigen-processing [94]. It was anticipated that in analogy with the induction of arthritis by heterologous collagen type II (CII), human cartilage glycoprotein (HCgp39) or proteoglycan aggregan, an autoimmune response to mFBG could be induced by normal or deiminated human FBG. Using mice with I-E MHCII molecules structurally similar to RA-susceptible (H-2^k and H-2^s) or non-susceptible (H-2^d and H-2^r) DR4 alleles, an interesting observation was made. The former type of mice produced 100-10,000 times higher titers of antibodies cross-reactive with mFBG, compared to the latter mice. Thus, there was a good correlation between autoimmune anti-mFBG responses in mice carrying I-E molecules similar to RA-susceptible HLA-DR alleles, and lack of autoimmunity to mFBG in mice carrying I-E molecules similar to RA-non-susceptible HLA-DR alleles. However, the high levels of anti-mFBG antibodies did not induce arthritis in the mice even after very long observation periods (more than 9 months). We observed no formation of antibodies against citrullinated FBG, ovalbumin (OA) or human serum albumin (HSA) (not shown). Then, we immunized high responder mice with citrullinated hFBG or mFBG. More than 600 genetically different mice were analyzed, and we found only traces of antibodies against citrulline structures when using deiminated hFBG, and none when using deiminated mFBG. In contrast, citrullination of hFBG induced no crossreactive anti-mFBG antibodies, a finding that may be related to fact that most arginine residues are found in the FBG sequences homologous between the two species. Finally, we immunized DR4*0401-transgenic mice with citrullinated hFBG. These mice produced high levels of anti-Citrulline antibodies but none of the mice developed arthritis [92].

A subsequent study established that the anti-FBG antibody responses were very tightly regulated, and they displayed very short time memory [93]. This was not due to induction of T_{reg} cells; rather it may be related to the multiple biological functions of fibrinogen and to the fact that T cells were relative independent of FBG-processing for T-cell activity. As described previously [92, 93] we did not succeed in producing T-cell lines or clones from FBG-immune spleen or lymph node populations. Therefore, we tried to produce T-cell hybridomas from FBG-immune cells [87]. The data in Table I demonstrate that we could produce such FBG-reactive T-cell hybridomas, and they reacted with either mFBG, hFBG or deiminated FBG:s presented by DC. However, there were several obligations for these reactions to occur: 1) the FBG preparations should be incubated with the DC:s for at least 24 hours, maximum loading was obtained after 48 hours. Other APC like macrophages or B cells were inactive; 2) "artificial" processing such as boiling, fibrinogen to fibrin conversion, treatment with trypsin-beads or presentation as FBG anti-FBG antibody complexes did not augment FBG-presentation. Furthermore, whether the T-cell hybridomas were produced from high or low responder mouse strains, the most frequent T-cell type was reacting specifically with hFBG. Only one hybridoma reacted against mFBG specifically, and three hybridomas reacted preferentially with citrullinated mFBG (out of 273 T-cell hybridomas analyzed).

Though there seems to be little doubt that anti-Citrulline antibodies may be a marker of RA in humans [91], citrulline-reactive T cells have not been demonstrated unequivocally in humans. The most clearcut effect of citrullination appears to be an enhanced binding of citrullinated peptides to MHCII molecules [95]. This could mean that either 1) citrulline is involved in the interaction with the MHC groove, and thereby inaccessible to T cells, or 2) that citrullination changes the overall structure of the peptide allowing it to interact better with MHCII molecules and phase the citrulline epitope towards the TCR; in this case, the T cells do not react with citrulline as such but against the new peptide structure induced by the citrulline residue. Our unpublished data on the attempt to use carrier-specific T cells to induce anti-citrulline antibody forming B cells in T-B cell collaboration experiments has been unsuccessful. Therefore, we believe that the mouse (and rat, unpublished experiments) is a poor model of RA induction by citrullinated self-proteins.

However, the data in this paragraph have clearly emphasized that self-tolerance is a matter of both the presence/reactivity of T cells emigrating from the thymus, and of the creation of different "self-epitopes" against which the peripheral T cells may or may not react. There is direct evidence for hapten-specific T cells [6, 96], so there is no reason that citrulline-specific T cells should not exist. At present, such T cells seem elusive. They may have been contra-selected, they may be strictly regulated, or they may have special activation requirements. It should be investigated whether the anti-citrulline antibodies produced in RA patients are T-cell dependent or independent antibodies; furthermore, it should be taken into consideration that large proteins may induce T-cell independent responses [94, 97].

Table I. Specicifity of FBG-Reactive T-Cell Hybridomas

	IL-2 production (IL-2 Units ± one SE)			
T-cell hybridoma	mFBG	citr-mFBG	hFBG	citr-hFBG
F3T6 (269)	54 ± 17	< 10	271 ± 38	243 ± 47
F3T20 (1)	162 ± 49	< 10	29 ± 9	< 10
F5T13 (3)	33 ± 14	87 ± 21	< 10	103 ± 26

T-cell hybridomas ($5x10^5$/ml) were cultured in quadruplicates with bone Marrow-derived dendritic cells (Ten day culture with GM-CSF + IL-4). The DC:s were pre-incubated with the different antigens for 48 hours before wash, addition to hybridoma cultures ($5x10^4$/ml), and incubated for 24 hours. Then, Supernatants were recovered and analyzed for IL-2 content by co-culture at different dilutions with CTLL-2 cells for 2 days, the last 24 hours in the presence of 1 μCi of ^{3}H-Thymidine.
FBG = fibrinogen; m = mouse, h = human, citr = citrullinated. DC:s were incubated with 100 μg/ml of protein. Citrullination was performed with rabbit skeletal muscle PAD (Sigma) for 3 h at 37°C.

4. Autoimmune, Type 1 Diabetes

a) Spontaneous T1D in NOD Mice

Type-1 Diabetes (T1D) is an autoimmune disease, where $CD4^+$ and $CD8^+$ T cells reacting with self components on the pancreatic islet β-cells induce auto-aggressive effector mechanisms leading to destruction of the β-islets. Consequently, the organism produces little or no Insulin, and hyperglycemia is induced and may cause death [98, 99]. This auto-reactivity happens in particular in susceptible individuals, where MHC molecules from susceptible loci present auto-antigens to developing thymocytes in such a way that auto-reactive T cells avoid negative selection and are permitted into the periphery. Normal individuals have either lower numbers or less efficient auto-reactive T cells, or more efficient regulator cells like NKT cells and T_{reg} cells coping with these auto-aggressive T cells [21, 100]. The balance between autoimmunity and normal immune status may be a question of quality and quantity of inducers and regulators [21, 100].

Since islet β-cells are $MHCI^+$ and $MHCII^-$, it seems unlikely that the autoimmune $CD4^+$ and $CD8^+$ T cells are activated directly by the β-cell peptides expressed on the β-cell MHC surface molecules. The first cells to enter the pancreatic β-islets are macrophages and DCs [101, 102]. Thus, it seems more likely that these phagocytic cells pick up autoantigen and migrate to the local pancreatic lymph nodes (PLN), where they present peptides from phagocytized β-islet membrane antigens associated with MHCI and MHCII to T cells. The latter pMHCII complexes activate auto-reactive $CD4^+$ T helper cells, which induce differentiation and maturation of β-islet specific, effector $CD8^+$ T cells or of activated macrophages [102]. NOD mice manifest spontaneous insulitis followed by T1D around 8-12 weeks of age. This is due to the expression of disease susceptible MHCII alleles, the $H\text{-}2^{g7}$ [98], to the deficient functions of NKT cells expressing an invariant TCR-Vα14/Jα281 chain [103], and to an inefficient function of CTLA-4 on T_{reg} cells caused by low expression of CD86 on NOD DC [104].

A number of genetically modified mice have been used to strengthen the data from NOD mice: 1) NOD mice deficient in expression of CD1d or Jα281 show exacerbated disease development [105, 106]; 2) NOD mice transgenic for CD1d expression on β-islets or for Vα14/Jα281 TCRα chain expression on NKT cells are protected from disease [105, 107-109]. The augmented presence of NKT cells in the PLN and islets suggest that they might interfere with the development of the autoimmune response in both tissues: 1) NKT cells could kill activated diabetogenic T cells, as NKT cells can kill via both Fas-FasL or perforin-mediated mechanisms. 2) NKT cells could influence T cell differentiation, driving effector cells toward a non-pathogenic Th2 profile [110]. 3) NKT cells could inhibit the development of an efficient Th1 response by interfering with the priming, differentiation and/or expansion of β-islet specific Th1 cells [111, 112].

The different DC subsets were pulsed overnight with vehicle (medium = white bars), αGal.Cer (black bars) or C20:2 (grey bars), washed and $5x10^4$ DC:s/200 μL culture were added $5x10^4$ DN32 NKT hybridoma cells (these cells were activated with PMA and Ionomycin as 100% control). After 24 hours of culture, the supernatants were analyzed for content of IL-2 by the CTLL-2 bioassay.

b) αGal.Cer or C20:2 Glycolipid-Pulsed DC as Therapy for T1D Protection

Mature NKT cells are activated by exogenous or endogenous glycolipids presented by CD1d [112-114]. These non-classical, non-polymorphic MHCI molecules bind the lipid chains in "tunnels" in the interior of the protein, and the sugar-head groups are presented to the NKT-TCR [7, 115]. The α-Gal.Cer glycolipid from marine sponges induce NKT cells to produce both Th1-type, inflammatory cytokines (IL-2, IFNγ) and Th2-type, immunomodulary cytokines (IL-4, IL-10). Conversely, other compounds with shorter acyl-chains containing unsaturated bonds (C20:2) stimulate better IL-4 than IFNγ synthesis [116]. The $CD4^+$ NKT cells produce preferentially Th2 type cytokines and $CD4^-CD8^-$ NKT cells release preferentially Th1 type cytokines [117, 118]. Recently, it was shown that the $CD4^+$ NKT cells use CD4 molecules as an anti-MHC receptor reacting with CD1d. In this way, some NKT cells can regulate the avidity of binding to $CD1d^+$ target cells [117, 118].

TCRαβ-transgenic mice such as BDC2.5 or AI14 contain antigen-specific Th, CTL, as well as T_{reg} cells [119, 120]. Recent data from the Delovitch laboratory have demonstrated that the T1D-preventive function of NKT cells in NOD mice may be regulated by $CD4^+CD25^+$ T_{reg} cells from wild-type or $CD1d^{-/-}$ NOD mice. Thus, treatment of NOD mice with anti-CD25 mAb before or during αGal.Cer activation inhibits the preventive effect of NKT cells [121]. All products which enhance $CD4^+CD25^+$ T_{reg} cell function decrease or eliminate T1D. Treatment with anti-TNFα antibodies augments $CD4^+CD25^+$ T_{reg} activity, and in particular $CD86^{high}$ DC induces strong $CD4^+CD25^+$ T_{reg} activity [121, 122].

A summary of the protection against T1D by transfer of DC into NOD mice. Four-six week old female NOD mice received 5-8x10^5 DC i.v. The DC:s were pulsed for 24 hours with either vehicle, αGal.Cer or C20:2 glycolipid. Data from mice receiving vehicle-pulsed or αGal.Cer-pulsed DC of either spleen or BM origin were pooled (= all).

αGal.Cer elicits very strong innate immune responses with possible side-effects such as transactivation of many other cell-types that NKT cells [98, 103, 121]. Therefore, we studied whether glycolipids other than αGal.Cer, e.g. C20:2 [116] could be valuable for T1D therapy. Opposing results have been obtained concerning eventual defects in the DC compartment of NOD mice. Some claims that DC development is deficient [124-127], others have found normal DC development in NOD mice compared to different inbred strains of mice [128, 129]. Previously, it has been shown that BM-derived or splenic DC could delay or abolish T1D in NOD mice, if transferred no later than at 6 weeks of age (124, 130-133). The mechanism(s) may be a change of the autoimmune response from a Th1 to a Th2 response (110, 134]. Injection of αGal.Cer or other glycolipids such as the C20:2 compound into NOD mice could prevent T1D [135]. We concentrated our efforts on a study of how DC transfer into NOD mice could intervene with the autoimmune response. In order to minimize subset differences among DC, we used either PDCA-1^+, $CD11c^+$ or PDCA-1^-, $CD11c^+$ splenic DC or BM-derived DC developed in the presence of GM-CSF and IL-4 (GM4-DC) or of Flt3L (F3L-DC) [136].

In contrast to αGal.Cer immunization, the T1D abolishing effect observed after immunization with C20:2 was not dependent on $CD4^+CD25^+$ T_{reg} cells (Ly, Rubin, Porcelli and Delovitch, in preparation). Therefore, we asked whether GM4-DC pulsed with either vehicle, αGal.Cer or C20:2 could inhibit T1D development in a similar way to the effect of αGal.Cer-pulsed GM4-DC enhancing B16 tumor cell immunity [137]. As can be seen in Figure 8, αGal.Cer- or C20:2-pulsed GM4-DC (but not vehicle pulsed GM4-DC) stimulated strong IL-2 production from the NKT cell hybridoma, DN32 [138].

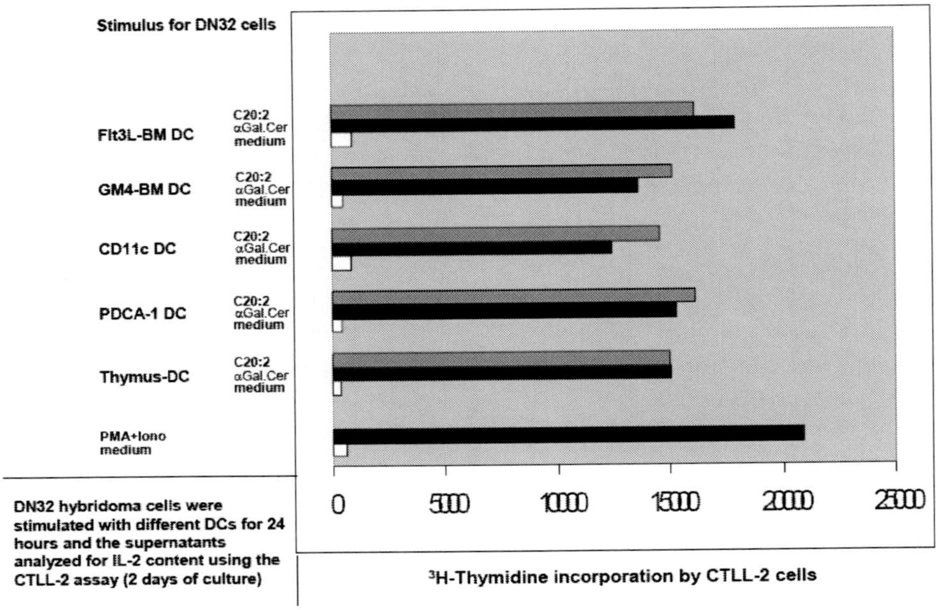

Figure 8. Presentation of αGal.Cer or C20:2 glycolipids to DN32 NKT hybridoma cells by different subsets of DC.

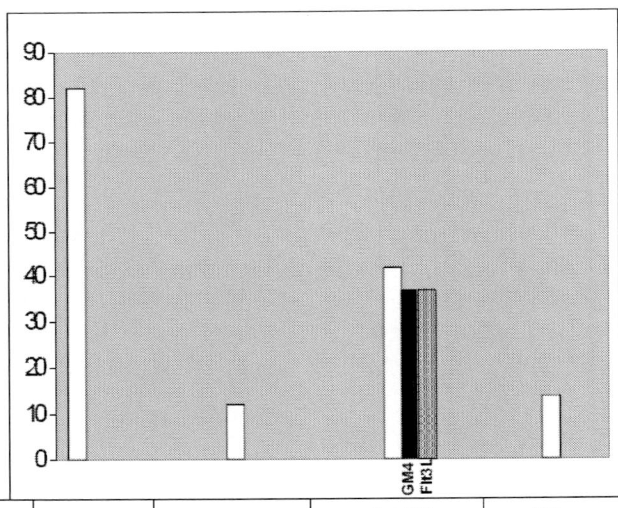

DC's origin	all	all	Spl BM	Spl
DC pulsed with	Vehicle	αGal.Cer	C20:2	IFNγ
Number of T1D mice/total mice	19/23	3/24	3/7 3/7 3/8	1/7

Figure 9. Transfer of glycolipid-pulsed DC decreases incidence of Type 1 Diabetes.

The data in Figure 9 show that αGal.Cer-pulsed GM4-DC protect the mice from T1D, whereas vehicle-pulsed GM4-DC does not protect and C20:2-pulsed GM4-DC protected partially. As shown before [131], injection of non-stimulated GM4-DC do not protect from T1D, whereas IFNγ activated splenic nDC do protect (Figure 9).

Injection of NOD mice with C20:2 protects against T1D, partially by induction of a shift from a Th1 response to a protective Th2 response [110, 134, 135], and this compound induces much less trans-activation (Ly et al. in preparation). The binding to CD1d molecules of αGal.Cer and C20:2 appears very similar; however, whereas αGal.Cer needs intracellular processing by DC or other APC, C20:2 seems to bind directly to surface CD1d molecules [116]. We analyzed whether there was any difference in NKT cell stimulatory capacity of αGal.Cer and C20:2. Spleen cells were depleted for $CD8^+$ and $CD19^+$ cells and cultured with different concentrations of αGal.Cer or C20:2 in the presence of $CD11c^+$ cells. There was no difference in NKT cell proliferative responses against the two compounds (not shown). C20:2 induced higher IL-4 and lower IFNγ responses compared to αGal.Cer (Figure 10).

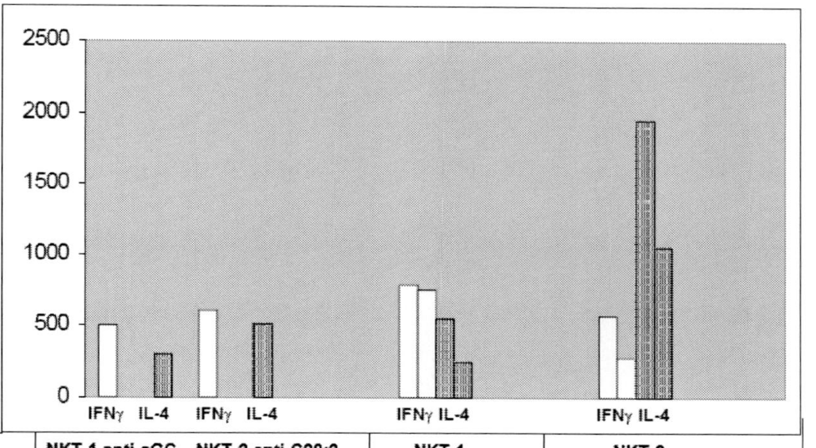

NKT cell line:	NKT-1 anti-aGC	NKT-2 anti-C20:2	NKT-1	NKT-2
1st stimulation: aGC C20:2	+ -	- +		
5th stimulation: aGC C20:2			+ - + - - + - +	+ - + - - + - +
% TCRβ+	34.7	31.2	93.3	97.6
% aGC/CD1d tetramer+	6.6	6.7	78.7	89.2

Figure 10. NKT cell activation by αGal.Cer or C20:2 glycolipids.

These characteristics were constant or accentuated during the development of NKT cell lines, where more than 60% of the T cells were αGal.Cer/CD1d tetramer-binding NKT cells (these NKT cell lines had no residual allo-reactivity). An interesting finding is that whereas αGal.Cer induces NSC to produce factor(s) that induce DC to become tolerogenic (and thereby T1D protective) [123], C20:2 did not induce NSC to produce significant amounts of the factor(s). However, as can be seen in Table II, NKT cell lines stimulated with αGal.Cer- or C20:2-pulsed, mitomycin C-treated DC release in the supernatant factors(s) which induces reduced IL-12 and increased IL-10 production in fresh DCs. In addition, these DCs showed increased expression of MHCII, CD40 and CD86, whereas CD8 expression was decreased indicating a tolerogenic DC phenotype [112-114, 123]. Thus it seems as if NKT cells need more repeated stimulations with C20:2 compared to αGal.Cer for differentiation factor(s) production.

Table II. Both αGal.Cer and C20:2 glycolipids stimulate NKT cell lines to produce DC maturation factor(s)

DC surface Marker	Supernatant from NKT cell cultures stimulated three days with Mitomycin C-treated CD11c$^+$ cells and the following glycolipids.		
	Vehicle	aGal.Cer	C20:2
CD40	12% ± 3	36% ± 8	39% ± 13
MHCII	8% ± 2	51% ± 11	50% ± 19
CD86	7% ± 2	42% ± 13	37% ± 12
CD8	11% ± 4	1% ± 1	2% ± 1
DC stimulation	pg/ml of IL-10 in DC supernatants		
Medium	<10	<10	<10
CpG	523 ± 39	1287 ± 123	1098 ± 251
	pg/ml of IL-12 in DC supernatants		
Medium	<10	<10	<10
CpG	1312 ± 437	153 ± 59	287 ± 73

5x10^6 NKT line cells (NKT-2 stimulated with C20:2 every week, the line was cultured for 12 weeks) were cultured with either Vehicle-, αGal.Cer- or C20:2-pulsed Mitomycin C-treated CD11c$^+$ splenic DCs for 3 days (6-well plates). Then the supernatant was harvested and added to fresh CD11c$^+$ DC. Three days later, the DC:s were analyzed in cellular ELISA for expression of CD40, MHCII, CD86 and CD8, or they were stimulated for 2 days with or without CpG (10μg/ml, and the supernatants analyzed for content of IL-10 or IL-12 by ELISA. Cytokine content is expressed as pg/ml of quadruplicates and the standard deviation. Similar results were obtained with 7 other NKT cell lines continuously stimulated with either αGal.Cer or C20:2 for 3-15 weeks.

NKT cell lines were produced by stimulating NKT cells (NOD spleen cells were incubated with anti-CD8 and anti-CD19 mAb beads and selected on magnetic columns) with αGal.Cer or C20:2 glycolipid (100ng/ml). Seven days later, surviving cells were analyzed for % TCRβ$^+$ and αGal.Cer/CD1d tetramer$^+$ cells (= 1st stimulation), and restimulated with αGal.Cer or C20:2 in the presence of splenic CD11c$^+$ DC that had been activated with CpG. After five such stimulations, the NKT cell lines contained highly selected tetramer$^+$/TCRβ$^+$ cells. In addition, the αGal.Cer-"specific" NKT-1 line produced much less IL-4 compared to the C20:2-"specific" NKT-2 line (line supernatant analyzed for cytokine content 48 hours after restimulation). Twelve analogous NKT cell lines gave the same results.

Multiple, low dose αGal.Cer regime was given to NOD mice in order to induce T1D protection [122]. Such a regime induces DCs to produce more IL-10 and less IL-12 [139]. We analyzed both multiple low dose and single high dose regimes with both αGal.Cer and C20:2 glycolipids: A single dose of αGal.Cer renders CD11c$^+$ DC highly sensitive to CpG or LPS activation of IL-12 production, whereas a single dose of C20:2 decreases IL-12 production in CD11c$^+$ DC upon stimulation with CpG or LPS. Production of IL-10 was identical in all groups. On the other hand, multiple dose treatment with αGal.Cer causes low production of IL-12 in CD11c$^+$ DC after stimulation with both CpG and LPS; the same treatment with C20:2 causes high IL-12 production with CpG and almost abolishes production of IL-12 in CD11c$^+$ DCs stimulated with LPS (not shown). Thus, all-together it appears that αGal.Cer is a much stronger stimulus for NKT cells compared to C20:2; however, repeated stimulations with C20:2 give the same end-result with much les trans-activation. In conclusion, a multiple low dose C20:2 regime may be more beneficial for induction of protection against T1D.

Conclusion

The present paper is based on the idea that MHC anti-MHC reactions play an important role in autoimmune reactions, and in whether or not these responses become beneficial for the body such as clearance of dying or dead cells and surveillance of tumor cell development or harmful, i.e. autoimmune diseases. In the previous paragraphs, we have discussed how these processes are intermingled with natural immunity, with post-translational modifications in self-protein structure, and with different degrees of interactions between the innate and adaptive immune systems. Many autoimmune diseases like multiple schlerosis (or the EAE model disease), rheumatoid arthritis, type 1 diabetes and thyroiditis are associated with multiple susceptibility genes. However, a common susceptibility gene is linked to MHCII genes in all species studied. This means that at a given stage in disease development, self-peptides are presented by MHCII molecules to T cells in a way that is different qualitatively and/or quantitatively from the presentation in the thymus. Thus, MHCII molecules play a central role in induction of autoimmune reactions. Self-peptides associate with MHCII molecules on the surface of professional APC like B cells, macrophages, and in particular, DC:s. Auto-reactive T cells mostly with low avidity receptors interact with such self-peptide-MHCII complexes via two anti-MHC receptors, the TCR against variable structures of the pMHCII complexes, and the CD4 molecules against constant structures of the MHCII. Consequently, the cumulative T-cell avidity against the pMHCII APC-surface molecules is increased and T-cell activation occurs.

Two other examples known for some time highlight the importance of MHC molecules in autoimmune reactions: 1) β_2-microglobulin deficient mice have no classical or non-classical MHCI molecules and very low CD8 T-cell activity. Such mice are highly vulnerable to tumor cell outgrowth and to autoimmune diseases; in the former case due to lack of $CD8^+$ T cells, and in the latter case due to lack of CD1d-mediated NKT-cell regulation [140]. 2) MHCII deficient mice [142] contain some $CD4^+$ T-cell reactivity, and as we have discussed above, this is associated with the reactivity of CD4 molecules with CD1d [117, 118]. Thus, the anti-MHC receptor, CD4, has at least two functions, to activate low-medium avidity $CD4^+$ Th cells in their reaction with MHCII, and to activate $CD4^+$ NKT cells in the interaction with CD1d, i.e. CD4 molecules are involved in both the innate and adaptive immune systems.

It has been discussed further that the T-cell repertoire, as measured by allogeneic T-cell proliferation, is the same in mice raised under SPF conditions as in a conventional environment. This means that the T-cell repertoire is independent on the environmental antigens, and that its maintenance is due to an internal network of interactions between random combinations of TCR-variable regions and self-peptide-MHC complexes [20, 45]. Consequently, genetically identical members of an inbred strain of mice living in the same cadge may have different T-cell repertoires.

NKT cells can be divided into $CD4^+$, $CD4^-CD8^-$ and $CD8^+$ cells. The most dominant type is restricted to CD1d molecules and via their invariant TCR (Vα14/Jα281 chains paired with mostly Vβ8, Vβ7 or Vβ2 chains), they react with exogenous or endogenous glycolipids. Thus, these innate immune cells use anti-MHC receptors (TCR) as activation receptors. The activity of these cells is controlled by other anti-MHC receptors, the killer cell inhibitory receptors (KIR). These receptors are present also on NK and mature $CD8^+$ T cells. KIRs interact with classical or non-classical MHCI molecules, and they display certain polymorphism exemplified by their reactivity against different haplotypes of classical MHCI molecules and different classical or non-classical MHCI molecules [4, 65]. It appears that KIRs control the activity of effector cells with high immediate effector function: NKT cells release high levels of IFNγ, IL-4 or IL-10 instantaneously upon activation, NK cells kill very efficiently and instantaneously $MHCI^{low}$ or negative target cells, and mature $CD8^+$ CTL have a very high cytotoxic potential.

We have discussed that NKT cells play an important role in the surveillance of tumor cells, and in the regulation of autoimmunity e.g. type 1 Diabetes. In response to tumor cells, NKT cells produce IFNγ, which increases MHC expression of $MHCI^{low}$ tumor cells and has damaging effects on tumor cells [80]. In addition, NKT cells activate DC to produce IL-12, which triggers activation of IFNγ production by NK cells. Whereas the NKT cells are often CD1d-restricted and carry invariant TCRαβ complexes, some NKT cells are independent on CD1d and carry variant TCRαβ heterodimers. The ligands for such cells are not clear at present [81].

$CD4^+CD25^+$ T_{reg} cells appear to have similar TCRαβ heterodimers as conventional Th and CTL; however, often their TCR has a higher avidity compared to Th or CTL [119, 120]. T_{reg} cells are dependent on MHCII on DC and relatively high concentrations of IL-2 for activation and maturation [119]. Such T_{reg} cells play an important role in the regulation of autoimmune reactions, and they play some sort of safety role against self-reactive T-cell clones in all of the autoimmune diseases described herein. The mechanism by which T_{reg} manifests their activity is not known but two extreme hypotheses suggest either consumption of IL-2 (and possible other cytokines) hindering autoimmune T cells to develop, or production of inhibitory cytokines such as TGFβ and IL-10 [142].

In conclusion, we have discussed how MHC anti-MHC receptor interactions initiate defensive immune responses as well as autoimmune reactions; these latter may be beneficial like anti-tumor cell responses or harmful as autoimmune disease reactions. Normally, self-peptides are presented in very high numbers and varieties but only, under very special conditions, in a high concentration of a particular self-peptide. Therefore, auto-reactive T cells with low-medium avidity TCR:s are either not activated or kept under control by $CD4^{+}CD25^{+}$ T_{reg} cells with medium-high avidity TCR:s. Autoimmune reactions abort because the TCR and CD4 anti-MHC receptors of T_{reg} cells have an advantage over those of $CD4^{+}$ T helper cells. In addition, NKT cells are activated by glycolipids associated with CD1d non-classical MHCI molecules, often with an impact from CD1d-CD4 anti-MHC reactions. These cells may initiate a series of events, which enhance anti-self T-cell responses against tumor cells and deviate anti-self autoimmune disease reactions to less harmful Th2 responses. Such responses trigger antibody-formation by B cells and thereby activate Fc receptors on B cells, macrophages, DC:s and NK/NKT cells for protection against autoimmune diseases.

Thus, not all is in the MHC, but the MHC molecules and the various anti-MHC receptors certainly both initiate, tune, and regulate defensive and pathogenic autoimmune reactions.

Acknowledgments

The present work was supported by the Centre Nationale de Recherche Scientifique (CNRS, France), Université Paul Sabatier (Toulouse, France), l'Association de Recherche contre le Cancer (ARC, France) and the National Diabetes Foundation (Canada). It is my pleasure to acknowledge my many collaborators in the experiments on which this review is based: J. Arnaud, M. Gonthier, and R. Llobera (CNRS UPR 2163, Toulouse), G. Sønderstrup (Stanford, USA), J.E.Gairin, J.Riond, L. Courtiade, N. Roullet (CNRS, UMR 2587, Toulouse), D. Ly and T. Delovitch (London, Ontario, Canada).

References

[1] Flajnik MF, Du Pasquier L. Evolution of innate and adaptive immunity : can we draw a line ? *Trends in Immunol.* 2004; 25: 640-4.

[2] Pancer Z, Cooper MD. The evolution of adaptive immunity. *Ann.Rev.Immunol.* 2006; 24: 497-518.

[3] Dissing S, Geisler C, Rubin B, Plesner T, Claesson MH. T-cell activation II. Activation of human T-lymphoma cells by crosslinking of their MHC class I antigens. *Cell. Immunol.* 1990; 126: 196-203.

[4] Vivier E, Anfossi N. Inhibitory NK-cell receptors on T cells: Witness of the past, actors of the future. *Nature Rev. Immunol.* 2004; 4: 190-8.

[5] Krogsgaard M, Davis MM. How T cells "see" antigen. *Nature Immunol.* 2005; 6: 239-45.

[6] Preckel T, Grimm, R, Martin S, Weltzien HU. Altered hapten ligands antagonize trinitrophenyl-specific cytotoxic T cells and block internalization of hapten-specific receptors. *J. Exp. Med.* 1997; 185: 1803-13.

[7] Borg NA, Wun KS, Kjer-Nielsen L, Wilce MCJ, Pellicci DG, Koh R, Besra GS, Bharadwaj M, Godfrey DI, McCluskey J, Rossjohn J. CD1d-lipid-antigen recognition by the semi-invariant NKT T-cell receptor. *Nature* 2007; 448: 44-9.

[8] Allison TJ, Winter CC, Fournié JJ, Bonneville M, Garboczi DN. Structure of a human γδ T-cell antigen receptor. *Nature* 2001; 411: 820-4.

[9] Li H, Llera A, Malchiodi EL, Mariuzza RA. The structural basis of T-cell activation by superantigens. Ann.Rev.Immunol. 1999; 17: 435-66.

[10] Naeher D, Daniels MA, Hausmann B, Guillaume P, Luescher I, Palmer E. A constant affinity threshold for T cell tolerance. *J. Exp. Med.* 2007; 204: 2553-9.

[11] Wilson SS, van den Elzen P, Maverakis E, Beech JT, Braciak TA, Kumar V, Sercarz, EE. Residual public repertoires to self. *J. Neuroimmunol.* 2000; 107: 233-9.

[12] Sakaguchi, S. Naturally arising $CD4^+$ regulatory T cells for immunological self-tolerance and negative control of immune responses. *Ann. Rev. Immunol.* 2004; 22: 531-62.

[13] Rubin B, Alibaud L, Huchenq-Champagne A, Arnaud J, Toribio ML. *Scand. J. Immunol.* 2002; 55: 111-8.

[14] Rudolph MG, Stanfield RL, Wilson IA. How TCRs bind MHCs, peptides, and coreceptors. *Ann. Rev. Immunol.* 2006; 24: 419-66.

[15] Rubin B, Knibiehler M, Gairin JE. Allosteric changes in the TCR/CD3 structure upon interaction with extra- or intra-cellular ligands. *Scand. J. Immunol.* 2007; 66: 228-37.

[16] Gil D, Schrum AG, Alarcon B, Palmer E. T-cell receptor engagement by peptide-MHC ligands induces a conformational change in the CD3 complex of thymocytes. *J. Exp. Med.* 2005; 201: 517-22.

[17] Becker AM, deFord-Watts L, Wuelfing C, van Oers NSC. The constitutive tyrosine phosphorylation of CD3ζ results from TCR-MHC interactions that are independent of thymic selection. *J. Immunol.* 2007; 178: 4120-8.

[18] Huseby ES, White J, Crawford F, Vass T, Becker D, Pinilla C, Marrack P, Kappler J. How the T cell repertoire becomes peptide and MHC specific. *Cell* 2005; 122: 247-60.

[19] Felix NJ, Donermeyer DL, Horvath S, Walters JJ, Gross ML, Suri A, Allen PM. Alloreactive T cells respond specifically to multiple distinct peptide-MHC complexes. *Nature Immunol.* 2007; 8: 388-97.

[20] Jerne NK. The somatic generation of immune regulation. *Eur. J. Immunol.* 1971; 1: 1-9.

[21] Aschenbrenner K, D'Cruiz LM, Vollmann EH, Hinterberger M, Emmerich J, Swee LK, Rolink A, Klein L. Selection of $Foxp3^+$ regulatory T cells specific for self antigen expressed and presented by $Aire^+$ medullary thymic epithelial cells. *Nature Immunol.* 2007; 8: 351-8.

[22] Krogsgaard M, Davis MM. How T cells "see" antigen. *Nature Immunol.* 2005; 6: 239-45.

[23] Graber M, Bockenstedt LK, Weiss A. Signaling via the inositol phospholipid pathway by T cell antigen receptor is limited by receptor number. *J. Immunol.* 1991; 146: 2935-43.

[24] Viola A, Lanzavecchia A. T cell activation determined by T cell receptor number and tunable thresholds. *Science* 1996; 273: 104-6.

[25] Germain RN. The T cell receptor for antigen: Signaling and ligand discrimination. *J. Biol. Chem.* 2001; 276: 35223-6.

[26] Huppa JB, Davis MM. T-cell antigen recognition and the immunological synapse. *Nature Rev. Immunol.* 2003; 3: 973-83.

[27] Montixi C, Langlet C, Bernard AM, Wurbel MA, Chauvin JP, Pierres M, He HT. Engagement of T cell receptor triggers its recruitment to low-density detergent-insoluble membrane domains. *EMBO J.* 1998; 17: 5334-48.

[28] van der Merwe PA, Davis SJ. Molecular interactions mediating T-cell antigen recognition. *Ann. Rev. Immunol.* 2003; 21: 659-84.

[29] Rodges W, Rose JK. Exclusion of CD45 inhibits activity of p56lck associated with glycolipid-enriched membrane domains. *J. Cell Biol.* 1996 135: 1515-23.

[30] Gordon S. Alternative activation of macrophages. *Nat. Rev. Immunol.* 2003; 3: 23-35.

[31] Moody DB, Porcelli S. Intracellular pathways of CD1 antigen presentation. *Nat. Rev. Immunol.* 2002; 3: 11-22.

[32] Schurr M, Chen Q, Shin A, Chen W, Toy T, Jenderek C, Green S, Miloradovic L, Drane D, Davis ID, Villadangos J, Shortman K, Maraskovsky E, Cebon J. Tumor antigen processing and presentation depend critically on dendritic cell type and the mode of antigen delivery. *Blood* 2005; 105: 2465-72.

[33] Blander JM, Medzhikov R. Toll-dependent selection of microbial antigens for presentation by dendritic cells. *Nature* 2006; 440: 808-12.

[34] Savina A, Amigorena S. Phagocytosis and antigen presentation in dendritic cells. *Immunol. Rev.* 2007; 219: 143-56.

[35] Graham DB, Stephenson LM, Lam SK, Brim K, Lee HM, Bautista J, Gilfillan S, Akilesh S, Fujikawa K, Swat W. An ITAM-signaling pathway controls cross-presentation of particulate but not soluble antigens in dendritic cells. *J. Exp. Med.* 2007; 204: 2889-97.

[36] Kalinski P, Moser M. Consensual immunity: success-driven development of Th1 and Th2 responses. *Nat. Rev. Immunol.* 2005; 5: 251-60.

[37] McKee A, Munks MW, Marrack P. How do adjuvants work? Important considerations for new generation adjuvants. *Immunity* 2007; 27: 687-90.

[38] Janeway CA. Jr Approaching the asymptote? Evolution andrevolution in immunology. *Cold Spring Harb. Symp. Quant. Biol.* 1989; 54: 1-13.

[39] Medzhitov R. Toll-like receptors and innate immunity. *Nature Rev.Immunol.* 2001; 1: 135-45.

[40] Carnaud C, Lee D, Donnars O, Park SH, Beavis A, Koezuka Y, Bendelac A. Cross-talk between cells of the innate immune system: NKT cells rapidly activate NK cells. *J. Immunol.* 1999; 163: 4647-50.

[41] Fernandez NC. et al Dendritic cells directly trigger NK cell functions: cross-talk relevant in innate anti-tumor immune responses in vivo. *Nature Med.* 1999; 5: 405-11.

[42] Smyth MJ, Godfrey DI. NKT cells and tumor immunity - a double-edged sword. *Nat. Immunol.* 2000; 1: 459-60.

[43] Kim KD, Zhao J, Auh S, Yang X, Du P, Tang H, Fu YX. Adaptive immune cells temper initial innate responses. *Nature Med.* 2007; 13: 1248-52.

[44] Avrameas S, Ternynck T, Tsonis IA, Lymberi P. Naturally occurring B-cell autoreactivity: A critical review. *J. Autoimmunity* 2007; 29: 213-8.

[45] Jerne NK. Idiotype networks and other preconceived ideas. 1984; 79: 5-24.

[46] Forni L, Coutinho A, Köhler G, Jerne NK. IgM antibodies induce the production of antibodies of the same specificity. *Proc. Natl. Acad. Sci. USA* 1980; 77: 1125-8.

[47] Goverman J, Woods A, Larson L, Weiner LP, Hood L, Zaller DM. Transgenic mice that express a myelin basic protein-specific T cell receptor develop spontaneous autoimmunity. *Cell* 1993; 72: 551-60.

[48] Lafaille JJ, Nagashima K, Katsuki M, Tonegawa S. High incidence of spontaneous autoimmune encephamyelitis in immunodeficient anti-myelin basic protein T cell receptor transgenic mice. *Cell* 1994; 78: 399-408.

[49] Wegener AMK, Holm B, Geisler C, Rubin B. Cellular and molecular characteristics of transformed T cells from antigen-specific T-cell line. *Scand. J. Immunol.* 1990; 31: 645-56.

[50] Gonthier M, Llobera R, Arnaud J, Rubin B. Self-reactive T cell receptor-reactive $CD8^+$ T cells inhibit T cell lymphoma growth in vivo. *J. Immunol.* 2004; 173: 7062-69.

[51] Cui Z, Willingham MC, Hicks AM, Alexander-Miller MA, Howard TD, Hawkins GA, Miller MS, Weir HM, Du W, DeLong CJ. Spontaneous regression of advanced cancer: identification of a unique genetically determined trait in mice. *Proc. Natl. Acad. Sci. USA* 2003; 100: 6682-7.

[52] Hicks AM, Willingham MC, Du W, Pang CS, Old LJ, Cui Z. Effector mechanisms of the anti-cancer immune response of macrophages in SR/CR mice. *Cancer Immunity* 2006; 6: 11-20.

[53] Prévost-Blondel A, Zimmermann C, Stemmer C, Kulmburg P, Rosenthal FM, Pircher, H. Tumor-infiltrating lymphocytes exhibiting high ex vivo cytolytic activity fail to prevent murine melanoma tumor growth in vivo. *J. Immunol.* 1998; 161: 2187-94.

[54] Cooke A, Zaccone P, Raine T, Phillips JM, Dunne, DW. Infection and autoimmunity: are we winning the war, only to lose the peace? *Trends in Parasitology* 2004; 20: 316-21.

[55] Smith KA, Efstathiou S, Cooke A. Murine gammaherpesvirus-68 alters self-antigen presentation and ntype 1 Diabetes onset in NOD mice. *J. Immunol.* 2007; 179: 7325-33.

[56] Zaccone P, Burton OT, Cooke A. Interplay of parasite-driven immune responses and autoimmunity. *Trends in Parasitology* 2007; in press.

[57] Vicente-Suares I, Takahashi Y, Cheng F, Horna P, Wang HW, Wang HG, Sotomayor EM. Identification of a novel negative role of flagellin in regulating IL-10 production. *Eur. J. Immunol.* 2007; 37: 3164-75.

[58] Lambert SL, Okada CY, Levy R. TCR vaccines against a murine T cell lymphoma: a primary role for antibodies of the IgG2c class in tumor protection. *J. Immunol.* 2004; 172: 929-36.

[59] Chang CC, Ferrone S. Immune selective pressure and HLA class I antigen defects in malignant lesions. *Cancer Immunol. Immunother*. 2007; 56: 227-36.

[60] Dunn GP, Old LJ, Schreiber RD The three aces of cancer immunoediting. *Ann. Rev. Immunol.* 2004; 22: 329-60.

[61] Carnaud C, Lee D, Donnars O, Park SH, Beavis A, Koezuka Y, Bendelak A. Cutting Edge: Cross-talk between cells of the innate immune system: NKT cells rapidly activate NK cells. *J. Immunol.* 1999; 163: 4647-50.

[62] Crowe NY, Coquet JM, Berzins SP, Kyparissousdis K, Keating R, Pellicci SG, Hayakawa Y, Godfrey DL, Smyth MJ. Differential antitumor immunity mediated by NKT cell subsets in vivo. *J. Exp. Med.* 2005; 202: 1279-88.

[63] Wu DY, Segal NH, Sidobre S, Kronenberg M, Chapman PB. Cross-presentation of Disialoganglioside GD3 to natural killer T cells; *J. Exp. Med.* 2003; 198: 173-81.

[64] Diefenbach A, Jamieson AM, Liu SD, Shastri N, Raulet, DH. Ligands for the murine NKG2D receptor: expression by tumor cells and activation of NK cells and macrophages. *Nature Immunol.* 2000; 1: 119-26.

[65] Kane KP, Silver ET, Hazes B. Specificity and function of activating Ly-49 receptors. *Immunol. Rev.* 2001; 181: 104-14.

[66] Cerwenka A, Lanier LL Natural killer cells, viruses and cancer. *Nat. Rev. Immunol.* 2001; 1: 41-9.

[67] Ganss R, Arnold B, Hämmerling GJ. Overcoming tumor-intrinsic resistance to immune effector function. *Eur. J. Immunol.* 2004; 34: 2635-41.

[68] Schüler T, Blankenstein T. $CD8^+$ effector T cells reject tumors by direct antigen recognition but indirect action on host cells. *J. Immunol.* 2003; 170: 4427-31.

[69] Seliger B, Wollscheid U, Momburg F, Blankenstein T, Huber C Characterization of the major histocompatibility complex class I deficiencies in B16 melanoma cells. *Cancer Res.* 2001; 61: 1095-9.

[70] Yee C, Greenberg P. Modulating T-cell immunity to tumors: new strategies for monitoring T-cell responses. *Nature Rev. Cancer* 2002; 2: 409-19.

[71] Tanigushi M, Seino KI, Nakayama T. The NKT cell system: Bridging innate and acquired immunity. *Nature Immunol.* 2003; 4: 1164-5.

[72] Tanaka K, Yoshioka T, Bieberich C, Jay G. Role of the major histocompatibility complex class I antigens in tumor growth and metastasis. *Ann. Rev. Immunol.* 1988; 6: 359-80.

[73] Ozato K, Wan YJ, Orrison BM. Mouse major histocompatibility class I gene expression begins at midsomite stage and is inducible in earlier-stage embryos by interferon. *Proc. Natl. Acad. Sci. USA* 1985; 82: 2427-31.

[74] Farrar MA, Schreiber RD. The molecular cell biology of interferon-γ and its receptor. *Ann. Rev. Immunol.* 1993; 11: 571-611.

[75] Lertmemongkolchai G, Cai G, Hunter CA, Bancroft GJ. Bystander activation of $CD8^+$ T cells contributes to the rapid production of IFNγ in response to bacterial pathogens. *J. Immunol.* 2001; 166: 1097-105.

[76] Taieb J, Chaput N, Ménard C, Apetot L, Ullrich E, Bonmort M, Péquignot M, Casares N, Terme M, Flament C, Opolon P, Lecluse Y, Métivier D, Tomasello E, Vivier E, Ghiringhelli F, Martin F, Klatzman D, Poynard T, Tursz T, Raposo G, Yagita H, Ryffel

B, Kroemer G, Zitvogel L. A novel dendritic cell subset involved in tumor immunosurveillance. *Nature Med.* 2006; 12: 214-9.

[77] Mocikat R, Braumüller H, Gumy A, Egeter O, Ziegler H, Reusch U, Bubeck A, Louis J, Mailhammer R, Riethmuller G, Koszinowski U, Rocken M. Natural killer cells activated by MHC class I^{low} targets prime dendritic cells to induce protective CD8 T cell responses. *Immunity* 2003; 19: 561-9.

[78] Böhm W, Thoma S, Leithäuser F, Möller P, Schirrmbeck R, Reimann J T cell-mediated, IFNγ-facilitated rejection of murine B16 melanomas. *J. Immunol.* 1998; 161: 897-908.

[79] Blohm U, Roth E, Brommer K, Dumrese T, Rosenthal FM, Pircher H. Lack of effector cell function and alrered tetramer binding of tumor-infiltrating lymphocytes. *J. Immunol.* 2002; 169: 5522-30.

[80] Rubin B, Riond J, Courtiade L, Roullet N, Gairin JE. The innate immune system recognizes and regulates MHCI expression on $MHCI^{low}$ tumor cells. *Cancer Immunity* 2008; (submitted).

[81] Gumperz JE, Roy C, Makowska A, Lum D, Sigita M, Podrebarac T, Koezuka Y, Porcelli SA, Caedell S, Brenner MB, Behar SM. Murine CD1d-restricted T cell recognition of cellular lipids. *Immunity* 2000; 12: 211-21.

[82] Velikovsky CA, Deng L, Chlewiski LK, Fernandez MM, Kumar V, Mariuzza RA. Structure of natural killer receptor 2B4 bound to CD48 reveals basis for heterophilic recognition in signalling lymphocyte activation molecule family. *Immunity* 2007; 27: 572-84.

[83] Kakuta S, Tagawa Y, Shibata S, Nanno M, Iwakura Y. Inhibition of B16 melanoma experimental metastasis by intereferon-γ through direct inhibition of cell proliferation and activation of anti-tumour host mechanisms. *Immunology* 2002; 105: 92-100.

[84] Ljunggren HG, Kärre K Host resistance directed selectively against H-2-deficient lymphoma variants. Analysis of the mechanism. *J. Exp. Med.* 1985; 162: 1745-59.

[85] Birnboim HC, Lemay AM, Lam DKY, Goldstein R, Webb JR. MHC class II-restricted peptides containing the inflammation-associated 3-nitrotyrosine evade central tolerance and elicit a robust cell-mediated immune response. *J. Immunol.* 2003; 171: 528-32.

[86] Herzog J, Maekawa Y, Cirrito TP, Illian BS, Unanue ER. Activated antigen-presenting cells select and present chemically modified peptides recognized by unique CD4 T cells. *Proc. Natl. Acad. Sci. USA* 2005; 102: 7928-33.

[87] Ireland J, Herzog J, Unanue ER. Unique T cells that recognize cittrullinated peptides are a feature of protein immunization. *J. Immunol.* 2006; 177: 1421-5.

[88] Veeraswamy RK, Cella M, Colonna M, Unanue ER. Dendritic cells process and present antigen across a range of maturation states. *J. Immunol.* 2003; 170: 5367-72.

[89] Rubin B, Wigzell H. The immune response to hapten-autologous protein conjugates in the mouse. III. Specificity of non-thymus processed (B) and thymus-processed (T) lymphocytes. *J. Exp. Med.* 1973; 137: 911-31.

[90] Claman HN, Miller SD, Sy MS, Moorhead JW. Suppressive mechanisms involving sensitization and tolerance in contact allergy. Immunol.Rev. 1980; 50: 105-39.

[91] Migliorini P, Pratesi F, Tommasi C, Anzilotti C. The immune response to citrullinated antigens in autoimmune diseases. *Autoimmunity Reviews* 2005; 4: 561-4.

[92] Rubin B, Sønderstrup G. Citrullination of self-proteins and autoimmunity. *Scand. J. Immunol.* 2004; 60: 112-20.
[93] Rubin B, Matron C. The mouse immune response to human fibrinogen reveals an autoimmune component against mouse fibrinogen. *Cell Immunol.* 2005; 233: 41-52.
[94] Lee P, Matsueda GR, Allen PM. T-cell recognition of fibrinogen. A determinant on the Aα-chain does not require processing. *J. Immunol.* 1998; 140: 1063-8.
[95] Hill JA, Southwood S, Sette A, Jevnikar AM, Bell DA, Cairns E. The conversion of arginine to citrulline allows for a high-affinity peptide interaction with the Rheumatoid Arthritis-associated HLA-DRB1*0401 MHC class II molecule. *J. Immunol.* 2003; 171: 538-41.
[96] Rubin B, Wigzell H. On the nature of hapten-reactive lymphocytes. *Nature* 1973; 242: 467-9.
[97] Sercarz EE, Maverakis E. MHC-guided processing: binding of large antigen fragments. *Nat. Rev. Immunol.* 2003; 3: 621-9.
[98] Delovitch TL, Singh B. The nonobese Diabetic mouse as a model of autoimmune Diabetes: Immune dysregulation gets the NOD. *Immunity* 1997; 7: 727-38.
[99] Hugues S, Mougneau E, Ferlin W, Jeske D, Hofman P, Homann D, Beaudoin L, Schrike C, Von Herrath M, Lehuen A, Glaisenhaus N. Tolerance to islet antigens and prevention from Diabetes induced by limited apoptosis of pancreatic β cells. *Immunity* 2002; 16: 169-81.
[100] Sakagushi S, Ono M, Setoguchi R, Yagi H, Hori S, Fehervari Z, Shimizu J, Takahashi T, Nomura T. Foxp3$^+$CD25$^+$CD4$^+$ natural regulatory T cells in dominant self-tolerance and autoimmune disease. *Immunol. Rev.* 2006; 212: 8-27.
[101] Dahlen E, Dawe K, Ohlsson L, Hedlund G. Dendritic cells and macrophages are the first and major producers of TNF-α in Pancreatic Islets in the nonobese diabetic mouse. *J. Immunol.* 1998; 160: 3585-93.
[102] Calderon B, Suri A, Unanue ER. In CD4+ T-cell induced diabetes, macrophages are the final effector cells that mediate islet β-cell killing. *Am. J. Pathol.* 2006; 169: 2137-47.
[103] Wilson SB, Delovitch TL. Janus-like role of regulatory iNKT cells in autoimmune disease and tumor immunity. *Nat. Rev. Immunol.* 2003; 3: 211-22.
[104] Dahlén E, Hedlund G, Dawe K. Low CD86 expression in the Nonobese diabetic mouse results in the impairment of both T-cell activation and CTLA-4 up-regulation. *J. Immunol.* 2000; 164: 2444-56.
[105] Kawano T, Cui J, Koezuka Y, Toura I, Kaneko Y, Motoki H, Ueno R, Nakagawa H, Sato E, Kondo H, Koseki H, Taniguchi M. CD1d-restricted and TCR-mediated activation of Vα14 NKT cells by glycosyl-ceramides. *Science* 1997; 278: 1626-9.
[106] Shi FD, Flodstrom M, Balasa B, Kim SH, van Gunst K, Strominger JL, Wilson SB, Sarvetnick N. Germ line deletion of the CD1 locus exacerbates diabetes in the NOD mouse. *Proc. Natl. Acad. Sci. USA* 2001; 98: 6777-82.
[107] Wang B, Geng YB, Wang CR. CD1-restricted NKT cells protect non-obese diabetic mice from developing Diabetes. *J. Exp. Med.* 2001; 194: 313-20.
[108] Falcone M, Facciotti F, Ghidoli N, Monti P, Olivieri S, Zaccagnino L, Bonifacio E, Casorati G, Sanvito F, Sarvetnick N. Up-regulation of CD1d expression restores the

immunoregulatory function of NKT cells and prevents autoimmune diabetes in NOD mice. *J. Immunol.* 2004; 172: 5908-16.

[109] Lehuen A, Lantz O, Beaudoin L, Laloux V, Carnaud C, Bendelac A, Bach JF, Monteiro RC. Overexpression of natural killer T cells protects Valpha14-Jalpha281 transgenic non-obese mice against Diabetes. *J. Exp. Med.* 1998; 188: 1831-39.

[110] Singh N, Hong S, Scherer DC, Serizawa I, Burdin N, Kronenberg M, Koezuka Y, van Kaer L. Cutting edge: Activation of NKT cells by CD1d and α-Gal.Cer directs conventional T cells to acquisition of a Th2 phenotype. *J. Immunol.* 1999; 163: 2373-7.

[111] Beaudoin L, Laloux V, Novak J, Lucas B, Lehuen A. NKT cells inhibit the onset of Diabetes by impairing the development of pathogenic T cells specific for pancreatic β cells. *Immunity* 2002; 17: 725-36.

[112] Naumov YN, Bahjat KS, Gausling R, Abraham R, Exley MA, Koezuka Y, Balk SB, Strominger JL, Clare-Salzer M, Wilson SB. Activation of CD1d-restricted T cells protects NOD mice from developing diabetes by regulating dendritic cell subsets. *Proc. Natl. Acad. Sci. (USA)* 2001; 98: 13838-43.

[113] Bezbradica JS, Stanic AK, Matsuki N, Bour-Jordan H, Bluestone JA, Thomas JW, Unutmaz D, Van Kaer L, Joyce S. Distinct roles of dendritic cells and B cells in Vα14Jα18 natural T cell in vivo. *J. Immunol.* 2005; 174: 4696-705.

[114] Cheng L, Ueno A, Cho S, Im JS, Golby S, Hou S, Porcelli SA, Yang Y. Efficient activation of Vα14 invariant NKT cells by foreign lipid antigen is associated with concurrent dendritic cell-specific self recognition. *J. Immunol.* 2007; 178: 2755-62.

[115] Scott-Browne JP, Matsuda JL, Mallewaey T, White J, Borg NA, McCluskey J, Rossjohn J, Kappler J, Marrack P, Gapin L. Germline-encoded recognition of diverse glycolipids by natural killer T cells. *Nat. Immunol.* 2007; 8: 1105-13.

[116] Yu KOA, Im JS, Molano A, Dutronc Y, Illarionov PA, Forestier C, Fujiwara N, Arias I, Miyake S, Yamamura T, Chang YT, Desra GS, Porcelli SA. Modulation of CD1d-restricted NKT cell responses by using N-acyl variants of α-galactosylceramides. *Proc. Natl. Acad. Sci. USA* 2005; 102: 3383-8.

[117] Thedrez A, de Lalla C, Allain S, Zaccagnino L, Sidobre S, Garavaglia C, Borsillino G, Dellabona P, Bonneville M, Scotet E, Casorati G. CD4 engagement by CD1d potentiates activation of $CD4^+$ invariant NKT cells. *Blood* 2007; 110: 251-8.

[118] Chen X, Wang X, Besra GS, Gumperz JE. Modulation of CD1d-restricted NKT cell responses by CD4. *J. Leuk. Biol.* 2007; 82: 1-11.

[119] Tarbell KV, Petit L, Zuo X, Toy P, Luo X, Mqadmi A, Yang H, Suthanthiran M, Mojsov S, Steinman RM. Dendritic cell-expanded, islet-specific $CD4^+CD25^+CD62L^+$ regulatory T cells restore normoglycemia in diabetic NOD mice. *J. Exp. Med.* 2007; 204: 191-201.

[120] Wong J, Obst R, Correia-Neves M, Losyev G, Mathis D, Benoit C. Adaptation of TCR repertoires to self-peptides in regulatory and nonregulatory $CD4^+$ T cells. *J. Immunol.* 2007; 178: 7032-41.

[121] Ly D, Mi QS, Hissain S, Delovitch TL. Protection from type 1 Diabetes by in,variant NK T cells requires the activity of $CD4^+CD25^+$ regulatory T cells. *J. Immunol.* 2006; 177: 3695-704.

[122] Wu AJ, Hua H, Munson SH, McDevitt H. Tumor necrosis factor-α regulation of $CD4^+CD25^+$ T cell levels in NOD mice. *Proc. Natl. Acad. Sci (USA)* 2002; 99: 12287-92.

[123] Chen YG, Choisy-Rossi CM, Holl TM, Chapman HD, Besra GS, Porcelli SA, Shaffer DJ, Roopenian D, Wilson SB, Serreze DV. Activated NKT cells inhibit autoimmune diabetes through tolerogenic recruitment of dendritic cells to pancreatic lymph nodes. *J. Immunol.* 2005; 174: 1196-204.

[124] Feili-Hariri M, Morel PA. Phenotypic and functional characteristics of BM-derived DC from NOD and Non-diabetes-prone strains. *Clin. Immunol.* 2001; 98: 133-42.

[125] Wicker LS, Miller BJ, Chai A, Terada M, Mullen Y. Expression of genetically determined diabetes and insulitis in nonobese diabetic (NOD) mice at the level of bone marrow-derived cells. *J. Exp. Med.* 1988; 167: 1801-10.

[126] Prasad SJ, Goodnow CC. Cell-intrinsic effects of non-MHC NOD genes on dendritic cell generation in vivo. *Int. Immunol.* 2002; 14: 677-84.

[127] Morel PA, Vasquez C, Feili-Hariri M. Immunobiology of DC in NOD mice. *J. Leuk. Biol.* 1999; 66: 276-80.

[128] Steptoe RJ, Ritchie JM, Harrison LC. Increased generation of dendritic cells from myeloid progenitors in autoimmune-prone nonobese diabetic mice. *J. Immunol.* 2002; 168: 5032-41.

[129] Chilton PM, Rezzoug F, Fugier-Vivier I, Weeter LA, Xu H, Huang Y, Ray MB, Ildstad ST. Flt3L treatment prevents diabetes in NOD mice. *Diabetes* 2004; 53: 1995-2002.

[130] Clare-Salzler MJ, Brooks J, Chai A, Van Herle K, Anderson C. Prevention of Diabetes in nonobese mice by dendritic cell transfer. *J. Clin. Invest.* 1992; 90: 741-8.

[131] Shinomiya M, Fazle Akbar SM, Shinomiya H, Onji M. Transfer of dendritic cells (DC) ex vivo stimulated with IFNγ down-modulates autoimmune diabetes in non-obese diabetic (NOD) mice. *Clin. Exp. Immunol.* 1999; 117: 38-43.

[132] Papaccio G, Nicoletti F, Pisanti FA, Bendtzen K, Galdieri M. Prevention of spontaneous autoimmune diabetes in NOD mice by transferring in vitro antigen-pulsed syngeneic dendritic cells. *Endocrinology* 2000; 141: 1500-5.

[133] Feili-Hariri M, Dong X, Alber SM, Watkins SC, Salter RD, Morel PA. Immunotherapy of NOD mice with Bone-marrow-derived dendritic cells. *Diabetes* 1999; 48: 2300-8.

[134] Feili-Hariri M, Falkner DH, Morel PA. Regulatory Th2 response induced following adoptive transfer of dendritic cells in prediabetic NOD mice. *Eur. J. Immunol.* 2002; 32: 2021-30.

[135] Forestier C, Takaki T, Molano A, Im JS, Baine I, Jerud ES, Illarionov P, Ndonye R, Howell AR, Santamaria P, Besra G, DiLorenzo TP, Porcelli SA. Improved outcomes in NOD mice treated with a novel Th2 cytokine-biasing NKT cell activator. *J. Immunol.* 2007; 178: 1415-25.

[136] Xu Y, Zhan Y, Lew AM, Naik SH, Kershaw MH. Differential development of murine dendritic cells by GM-CSF versus Flt3 ligand has implications for inflammation and trafficking. *J. Immunol.* 2007; 179: 7577-84.

[137] Fujii SI, Shimizu K, Kronenberg M, Steinman RM. Prolonged IFNγ-producing NKT response induced with α-galactosylceramide-loaded DCs. *Nat. Immunol.* 2002; 3: 867-74.

[138] Lantz O, Bendelac A. An invariant T cell receptor α chain is used by a unique subset of major histocompatibility complex class I-specific CD4+ and CD4-8- T cells in mice and humans. *J. Exp. Med.* 1994; 180: 1097-106.

[139] Kojo S, Seino KI, Harada M, Watarai H, Wakao H, Uchida T, Nakayama T, Taniguchi M. Induction of regulatory properties in dendritic cells by Vα14 NKT cells. *J. Immunol.* 2005; 175: 3648-55.

[140] Zijlstra M, Bix M, Simister NE, Loring JM, Raulet DH, Jaenisch R. β2-microglobulin deficient mice lack $CD4^{-}CD8^{+}$ cytolytic T cells. *Nature* 1990; 344: 742-6.

[141] Cardell S, Tangri S, Chan S, Kronenberg M, Benoist C, Mathis D. CD1-restricted $CD4^{+}$ T cells in major histocompatibility complex class II-deficient mice. *J. Exp. Med.* 1995; 182: 993-1004.

[142] Scheffold A, Murphy KM, Höfer T. Competition for cytokines: Treg cells take all. *Nature Immunol.* 2007; 8: 1285-7.

In: Autoimmunity: Role, Regulation and Disorders
Editor: Fynn L. Vogel and L. F. Zimmermann
ISBN 978-1-60456-833-2

Chapter 10

Thyroid, Autoimmunity and Pregnancy

Roberto Negro*
Ospedale "V. Fazzi"
Piazza F. Muratore; 73100, Lecce, Italy

Introduction

Multiple and complex are the interactions involving the thyroid gland and the reproductive sphere, before and during pregnancy. The most common thyroid dysfunction in women of reproductive age is hypothyroidism due to thyroid autoimmunity (TAI), and widely identified are the complications due to hypothyroidism before and during pregnancy. Hypothyroidism increases the risk of menstrual irregularities, infertility and pregnancy morbidity. Furthermore, also isolated TAI is associated with infertility, and increased rate of miscarriage. But while the pathological mechanisms which link hypothyroidism and obstetrical complications are well known, the ones which link TAI and infertility, for example, remain largely speculative. In a condition where TAI and hypothyroidism are so strictly associated, these two entities can not be clear cut and represent the two sides of the same coin. Then, the hypothesized mechanisms which underlie obstetrical complications namely, autoimmunity *per se* and thyroid impairment, appear to be not mutually exclusive. Finally, among the complications due to TAI and hypothyroidism, of particular interest are the ones associated with the impaired neural development in the fetus and the following reduced intelligence quotient in the offspring.

Infertility

Infertility is the absolute inability to conceive after one year of regular intercourse without contraception and its overall prevalence ranges from 10-15 % [1, 2]. Female causes

* Tel. +390832661680; Fax +390832661911; e-mail robnegro@tiscali.it

of infertility account for 35% of couples, with the remaining causes due to a male factor in 30%, a combination of both in 20 %, and finally idiopathic one in 15% of cases [3]. Therapeutic approaches include the induction of ovulation in women with ovulatory dysfunction, endoscopic/surgical procedures to alleviate tubal obstruction, ablation of endometriosis, and intrauterine insemination (IUI) with donor or partner sperm. Other than the abovementioned techniques, assisted reproductive technologies (ART) may be used: *in vitro* fertilisation (IVF) or intra-cytoplasmic sperm injection (ICSI) [4]. Success rate of ART may be presented *per* cycle started, as the number of oocytes retrieved, or *per* embryo transferred, and finally as the rate of pregnancy at term (newborns). A major determinant of success after ART is woman's age, since both ovarian reserve and quality of oocytes decline fast from 35 years onwards. The average live birth rate, after one ART cycle in the 30-35 yr age group, ranges between 25 and 30% [5].

Thyroid Autoimmunity and Infertility

The prevalence of TAI is 5- to 10-fold higher in women than in men, and the reason for this higher prevalence is not known. A combination of genetic factors, estrogen-related effects, and chromosome X abnormalities have been postulated as possible causes [6, 7]. TAI is the most common autoimmune disorder, affecting about 10 % of women in the childbearing period [8]. TAI is also the main cause of thyroid dysfunction, even though thyroid autoimmunity can be present without hormonal dysfunction. In the last 10 years, several studies have investigated the prevalence of TAI in women with infertility. In particular, since 1996 to 2007, 9 studies have been published, trying to clarify if an association between TAI and infertility exists [9-17]. The global interpretation of the data reported in these studies is quite difficult because they are sometimes very different one from another. The studies vary for selection criteria, interfering factors, infertility causes, study design, control groups, sample size and type of assays employed for measurement of thyroid autoantibodies. In some studies, for example, a positive association between TAI, endometriosis and ovarian failure was found. Poppe *et al.,* published a case-controlled prospective study, in which 438 women of infertile couples were compared with 100 age-matched fertile women: a significantly increased relative risk was found for presence of TAI in women with endometriosis [14]. Two other studies have also reported a positive association between TAI and endometriosis, by Gerhard (44 % TAI in women with endometriosis *vs* 9 % in control women) and by Abalovich (25 % *versus* 14 % TAI) [16, 18]. In a recent study from Brazil aiming specifically at investigating a possible association between TAI and endometriosis, such association could not be confirmed. It should, however, be mentioned that the prevalence of TAI in their control group was much higher (reaching 25%) than in most other studies [17]. Endometriosis has frequently been associated with a variety of immunological changes, such as the presence of auto-antibodies to endometrial antigens, complement deposits, NK-cell depression, and cytotoxicity against autologous endometrium [19]. One other particular association between TAI and infertility has been observed in women with ovarian causes of infertility. In a study by Janssen, this was shown to be the case in women with PCOS, in whom 27% had TAI compared with only 8%

in women without PCOS [15]. According to the authors, the association was partly correlated with an increased estrogen to progesterone ratio characteristic of the syndrome. More recently in a study by Abalovich, an association was found between TAI and women with premature ovarian failure, which may have been due to a shared autoimmune etiology of the disorder [16].

Even taking into account the differences between these studies, when pooling their data, a significant association between TAI and infertility is present, with a TAI prevalence of 18% in infertile patients *vs* 7% in controls (P<0.001; RR 95% CI: 2.5). Underlying pathogenic mechanisms to explain associations between TAI and infertility remain largely speculative. It is plausible that several mechanisms coexist, as the various causes of female infertility encompass markedly different and heterogeneous diseases. It is not known whether thyroid antibodies are directly involved in the pathogenesis of infertility or they represent just innocent bystanders, being a marker of an unfavourable autoimmune environment. It should not be disregarded that a subtle thyroid dysfunction may be present in women with TAI, as in studies published by now, usually these patients, beneath in a condition of euthyroidism, display higher TSH values in respect to controls; furthermore, women with TAI are usually older than TAI-negative ones, a condition which is associated with an increased risk of infertility [20-22].

Autoimmune Hypothyroidism and Infertility

The prevalence of hypothyroidism in women in reproductive age varies between 2-4%, and is mostly caused by TAI [8]. Hypothyroidism is frequently associated with menstrual irregularities. The prevalence of oligomenorrhea is higher in hypothyroid women compared to controls (23% *vs* 8%) and the severity of menstrual abnormalities is associated with the elevation of TSH levels [23]. Hypothyroidism is also associated with menorrhagia, due to altered production of coagulation factors [24]. As thyroid hormones exert numerous interactions with the female reproductive system, hypothyroidism profoundly affects ovulatory function. Thyroid hormone receptors have been described in human oocytes, where they synergize with the FSH-mediated LH/hCG receptor to exert direct stimulatory effects on granulosa cell function (i.e. progesterone production) and on trophoblastic differentiation [25, 26]. In women with infertility, Cramer showed that serum TSH was a significant predictor of IVF failure, with TSH concentrations being significantly higher among women who produced oocytes that failed to achieve fertilization [27]. Furthermore, hypothyroidism can alters the pituitary-ovarian axis, by decreasing the binding activity of sex hormone-binding globulin (SHBG) resulting in increased serum free testosterone and estradiol. Also, elevated thyrotrophin-releasing hormone (TRH) levels due to hypothyroidism is often associated with increased prolactin levels, and a delayed LH response to LH-releasing hormone (LHRH) [28-30].

Several studies examined the prevalence of overt and subclinical hypothyroidism in infertile women. Among infertile females 2-6% was found to be affected by hypothyroidism, a prevalence that is not significantly different from the general population of women in childbearing age [31-33]. The prevalence of subclinical hypothyroidism shows a wide variation among the study published. It ranges from 0.7% in the study of Shalev to 43% in the study of Gerhard [14, 16, 18, 33-37]. These studies are hardly comparable because of differences in study design, size of sample, causes of infertility, and diagnosis criteria. Some authors considered affected by subclinical hypothyroidism those women presenting a TSH value higher than 5.5 mIU/l while others considered abnormal a TSH value higher than 3.0 mIU/l; furthermore, some studies considered as subclinical hypothyroid, those patients with altered TSH response to TRH stimulation test. From careful scrutiny of the data, the main trend was that SCH appeared to be more frequent in women with ovulatory disorders.

Thyroid Autoimmunity and Pregnancy

The state of pregnancy is characterized by a condition of tolerance of the maternal immune system to avoid a possible rejection of the semi-allogeneic fetal graft with its paternal antigens. In this view, women with and without TAI show similar pregnancy rates as demonstrated in women undergoing ART [38, 39]. Then, TAI *per se* does not seem to alter implantation of the embryo. Different studies, however, support an association between (recurrent) miscarriage and the presence of non-organ specific autoantibodies as well as organ specific autoimmunity. Nineteen studies have been published since 1990. The study which described such association was by Stagnaro-Green [40]. After screening 552 pregnant women for the presence of thyroid antibodies in first trimester, the authors found a double rate of miscarriages in TAI-positive compared with TAI-negative women. The increased miscarriage rate was independent of demographic data, serum TSH, thyroid antibody titers, prior obstetrical history, maternal age or presence of anti-cardiolipin antibodies. The authors mentioned however that TSH levels were abnormal in 6 out of 17 TAI-positive women who miscarried. Thereafter, an impressive number of studies have been published on the same issue and, altogether, allow to firmly conclude that TAI (without overt thyroid dysfunction) is significantly associated with a 3-fold to 5-fold increase in overall miscarriage rate, independently of the presence of antinuclear and anticardiolipin antibodies [11, 38, 39, 41-55]. Despite the heterogeneity of the studies investigating the association between TAI and pregnancy loss, it is remarkable that 15 out 19 studies confirmed this association. Finding an association does not necessarily imply a causal relationship and in this complex picture three hypotheses have been proposed to explain this association. The first hypothesis assumes that the increased risk of miscarriage is not directly due to the presence of thyroid antibodies, but these latter may just represent a marker of an unfavourable autoimmune environment, which in turn should be responsible for the rejection of the fetal graft. Women with recurrent abortions have an increased number of CD5/20-positive B cells, compared to women with no or only 1 abortion [56]. Moreover, abnormal T-lymphocyte function has been reported in women with TAI, including a higher number of endometrial T-cells [57]. Animal models favour a possible role for thyroid microchimerism (i.e. the presence of fetal cells of paternal origin in the maternal thyroid) to facilitate fetal loss. Finally, aberrant immune recognition of thyroglobulin (Tg) and placental antigens by anti-Tg antibodies has been demonstrated in mice immunized with human Tg, who then experienced a decrease in fetal and placental weights [58]. The second hypothesis assumes that women suffering from TAI display a subtle thyroid insufficiency, which worsens during pregnancy. In fact pregnant women with TAI have a reduced functional reserve, usually display higher TSH values before and during pregnancy in respect to TAI-negative ones, and are prone to develop subclinical hypothyroidism during pregnancy [55, 59, 60]. Data to support this hypothesis were obtained from women with threatened abortion, in whom significantly lower thyroid hormone levels were observed only in women who subsequently actually had miscarriage, compared to those women who delivered successfully [61]. Women with TAI, compared with controls, show significantly reduced TSH levels throughout trimesters of pregnancy and lower FT4 values from midgestation onward [60, 62]. The pattern of changes in thyroid hormones in pregnancies following ART shows an even clearer dissociation between serum TSH (higher) and free T4 (lower) in women with TAI, compared to those without TAI [63]. Futhermore, in a study by Bagis, only those women positive for TAI and who had a miscarriage showed a difference in median serum TSH and free T4, compared to women without TAI [53]. Finally, a third hypothesis is based on the relatively higher age of women with TAI compared with healthy controls. The speculation relies on the notion that women with TAI have a subtle underlying fertility problem. Because TAI is associated with infertility, this may lead women to conceive at a later age (3-4 years older, on the average) [64]. Overall, these hypotheses do not contradict one another, and it remains plausible that the increased risk of pregnancy loss associated with TAI results from a combination of several independent deleterious factors.

Medical intervention to reduce the miscarriage risk in women with TAI is based on immuno-modulation or thyroxine administration. Successful modulation of the immune system was reported in patients with TAI with the use of immunoglobulins with (or without) additional heparin or aspirin [65, 66]. Although these treatments were beneficial in terms of pregnancy outcome, the studies included only a small number of patients, as well as women who had other autoantibodies (besides thyroid antibodies), and finally often lacked appropriate controls. In the study by Vaquero, a comparison was made between the beneficial effects of immunoglobulins and thyroid hormone extracts (started before conception and continued until mid-gestation) on the outcome of pregnancy in women with TAI with a history of recurrent miscarriage. In the 16 women treated with thyroid hormones, there was a significant improvement in live-birth rate, compared with the 11 women who received immunoglobulins (81% *vs* 51 %) [67]. Criticism to the study was the small number of patients and also that thyroid hormone extracts were started already before conception. Another study by Stricker, evaluated the efficacy of low-dose intravenous immunoglobulin treatment in older women (37 years) with different immunologic abnormalities and recurrent spontaneous abortion. Of the 47 patients enrolled, 53% were TAI-positive. A subgroup (11 patients) refused immunoglobulin treatment, and results showed that the treated group gave live births in a significantly higher number of cases [68]. Recently, two studies, by Negro, investigated the chance that treatment with thyroxine may be beneficial in reducing pregnancy loss; the first study was in an ART setting, while the second one in spontaneous pregnancies. In the first study, the authors showed that the miscarriage rate was reduced to 33% in thyroxine-treated women, compared with 52% in placebo-treated group [39]. The data failed to reach statistical significance, probably because of the small number of patients. In the second study, the investigators followed a large group of pregnant women, among whom 12% were TAI-positive [62]. One half of the latter group was treated with thyroxine during gestation, while the other half was left untreated. The end points of the study were to assess the outcome of pregnancy and changes in thyroid function, by comparing the group of TAI-positive women without treatment to those who were treated and also to healthy pregnant controls. Concerning pregnancy outcome, the results showed a drastic reduction in the rates of both spontaneous miscarrriage (a 75% decrement) and premature delivery (a 69% decrement) in TAI-positive women who received thyroxine since early gestation and throughout pregnancy. Concerning thyroid function, and as expected, thyroxine administration allowed to maintain normal thyroid function tests in women with TAI, while serum free T4 decreased by 30% and TSH levels increased progressively during gestation in the untreated group: 19% of these women became subclinically hypothyroid at the time of parturition. Despite some criticism because the study was not placebo-controlled nor double-blinded, and also because the mean serum TSH was already significantly higher before medical intervention in women with TAI (compared with controls), the study had the great merit of representing the first prospective randomized trial to confirm the efficacy of thyroxine administration in pregnant women with autoimmune features and who present a euthyroid status [69]. This study also has implications both for screening programmes and medical intervention proposals. However, before systematically administering thyroxine to all euthyroid women with TAI, it will first be necessary to confirm the beneficial results already obtained in other large double-blind placebo controlled trials.

Autoimmune Hypothyroidism and Pregnancy

The main cause of hypothyroidism during pregnancy is chronic autoimmune thyroiditis, at least in countries where the iodine intake in the population is adequate. In both prospective and retrospective studies of unselected pregnant women with hypothyroidism, thyroid autoantibodies can be found in 25-77% of the cases, with an average prevalence of 46%. In the studies where sufficient epidemiological information is available on control pregnant women, TAI is 5-fold more prevalent in pregnant women with a diagnosis of hypothyroidism. In women with TAI who maintain a euthyroid status in early gestation, pregnancy frequently triggers progression to hypothyroidism because the maternal thyroid needs to produce more thyroid hormone during gestation and TAI-positive women are less able to sustain this indispensable increase owing to their reduced thyroidal functional reserve. Therefore, progressive hypothyroidism often develops or worsens as gestation progresses [60]. Pregnant women with hypothyroidism have a greater risk of early and late obstetric complications, namely miscarriage, anemia, gestational hypertension, placental abruption, premature delivery, postpartum haemorrhage, and admission of their newborn to neonatal intensive care (particularly for respiratory distress syndromes) [70, 71]. Obstetric complications are associated with overt hypothyroidism as well as SCH, and thyroxine treatment with subsequent restoration of normal thyroid function greatly reduces the frequency of these complications [72].

Besides obstetrical complications, maternal thyroid deficiency is also detrimental for fetal development. It is presently accepted that the fetal effects depend upon the severity and early onset of a reduced availability of maternal thyroid hormone. Recent studies have indicated that undiagnosed (and hence untreated) hypothyroidism occurring during the 1st half of pregnancy is associated with a risk of a poorer neuro-developmental outcome in the progeny [73, 74]. Severe impairment of fetal neurodevelopment is thought to require prolonged maternal hypothyroidism. The study by Haddow in 1999 showed that when maternal hypothyroidism was mainly due to chronic autoimmune thyroiditis, the offspring of untreated women were at risk for clinically relevant cognitive deficits [75]. Even isolated hypothyroxinaemia during early gestation (defined as serum free T4 value near the lower limit of normality with a normal serum TSH and no detectable thyroid antibodies) may be associated with a lower psycho-developmental index in the offspring [76]. A very interesting study has been recently published, concerning maternal thyroid status and fetal neurodevelopment. In particular, the authors investigated the relationship between TPOAb and sensorineural hearing loss (SNHL) [77]. They tested stored third-trimester maternal serum specimens of 1,736 children for TPOAb. An audiology examination was administered to the children at 8 years of age and was used to identify cases of SNHL. Compared with 4.3% of the other children, 22.7% of the children whose mothers had elevated TPOAb had SNHL ($p<0.05$; OR: 7.5, 95% confidence interval: 2.4-23.3). These data suggest that antenatal exposure to maternal TPOAb during pregnancy is associated with impaired auditory development. A limitation in this study derive from the fact that dosages for TSH and FT4 were not performed, then we can not be sure that SNHL is due to gestational thyroid impairment. Anyway it is reasonable to hypothesize that thyroxine deficit, even if mild and transient may adversely affect the neurodevelopment of the acoustic system. Delay of the foetal brain development seems to be the only adverse consequence of maternal hypothyroxinemia. A recently published paper by Casey *et al.* evaluated if isolated maternal hypothyroxinemia (FT4 < 0.86 ng/dl) in the first half of gestation may affect the perinatal outcome [78]. The authors evaluating 17,289 women who presented for prenatal care during the first 20 weeks of gestation, identified three groups to be studied, i.e. pregnant women with normal thyroid function, with subclinical hypothyroidism, and with isolated hypothyroxinemia. Women suffering from subclinical hypothyroidism when compared with the other two groups, showed increased risk of developing gestational diabetes, placental abruption and, pre-term delivery. Babies born from mothers with subclinical hypothyroidism when compared with the other two groups displayed increased risk of admission to intensive care unit, low APGAR score, and respiratory distress syndrome. No differences were found concerning the abovementioned complications between euthyroid and hypothyroxinemic women. Notably, the prevalence of TPOAb was similar in woman with and without hypothyroxinemia (5% and 4%, respectively), while was higher in women with subclinical hypothyroidism (31%); these latter results may lead to suppose that isolated hypothyroxinemia is mainly due to iodine deficiency, while high TSH values to thyroid autoimmunity. Further explanations about these matters will come from the ongoing research by JH Lazarus. The prospective and randomized study, called "Controlled Antenatal Thyroid Screening Study" (CATS), consists in the supplementation with thyroxine in a group of pregnant women who, within the 16th week of gestation, display FT4 values lower than the 2.5th percentile and/or TSH values above the 97.5th percentile. The study will produce two groups of women (treated and untreated) whose newborns will be tested for neuropsychological development at an age of 3 years. Preliminary data from this study suggests that utilizing both parameters results in two abnormal pregnant populations – namely, about half with a low T4 and an equal number with a high TSH, with very few having both a low T4 and a high TSH. The principal scope of the study is to ascertain if the offspring of mothers with high-normal TSH and/or low-normal FT4 values has a delayed neuropsychological development and if this condition may be prevented with thyroxine treatment. Another study sponsored by the Maternal-Fetal Medicine Units Network of the National Institute of Child Health and Human Development started in 2006. It is a randomized, placebo-controlled treatment trial, involving 120,000 pregnant women; aim of this study is to look at the effects of thyroxine treatment on intellectual function in 1,000 5-year-old children of mothers diagnosed with subclinical hypothyroidism during the first half of pregnancy. If these trials will definitively demonstrate that subclinical hypothyroidism and/or hypothyroxinemia exert detrimental effects on pregnancy and offspring and that these complications may be prevented by the use of thyroxine, there will be a valid reason to sustain the screening for thyroid function at the beginning of pregnancy.

References

[1] Wang X *et al.* (2003) Conception, early pregnancy loss, and time to clinical pregnancy: a population-based prospective study. *Fertil Steril.* 79: 577-84

[2] Gnoth C *et al.* (2003) Time to pregnancy: results of the German prospective study and impact on the management of infertility. *Hum. Reprod.* 18: 1959-66.

[3] Healy DL *et al.* (1994) Female infertility: causes and treatment. *Lancet* 343: 1539-44.

[4] Braude P and Rowell P (2003) Assisted conception. In vitro fertilisation and intracytoplasmic sperm injection. *BMJ* 327: 852-5.

[5] Osmanagaoglu K *et al.* (2002) Cumulative delivery rates after ICSI in women aged >37 years. *Hum. Reprod.* 17: 940-4.

[6] Tomer Y and Davies TF (2003) Searching for the autoimmune thyroid disease susceptibility genes: from gene mapping to gene function. *Endo. Rev.* 24: 694-717.

[7] Prummel MF *et al.* (2004) The environment and autoimmune thyroid diseases. *Eur. J. Endocrinol.* 150: 605-18.

[8] Hollowell JG *et al.* (2002) Serum TSH, T4, and thyroid antibodies in the United States population (1988 to 1994): National Health and Nutrition Examination Survey (NHANES III). *J. Clin. Endocrinol Metab* 87: 489-99.

[9] Roussev RG *et al.* (1996) Laboratory evaluation of women experiencing reproductive failure. *Am. J. Reprod. Immunol.* 35: 415-20.

[10] Geva E *et al.* (1997) The presence of antithyroid antibodies in euthyroid patients with unexplained infertility and tubal obstruction. *Am. J. Reprod. Immunol.* 37: 184-6.

[11] Kutteh WH *et al.* (1999) Increased prevalence of antithyroid antibodies identified in women with recurrent pregnancy loss but not in women undergoing assisted reproduction. *Fertil Steril.* 71: 843-8.

[12] Kaider AS *et al.* (1999) Immunodiagnostic evaluation in women with reproductive failure. *Am. J. Reprod. Immunol.* 42: 335-46.

[13] Reimand K *et al.* (2001) Autoantibody studies of female patients with reproductive failure. *J. Reprod. Immunol.* 51: 167-76.
[14] Poppe K *et al.* (2002) Thyroid dysfunction and autoimmunity in infertile women. *Thyroid* 12: 997-1001.
[15] Janssen OE *et al.* (2004) High prevalence of autoimmune thyroiditis in patients with polycystic ovary syndrome. *Eur. J. Endocrinol.* 150: 363-9.
[16] Abalovich M *et al.* (2007) Subclinical hypothyroidism and thyroid autoimmunity in women with infertility. *Gynecol. Endocrinol.* 23: 279-83.
[17] Petta CA *et al.* (2007) Thyroid autoimmunity and thyroid dysfunction in women with endometriosis. *Hum. Reprod.* 22: 2693-7.
[18] Gerhard I *et al.* (1991) Thyroid and ovarian function in infertile women. *Hum. Reprod.* 6: 338-45.
[19] Matarese G *et al.* (2003) Pathogenesis of endometriosis: natural immunity dysfunction or autoimmune disease? *Trends Mol. Med.* 9: 223-8.
[20] Menken J *et al.* (1986) Age and Infertility. *Science* 233:1389-94.
[21] van Noord-Zaadstra B *et al.* (1991) Delaying childbearing: effect of age on fecundity and outcome of pregnancy. *Br. Med. J.* 302:1361-5.
[22] Tatone C. (2008) Oocyte senescence: a firm link to age-related female subfertility. *Gynecol. Endocrinol.* 24:59-63.
[23] Krassas GE *et al.* (1999) Disturbances of menstruation in hypothyroidism. *Clin. Endocrinol.* 50: 655-9.
[24] Weeks AD. (2000) Menorrhagia and hypothyroidism. Evidence supports association between hypothyroidism and menorrhagia. *BMJ* 320:649.
[25] Wakim AN *et al.* (1993) Thyroid hormones in human follicular fluid and thyroid hormone receptors in human granulosa cells. *Fertil. Steril.* 59: 1187-90.
[26] Maruo T *et al.* (1991) Thyroid hormone as a biological amplifier of differentiated trophoblast function in early pregnancy. *Acta Endocrinol.* 125: 58-66.
[27] Cramer DW *et al.* (2003) Serum prolactin and TSH in an in vitro population: is there a link between fertilization and thyroid function? *J. Assist. Reprod. Genet.* 20: 210-15.
[28] Thomas R and Reid RL (1987) Thyroid disease and reproductive dysfunction: a review. *Obstet. Gynecol.* 70: 789-98.
[29] Trokoudes KM *et al.* (2006) Infertility and thyroid disorders. *Curr. Opin. Obstet Gynecol.* 18:446-51.
[30] Krassas GE (2000) Thyroid disease and female reproduction. *Fertil. Steril.* 74:1063-70.
[31] Joshi JV *et al.* (1993) Menstrual irregularities and lactation failure may precede thyroid dysfunction or goitre. *J. Postgrad. Med.* 39:137-41.
[32] Lincoln SR *et a.l* (1999) Screening for hypothyroidism in infertile women. *J. Reprod. Med.* 44:455-7.
[33] Arojoki M *et al.* (2000) Hypothyroidism among infertile women in Finland. *Gynecol. Endocrinol.* 14: 127-31.
[34] Bohnet HG *et al.* (1981) Subclinical hypothyroidism and infertility. *Lancet* 5: 1278.
[35] Shalev E *et al.* (1994) Routine thyroid function tests in infertile women: are they necessary? *Am. J. Obstet. Gynecol.* 171: 1191-2.

[36] Grassi G *et al.* (2001) Thyroid autoimmunity and infertility. *Gynecol. Endocrinol.* 15: 389-96.

[37] Raber W *et al.* (2003) Thyroxine treatment modified in infertile women according to thyroxine-releasing hormone testing: 5 year follow-up of 283 women referred after exclusion of absolute causes of infertility. *Hum. Reprod.* 18: 707-14.

[38] Poppe K *et al.* (2003) Assisted reproduction and thyroid autoimmunity: an unfortunate combination? *J. Clin. Endocrinol. Metab.* 88: 4149-52.

[39] Negro R *et al.* (2005) Levothyroxine treatment in thyroid peroxidase antibody-positive women undergoing assisted reproduction technologies: a prospective study. *Hum. Reprod.* 20: 1529-33.

[40] Stagnaro-Green A *et al.* (1990) Detection of at-risk pregnancy by means of highly sensitive assays for thyroid autoantibodies. *JAMA* 264: 1422-5.

[41] Glinoer D. (1991) Pregnancy in patients with mild thyroid abnormalities: maternal and neonatal repercussions. *J. Clin. Endocrinol. Metab.* 73: 421-7.

[42] Lejeune B *et al.* (1993) Antithyroid antibodies underlying thyroid abnormalities and miscarriage or pregnancy induced hypertension. *Br. J. Obstet. Gynaecol.* 100: 669-72.

[43] Pratt DE *et al.* (1993) The association of antithyroid antibodies in euthyroid nonpregnant women with recurrent first trimester abortions in the next pregnancy. *Fertil. Steril.* 60: 1001-5.

[44] Singh A *et al.* (1995) Presence of thyroid antibodies in early reproductive failure: biochemical versus clinical pregnancies. *Fertil. Steril.* 63: 277-81.

[45] Bussen S and Steck T. (1995) Thyroid autoantibodies in euthyroid non-pregnant women with recurrent spontaneous abortions. *Hum. Reprod.* 10: 2938-40.

[46] Iijima T *et al.* (1997) Effects of autoantibodies on the course of pregnancy and fetal growth. *Obstet. Gynaecol.* 90: 364-9.

[47] Esplin MS *et al.* (1998) Thyroid autoantibodies are not associated with recurrent pregnancy loss. *Am J. Obstet. Gynecol.* 179: 1583-6.

[48] Kim CH *et al.* (1998) Influence of antithyroid antibodies in euthyroid women on in vitro fertilization-embryo transfer outcome. *Am. J. Reprod. Immunol.* 40: 2-8.

[49] Muller AF *et al.* (1999) Thyroid autoimmunity and abortion: a prospective study in women undergoing in vitro fertilization. *Fertil. Steril.* 71: 30-4.

[50] Bussen S *et al.* (2000) Increased prevalence of thyroid antibodies in euthyroid women with a history of recurrent in-vitro fertilization failure. *Hum. Reprod.* 15: 545-8.

[51] Dendrinos S *et al.* (2000) Thyroid autoimmunity in patients with recurrent spontaneous miscarriages. *Gynecol. Endocrinol.* 14: 270-4.

[52] Rushworth FH *et al.* (2000) Prospective pregnancy outcome in untreated recurrent miscarries with thyroid autoantibodies. *Hum. Reprod.* 15: 1637-9.

[53] Bagis T *et al.* (2001) Autoimmune thyroid disease in pregnancy and the postpartum period: relationship to spontaneous abortion. *Thyroid* 11: 1049-53.

[54] Sieiro Netto L *et al.* (2004) Influence of thyroid autoimmunity and maternal age on the risk of miscarriage. *Am. J. Reprod. Immunol.* 52: 312-6.

[55] Negro R *et al.* (2007) Euthyroid women with autoimnmune disease undergoing assisted reproduction technologies: The role of autoimmunity and thyroid function. *J. Endocrinol. Invest* 30: 3-8.

[56] Roberts J *et al.* (1996) Recurrent miscarriage is associated with increased numbers of CD5/20 positive lymphocytes and an increased incidence of thyroid antibodies. *Eur. J. Endocrinol* 134: 84-6.

[57] Matalon ST *et al.* (2001) The association between anti-thyroid antibodies and pregnancy loss. *Am. J. Reprod. Immunol.* 45: 72-7.

[58] Matalon ST *et al.* (2003) The pathogenic role of anti-thyroglobulin antibody on pregnancy: evidence from an active immunization model in mice. *Hum. Reprod.* 18: 1094-9.

[59] Pearce EN *et al.* (2008) Association of first-trimester thyroid function test values with thyroperoxidase antibody status, smoking, and multivitamin use. *Endocr. Pract.* 14:33-9.

[60] Glinoer D *et al.* (1994) Risk of subclinical hypothyroidism in pregnant women with asymptomatic autoimmune thyroid disorders. *J. Clin. Endocrinol. Metab.* 79:197-204.

[61] Maruo T *et al.* (1992) The role of maternal thyroid hormones in maintaining early pregnancy in threatened abortion. *Acta Endocrinol.* 127: 118-22.

[62] Negro R *et al.* (2006) Levothyroxine treatment in euthyroid pregnant women with autoimmune thyroid disease: effects on obstetrical complications. *J. Clin. Endocrinol. Metab.* 91: 2587-91.

[63] Poppe K *et al.* (2004) Impact of ovarian hyperstimulation on thyroid function in women with - and without thyroid autoimmunity. *J. Clin. Endocrinol. Metab.* 89: 3808-12.

[64] Prummel MF and Wiersinga WM. (2004) Thyroid autoimmunity and miscarriage. *Eur. J. Endocrinol* 150: 751-5.

[65] Kiprov DD *et al.* (1996) The use of intravenous immunoglobulin in recurrent pregnancy loss associated with combined alloimmune and autoimmune abnormalities. *Am. J. Reprod. Immunol.* 36: 228-34.

[56] Sher G *et al.* (1998) The use of combined heparin/aspirin and immunoglobulin G therapy in the treatment of in vitro fertilization patients with antithyroid antibodies. *Am. J. Reprod Immunol.* 39: 223-5.

[67] Vaquero E *et al.* (2001) Pregnancy outcome in recurrent spontaneous abortion associated with anti-phospholipid antibodies: a comparative study of intravenous immunoglobulin versus prednisone plus low-dose aspirin. *Am. J. Reprod. Immunol.* 45: 174-9.

[68] Stricker RB *et al.* (2000) Successful treatment of immunologic abortion with low-dose intravenous immunoglobulin. *Fertil. Steril.* 73:536-40.

[69] Glinoer D (2006) Miscarriage in women with positive anti-TPO antibodies: is thyroxine the answer? (Editorial) *J.Clin. Endocrinol. Metab.* 91: 2500-2.

[70] Mandel SJ (2004) Hypothyroidism and chronic autoimmune thyroiditis in the pregnant state: maternal aspects. *Best Pract. Res. Clin. Endocrinol Metab* 18: 213-24.

[71] Casey BM *et al.* (2005) Subclinical hypothyroidism and pregnancy outcomes. *Obstet Gynecol.* 105: 239-45.

[72] Abalovich M *et al.* (2002) Overt and subclinical hypothyroidism complicating pregnancy. *Thyroid* 12: 63–8

[73] Glinoer D and Delange F (2000) The potential repercussions of maternal, fetal, and neonatal hypothyroxinemia on the progeny. *Thyroid* 10: 871-87.

[74] Morreale GM *et al.* (2004) Maternal thyroid hormones early in pregnancy and fetal brain development. *Best Pract Res. Clin. Endocrinol Metab.* 18: 225-48.

[75] Haddow JE *et al.* (1999) Maternal thyroid deficiency during pregnancy and subsequent neuro-psychological development of the child. *N. Engl. J. Med.* 341: 549-55.

[76] Pop VJ *et al.* (2003) Maternal hypothyroxinaemia during early pregnancy and subsequent child development: a 3-year follow-up study. *Clin. Endocrinol.* 59: 282-8.

[77] Wasserman EE *et al.* (2008) Maternal thyroid autoantibodies during the third trimester and hearing deficits in children: an epidemiologic assessment. *Am. J. Epidemiol.* 167:701-10.

[78] Casey BM *et al.* (2007) Perinatal significance of isolated maternal hypothyroxinemia identified in the first half of pregnancy. *Obstet. Gynecol.* 109:1129-35.

In: Autoimmunity: Role, Regulation and Disorders
Editor: Fynn L. Vogel and L. F. Zimmermann
ISBN 978-1-60456-833-2

Chapter 11

Autoantibody Profiles of an Asbestos-Exposed Population

Jean C. Pfau*[*1], David J. Blake[2] and Marvin J. Fritzler[3]
[1]Department of Biomedical and Pharmaceutical Sciences,
University of Montana, Missoula MT
[2]Johns Hopkins University, Baltimore MD
[3]Department of Medicine, University of Calgary, Calgary, Alberta

Abstract

Asbestos exposure is associated with autoimmune responses including increased serum immunoglobulins, positive autoantibody tests and immune complex deposition. Occupational and environmental asbestos exposures continue to occur world-wide, making this a current human health issue. The premise that asbestos exposure exacerbates autoimmunity is supported by recent studies from an asbestos exposed population in Libby, Montana, USA. Residents of Libby have experienced significant exposures to amphibole asbestos due to the mining of asbestos-contaminated vermiculite near the community over several decades. This community exhibits higher frequencies of positive anti-nuclear antibody (ANA) tests compared to an unexposed control population and what would be expected based on epidemiological data.

Systemic autoimmune diseases are characterized by autoantibody profiles that correspond to specific sets of intracellular components. These profiles can be used to help predict disease, establish a diagnosis as well as assess clinical progression. At this time, it is not known whether a discrete clinical or sub-clinical autoimmune entity is associated with amphibole asbestos exposure. However, asbestos exposure leads to clinical manifestations similar to systemic lupus erythematosus (SLE) in asbestos exposed mice. Therefore, we hypothesized that features of certain autoimmune diseases may be associated with asbestos exposure in humans. The purpose of this study was to determine whether a serological signature exists in this asbestos-exposed population, and

[*] Contact Information: Jean C. Pfau, Ph.D. Skaggs 283, Department of Biomedical and Pharmaceutical Sciences, University of Montana, Missoula MT 59812, (406) 243-4529. jean.pfau@umontana.edu

to compare this profile with other known systemic autoimmune disease autoantibody profiles.

Our results indicate that autoantibodies from individuals exposed to amphibole asbestos primarily recognize chromatin, histone and Ro52, similar to patients with systemic lupus erythematosus (SLE). Anti-dsDNA and anti-Ro52 antibodies are also generated in a murine model of asbestos induced autoimmunity, which suggests that asbestos may drive similar immune phenomena in both humans and mice. In addition, we show that an unexpected number of subjects expressed the Scl-topoisomerase I (topo I: also referred to as Scl-70) antibody, typically seen in scleroderma. The subjects with anti-topo I tended to have higher levels of asbestos exposure and more severe lung disease compared to those without topo I, whereas there was no association with exposure or lung disease among people with anti-RNP (antibodies to ribonucleoprotein, common in SLE). Finally, we show that some Libby serum samples contained antibodies that bound fibroblasts, a phenomenon that is also seen in scleroderma. By comparison, neither rheumatoid factor (RF) nor anti-cyclic citrullinated peptide (CCP), markers for rheumatoid arthritis (RA), was substantially elevated in the Libby sample set. This information could be extremely valuable for improved screening of exposed populations. In addition, certain autoantibody profiles may serve as diagnostic or prognostic markers relative to asbestos exposure.

Introduction

Occupational and environmental exposures to biologically active forms of silicon oxides such as crystalline silica and amphibole fibers (asbestos and asbestiform minerals) continue to occur and pose serious health risks because of their abundance in the earth's crust and their use in many materials in developed and developing nations. Studies regarding health effects from these exposures are critical at many levels, from epidemiological data to exploring cellular and molecular mechanisms, so that the information can be used in setting regulatory exposure standards, minimizing exposure risks, screening exposed populations, anticipating healthcare costs in industry, and exploring preventive and therapeutic modalities. While acknowledging the impact and severity of the cancers and fibrotic disorders associated with silica and asbestos, this chapter focuses on the complex, enigmatic, and often devastating systemic autoimmune disorders.

As early as 1914, an association between occupational exposures of inhaled crystalline silica[1] and autoimmunity was suggested when Bramwell reported increased frequencies of diffuse systemic sclerosis (SSc) in stone masons [1]. However, documented reports of the increased prevalence of SLE in workers occupationally exposed to silica first appeared in the 1990's [2, 3]. Case reports and population-based studies have continued to enrich and strengthen the data supporting the association between crystalline silica and SLE. The historical literature linking silica exposure with autoimmune diseases is summarized in recent reviews [4-6]. While the background literature regarding silica is fairly extensive, studies regarding asbestos exposures and autoimmunity have been more limited. Studies of the humoral responses following asbestos exposure appear in the literature beginning around

[1] A distinction is made between crystalline silica and either amorphous silica or silicone, as the immunological effects of the latter two have not been established and remain controversial.

1965 when the presence of rheumatoid factor (RF) and antinuclear antibodies (ANA) were reported in asbestos workers [7, 8]. Interestingly, despite clear associations between silica exposure and systemic autoimmune diseases (SAID) such as systemic lupus erythematosus (SLE), SSc and rheumatoid arthritis (RA), asbestos exposure has not yet been linked with any particular autoimmune or connective tissue disorder. There are several possibilities for this knowledge gap, including a lack of statistical power due to relatively small or diffuse exposure cohorts, difficulties in exposure assessment, mild or sub-clinical entities that remain undetected or masked by other pathology, or alternatively, an absence of any associated autoimmune pathology despite the presence of the autoantibodies. In addition, because of the latency and complexity of diseases such as SLE [9], establishing an association between exposure and actual clinical disease is difficult.

Asbestos exposure in humans is associated with the development of malignant and nonmalignant diseases including lung cancer, pulmonary fibrosis (asbestosis) as well as an increased frequency of autoantibody production. Although the commercial use of asbestos has decreased in the United States since the 1970s, asbestos exposure remains a major environmental health concern. More than 30 million tons of asbestos have been mined in the US alone [10] and more than 27 million people were exposed to asbestos between 1940 and 1979 [11]. As late as 1989, the use of asbestos products in the U.S. exceeded 55,000 tons per year. Developed countries have restricted the use of asbestos because of its harmful public health effects. However, asbestos is now a major concern in developing countries due to increased marketing and commercial use [12, 13]. Additionally, in 2002 the vermiculite mine and community of Libby, MT were designated by the Environmental Protection Agency (EPA) as Superfund sites due to the amphibole asbestos contamination of vermiculite, which led to exposure throughout the mine site and surrounding area. Significant health issues have become evident in Libby and many other sites where the vermiculite was shipped for processing [14]. Hence, asbestos exposure remains an immediate environmental health concern not only in Libby but throughout the United States and in developing countries.

Amphibole Asbestos Contamination in Libby, MT

From 1924 to 1990, Zonolite mountain near Libby, Montana was the site of a vermiculite mining operation. In 1963, W.R. Grace bought the Zonolite mining operations, which subsequently provided approximately 80% of the world's supply of vermiculite [15]. Unfortunately the vermiculite extracted from the Libby mine was contaminated with naturally-occurring asbestos fibers. The mine closed in 1990 after almost 60 years of operation. The first emergency response team from the EPA was sent to Libby in November 1999. The EPA began collecting air, soil and insulation samples. In October of 2002 the vermiculite mine and surrounding community of Libby were designated as EPA Superfund sites due to the asbestos contamination of vermiculite. The various mining, transportation, and processing activities as well as the personal and commercial use of vermiculite in the community led to widespread environmental exposures in the Libby area, which resulted in significant asbestos-related diseases even in residents with short exposure times of less than a year [16]. The extensive asbestos exposure has led to considerable health problems in the community including reduced pulmonary function, enhanced autoimmune responses and increased mortality from lung cancer, malignant mesothelioma and fibrosis [17, 18]. The asbestos-related disease (ARD) observed in patients from Libby include interstitial fibrosis, pleural plaques, and mesothelioma, with a subset of patients developing rapid progression of disease.

The asbestos contamination of Libby vermiculite has been characterized as both regulated asbestos fibers (e.g., tremolite and other amphibole forms) and unregulated fibers (e.g., winchite and richterite) [19]. The mixture of amphibole fibers in the Libby amphibole sample differs in terms of fiber length and metallic cations adhered to the fiber surface. Moreover, these amphibole fibers are thought to be more pathogenic than serpentine asbestos fibers because the longer amphibole fibers cannot be readily cleared from the lung [20].

The premise that asbestos exposure exacerbates autoimmune responses in humans is supported by two recent studies of the asbestos exposed population in Libby. According to data from these studies, exposure to Libby amphibole asbestos increases the risk for SAID by more than 50% [21]. Moreover, residents of Libby have higher frequencies of positive ANA tests compared to those from an unexposed control population [22]. Anecdotal concerns have been raised by the residents regarding SLE or SLE-like connective tissue disease, and at a recent conference in Denver, Colorado addressing the epidemiology of asbestos-related diseases related to the Libby vermiculite[2], physicians present agreed that autoimmune/connective tissue diseases needed to be included in a thorough evaluation of asbestos-related pathologies. This is particularly important due to reports that those individuals who manifest positive ANA tests and/or rheumatic symptoms may experience more severe pulmonary complications ([22], and personal communication, B. Black, M.D., Libby Center for Asbestos Related Disease).

An analysis of the specific targets of autoantibodies (AA) from residents in Libby, MT can provide insight and help define the clinical diagnoses in this exposed population. The spectrum of AA related to amphibole asbestos exposure may have implications in elucidating the immunologic response to asbestos and provide a biomarker for clinical screening. The objective of this study was to characterize the specific AA found in serum samples from the Libby cohort and to determine if the presence of AA correlated with a particular clinical pattern.

Materials and Methods

Human samples. All samples were acquired according to approved University of Montana Institutional Review Board protocols intending to protect the well-being and confidentiality of all subjects. The recruitment and collection of samples described in this chapter have been reported previously [21, 22], and include subjects from both Libby and

[2] July 23-24, 2007. Sponsored by the Environmental Protection Agency, with participation from Centers for Disease Control, Agency for Toxic Substances and Disease Registry, NIOSH, several university researchers, the Montana Department of Environmental Quality, and the community of Libby MT. For more information: www.epa.gov/region8/toxics_pesticides/asbestos/

Missoula MT, with Missoula as the unexposed reference population. Wherever data is compared between Libby and Missoula, sample sets were matched by age and sex.

Missoula is similar to Libby in being located in a mountain valley, subject to similar climatic conditions, including winter inversions, dry summers, and exposure to smoke from forest fires and wood burning. Because prevailing winds in Missoula are from the west and Libby is well to the north, there is no detectable transfer of asbestos from the Libby airshed to the Missoula airshed. Therefore, on a relative basis, while one cannot exclude the possibility that there could have been some minimal asbestos exposure by the Missoula population, it is an acceptable reference population for the Libby subjects who were definitely exposed to asbestos. Subjects in both communities are fairly homogeneous in terms of ethnicity; the majority of residents are of northern European descent, with 94.7% Caucasian in Lincoln County and 93.6% Caucasian in Missoula County according to Montana census data. The presence of physician-diagnosed autoimmune disease among Libby subjects was not assessed in the screening. None of the Missoula subjects recruited had diagnosed SAID, although this was not a criterion for exclusion. Subjects were excluded when data indicated that they were currently using medications that are known to be associated with positive ANA tests and drug-induced lupus (DIL), specifically chlorpromazine, hydralazine, isoniazid, methyldopa, minocycline, procainamide, quinidine. However, many other drugs may be associated with DIL but were not among the exclusion criteria used for this study.

Sample and Data Collection

The blood samples were collected, and serum samples were obtained and frozen by standardized clinical methods to prevent differences due to handling. The samples were blinded with only sex and age noted, and stored at -80°C until assayed. Coded information regarding disease status and exposure was obtained from a questionnaire and screening data from the Agency for Toxic Substances and Disease Registry (ATSDR), which performed a screening in Libby during 2000-2001 [23].

ARD and asbestos exposure rankings. The lung diseases reported in Libby have been previously described [24, 25], and include primarily pleural and some interstitial abnormalities. In our Libby sample set, Asbestos-Related Disease (ARD) status, based on data recorded in the database primarily as a result of the ATSDR screenings, was ranked on a scale of 0 – 3 as previously described [22]. The rankings combine pleural and interstitial abnormalities, and were intentionally simplified, based on radiographic evidence of single versus extensive plaques or interstitial abnormalities, as well as spirometric evidence of functional deficits. For example, a subject with single-lobe pleural plaques and no functional deficit would be scored at 1, subjects with more extensive plaques or fibrosis but without functional deficits received a score of 2, whereas a subject with bilateral plaques and/or fibrosis with effects on spirometry was scored at 3. To further stratify the sample sets by disease types would have made the subsets too small for statistical analysis. Exposure status was ranked on a scale of 0 – 4, where zero means no known exposure, 1 = 1-2 routes of exposure for less than 5 years, 2 = 3 or more routes of exposure for less than 5 years, 3 = 1-2 routes of exposure for ≥ 5 years, and 4 = 3 or more routes of exposure for ≥ 5 years [22].

Detection of Serum Autoantibodies

A clinical test for autoantibodies to nuclear antigens (ANA assay) was performed at a screening dilution of the sera. All serum samples were diluted 1:40 in phosphate-buffered saline (PBS) and tested by indirect immunofluorescence (IIF) on a commercially prepared and fixed HEp-2 cell substrate (ImmunoConcepts Inc., Sacramento, CA), according to manufacturer's instructions. The staining pattern and relative fluorescence intensity were compared with known positive and negative controls using a Zeiss fluorescence microscope with 40x objective and recorded as positive (1+ to 4+) or negative (0). The staining pattern was also noted and recorded. The same microscope and settings were used for all samples, and the slides were read by two independent readers.

Addressable Laser Bead Immunosorbent Assay (ALBIA)

Analyses of antibodies to eight extractable nuclear antigens (ENAs) commonly seen in SAID (Sm, RNP, Ro52, SS-A60, SS-B, topo I, Jo-1, Ribosomal P, chromatin) were performed using an ALBIA kit (QUANTA Plex™ SLE Profile 8; INOVA Diagnostics) according to the manufacturer's instructions, on a Luminex multiplex system (MiraiBio, Alameda, CA). The values were compared using Starstation 2.0 software (Applied Cytometry Systems, Sacramento, CA) to negative and graduated positive control reagents provided with the kit, and determined to be low or high positive, or negative.

Quantification of IgM Rheumatoid factor (RF), Anti-Cyclic Citrullinated Peptide (CCP), Topo I, and Histone by ELISA

IgM RF, anti-CCP, anti-topo I, and anti-histone antibodies in the serum samples were measured by ELISA according to the manufacturer's protocol (Quanta Lite™, INOVA Diagnostics). The plates were read on the SpectraMax plate reader (Molecular Devices, Sunnyvale, CA). Optical density (OD) values were compared with known controls provided with the kit and rated as negative or positive (low or high).

Cell-Based ELISA for Anti-Fibroblast Antibodies

MRC-5 human lung fibroblast cells (American Type Culture Collection, ATCC) were plated to 96-well plates at 10,000 cells per well in DMEM media containing 10% fetal calf serum and antibiotics, and allowed to adhere and grow for 48 hr at 37°C in a 5% CO_2 incubator. The cells were washed with warm PBS and then blocked in PBS containing 5% goat serum with 0.5% Tween-20 for 1 hr at 37°C. Serum samples were applied as the primary antibody at 1:100 dilution and allowed to stain the cells for 1 hr at 37°C with occasional gentle rocking of the plate by hand. After gentle washing with blocking buffer, the secondary antibody (HRP-Goat anti-human IgG) was applied at 1:5000 dilution in blocking buffer, and again allowed to stain for an hour as above. After gentle washing 2x with blocking buffer,

HRP-TMB substrate (Sigma) was added to the wells and allowed to develop color. The plates were read on a microtiter plate reader at 450 nm.

Statistical Analysis

Serum samples that recognized one of the nine autoantigens as described above were classified as positive and treated as ordinal data. Alternatively, serum samples that were unreactive to the autoantigens were classified as negative. Extent of lung disease or exposure was classified as ordinal data as 4 or 5 point levels, respectively. Data was analyzed non-parametrically through two approaches. Data was analyzed using contingency tables using subject scores through the chi-square test. Data was also analyzed using Mann-Whitney analysis using subject scores. Where appropriate, a one-way ANOVA analysis was used to observe trends among multiple groups of data. Statistical significance was established as a two-tailed probability of type I error occurring at less than 5%. Analysis was performed on Prism 4.0 software (GraphPad, San Diego, CA).

Results

Frequency of Antinuclear Antibodies

Seventy randomly chosen serum samples from Libby, MT were tested by IIF for ANA and were determined to be positive or negative based on known controls. Fifty of the 70 serum samples (70%) were ANA positive, which is consistent with previously published results for this population (16). The intensity and the staining patterns visible on the ANA tests were also recorded (Table I). The staining patterns that were the most prevalent were homogeneous (indicative of antibodies to chromatin components), nucleolar and speckled staining patterns (Figure 1). The most common ANA pattern from Missoula was the speckled pattern, consistent with data from normal populations, in which approximately 30-32% screen positive for ANA at a 1:40 dilution of the serum [26]. In addition, nine Libby samples showed a filamentous cytoplasmic pattern indicative of cytoskeletal staining (indicated as "cytosk" in Table I), and one had a cytoplasmic speckled staining pattern (indicated as "cytosp" in Table I, subject # 70).

Autoantibody Characterization

The ALBIA, which detects reactivity to nine autoantigens commonly targeted in SAID, was used to characterize the specific target antigens of the autoantibodies found in the Libby cohort. Sixteen of the 70 total Libby serum samples (23%) had positive ALBIA tests and most were reactive to a single target antigen (Table I). The most common autoantibodies detected in the Libby serum samples were autoantibodies to chromatin (44% of the positive samples) and autoantibodies to Ro52 (19% of the positive samples). Serum samples that had antibodies to chromatin were further analyzed on a histone ELISA. Of the seven samples that were positive against chromatin, five samples tested positive against histones (71%). No serum samples reacted with Jo-1, Sm or Ribo P. Figure 2 shows the distribution of positive tests against the target antigens.

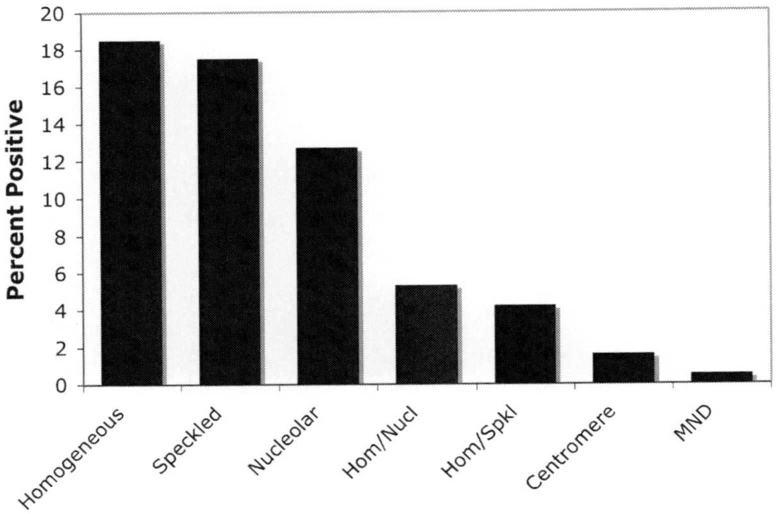

Figure 1. Percentages of ANA IIF patterns for Libby samples. A total compilation of the ANA staining patterns at screening dilution 1:40 of 189 Libby serum samples is shown as a percent of the total. Mean age = 57 ± 39.5 years. MND= Multiple Nuclear Dot.

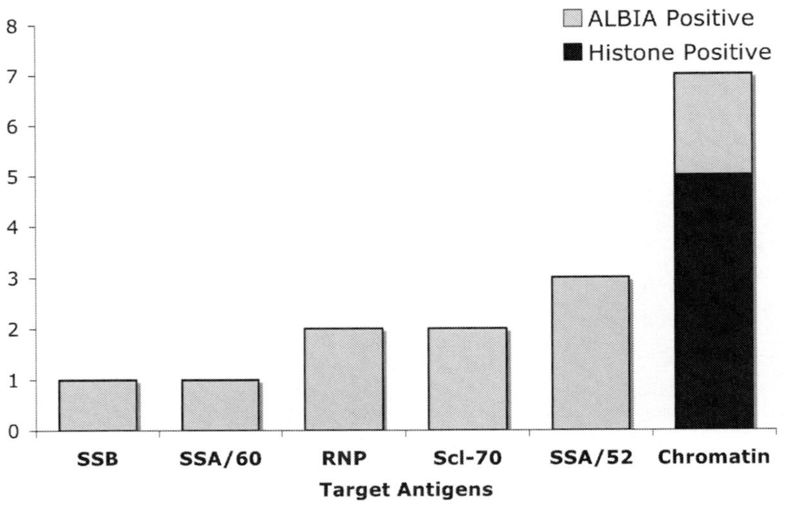

Figure 2. Frequencies of specific autoantibodies in Libby serum samples by ALBIA. The specific targets recognized by AAs from Libby serum samples were characterized with an addressable laser bead immunoassay as described in Materials and Methods. Samples that tested positive for chromatin were further analyzed for reactivity against H2/H3/H4 histones by ELISA.

Topo-I antibodies were also analyzed by ELISA, which detected not only the two samples positive by ALBIA, but also an additional 6 samples. The ELISA data had a better correlation with the ANA positive status of the samples, especially nucleolar and homogeneous staining patterns. The total positive for Scl-70 was 8 of 70 (11%).

IgM RF and Anti-CCP Frequency

RF is an autoantibody directed at the Fc region of IgG and is usually of IgM isotype. RF is associated with a number of inflammatory diseases and is not specific for RA (10). The presence of these autoantibodies may contribute to disease by the formation of immune complexes in tissues. In a separate set of 45 randomly selected Libby samples, the presence of anti-CCP was also measured, due to the sensitivity and specificity of this test for RA [27]. Both antibodies were measured semi-quantitatively by ELISA. Twenty-four of the seventy total Libby serum samples (34%) were positive for RF IgM (Table I), which is consistent with previously published results [22]. None of the samples tested higher than 25 RF units in this assay, suggesting a low titer. Three of 45 samples (6.6%) were positive for anti-CCP, with two in the low positive range and one in the high positive range for this assay (Data not shown).

Correlation of Autoantibodies with Extent of Exposure and ARD

To determine whether an association existed between the presence of a positive ALBIA test (Figure 2) and the extent of exposure (ranked by years of exposure as well as number of pathways), the presence or absence of AA to one of the nine autoantigens was classified as ordinal data and designated as positive or negative, respectively. The data were analyzed using a chi-square test and a non-parametric Mann-Whitney U-test. No significant association was observed between the presence of these autoantibodies and the extent of exposure. Subjects with positive ALBIA tests had a slightly higher exposure status, but this difference was not statistically significant (Figure 3a) ($P = 0.1312$). The presence of individual autoantibody specificities was also generally not correlated with extent of exposure, represented here by samples positive for anti-RNP (Figure 3b).

Because pulmonary abnormalities are common in SAID, it was important to determine whether the presence of particular autoantibodies was associated with the severity of asbestos-related lung disease (ARD). The only autoantibody specificity that showed a significant association with ARD score was topo-I as measured by ELISA (Figure 3c). The association of anti-topo-I with extent of exposure and with ARD was only found to be significant when all eight samples were used in the analysis, to include those positive by ELISA, as described above. This raises the possibility that the lack of association for the other autoantibodies could be attributed to the limited size of the groups analyzed.

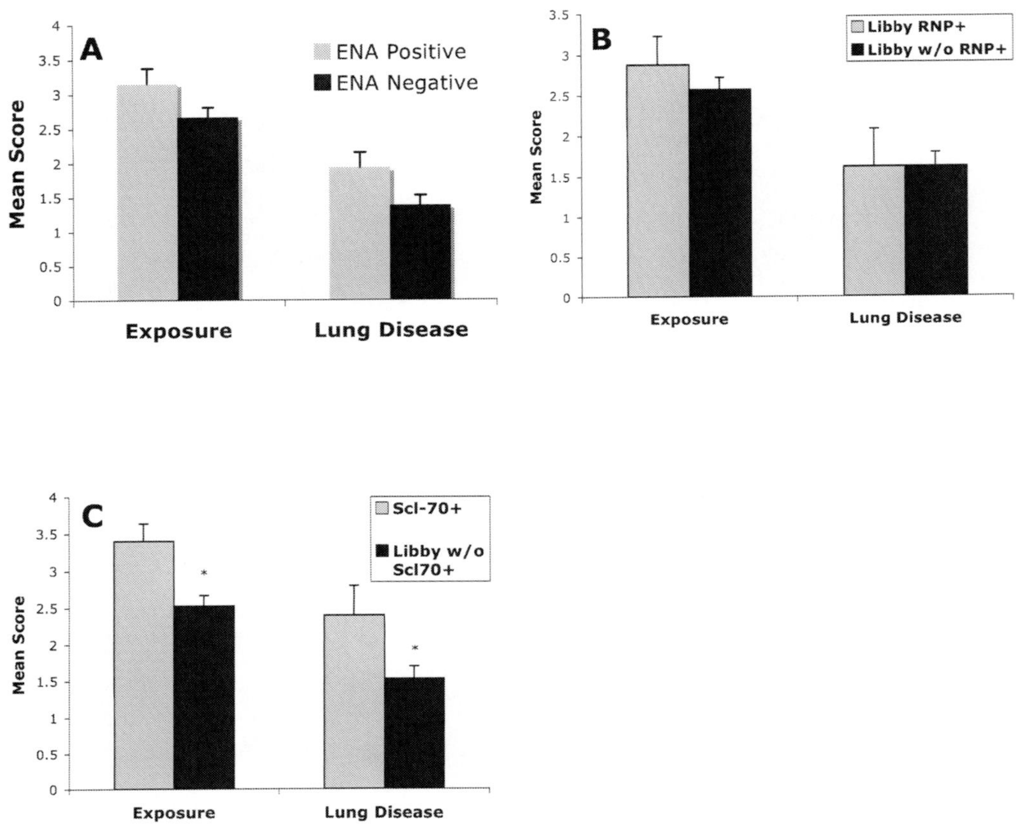

Figure 3. Asbestos exposure and lung disease scores for subjects with and without antibodies to ENA. Using a scoring system applied to exposure and lung disease data for each of the Libby subjects, the mean scores for subjects with and without these antibodies are shown. There was no significant difference in exposure or disease scores for subjects positive for any ENA Ab (A), nor for anti-RNP alone (B). C. DNA Topo 1 positive subjects had a significantly higher score for both parameters, suggesting that these antibodies are associated with higher exposure and more severe lung disease. (* = $p< 0.05$ by Mann-Whitney non-parametric U test).

Presence of Antibodies to Fibroblasts

Patients with SAID also have been shown to produce autoantibodies against non-nuclear antigens, such as cell surface proteins of fibroblasts. The presence of anti-fibroblast antibodies (AFA) was assessed using a cell-based ELISA, measuring the binding of serum antibodies to MRC-5 human fibroblasts. Figure 4a shows that several of the Libby serum samples contain antibodies that bind fibroblasts, increasing the mean optical density (OD) of the Libby samples to a value significantly higher than the mean OD of the Missoula samples. The majority of the high binding samples appear to occur among those who were positive for anti-topo-I by ELISA (Figure 4b).

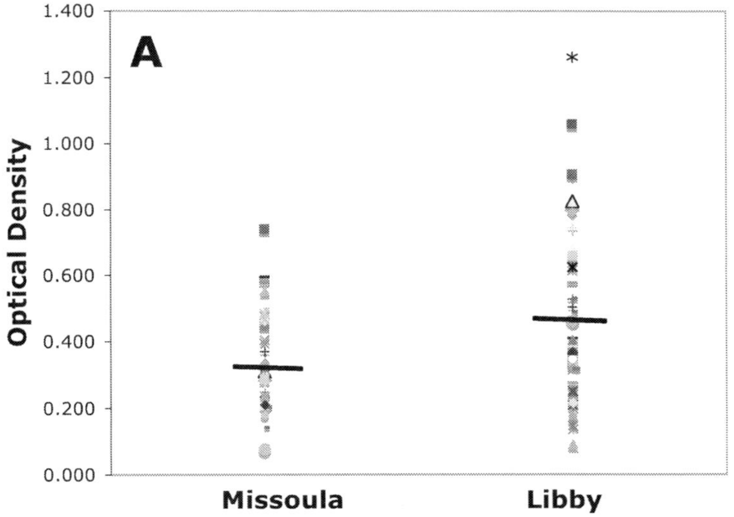

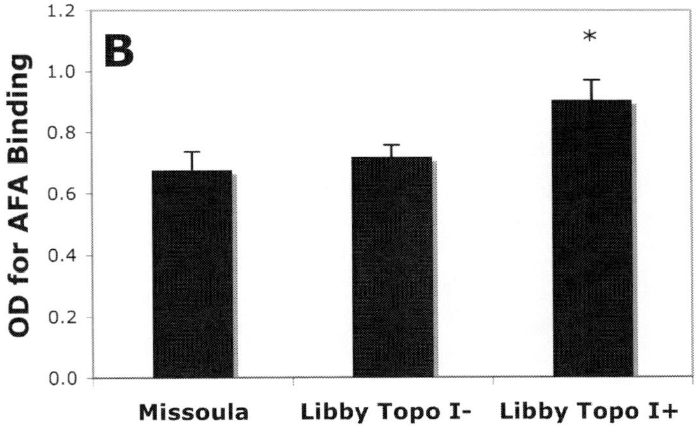

Figure 4. Antifibroblast antibodies in Libby serum samples. Serum samples from Missoula and Libby were analyzed by cell-based ELISA for anti-fibroblast antibodies (AFA). A. At least a subset of the Libby samples had quite high binding, making the mean OD significantly higher than for Missoula. B. High AFA binding occurred in the Scl-70+ group. * = $p < 0.05$ by unpaired t test.

Discussion

The ubiquitous nature of silicon oxides as a major elemental component of our planet poses tremendous challenges for identifying and tracking exposures. High exposures primarily occur occupationally during mining and sandblasting as well as the manufacture of pottery, insulation, ceramics, glass, absorbents, dessicants, filler, and abrasive cleaners. In many of these cases, the biologically active component is crystalline silica, as a result of charge interactions with silicon oxide radicals that form during fracturing processes [28].

Additionally, fibrous silicates such as amphibole asbestos fibers remain significant health hazards. Asbestos is a general term for hydrated silicate fibers that are strong and heat-resistant. Because of its high tensile strength and ability to absorb heat, asbestos has been used extensively as building materials in roofing, siding, fire protection material, heating and electrical wire insulation, appliance components, sheet flooring, ceiling and floor tiles, and drywall.

Asbestos fibers are categorized into two separate families based on morphology. Amphibole fibers are straight rod-like fibers that include fibers such as amosite, tremolite, crocidolite and Libby amphibole asbestos (Figure 5). In contrast, serpentine fibers are curved pliable fibers. The serpentine fiber family includes a single fiber type, chrysotile, which accounts for much of the world's asbestos consumption. Asbestos fibers can remain airborne in contaminated areas and eventually settle into soil, sediment and tree bark [29, 30]. Therefore, the toxic potential of asbestos fibers remains for long periods in contaminated areas once they are introduced into the environment.

Although there appear to be some similarities between silica and asbestos in terms of induction of autoantibodies and immune complexes, the pathologies associated with crystalline versus fibrous silicates appear to be somewhat unique, necessitating the separate study of these two silicate families. In particular, the pulmonary manifestations of silicosis versus asbestosis are readily distinguishable and classified separately [31, 32]. Although several studies show increased frequencies and titers of autoantibodies with asbestos exposure, published studies indicate that asbestos is more commonly associated with cancer rather than SAID, possibly due to differential effects on the activation of T cells, though the mechanism of this difference remains unclear [33, 34].

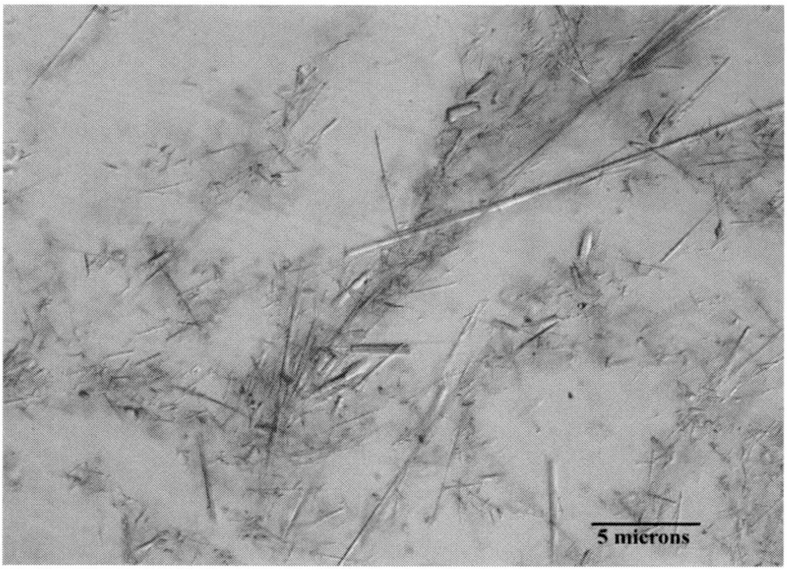

Figure 5. Light micrograph of Libby amphibole mixture. This material, collected from six sites around the Libby vermiculite mine has been labeled as "Libby Six-Mix" by U.S. Geological Survey who kindly provided the sample [19].

This is further complicated by the fact that there are many forms of asbestos that vary in terms of surface charge and adsorbed ions, leading to different biological effects [35, 36]. Nevertheless, since both mineral silicates cause apoptosis and oxidative stress in various cell types and both are considered to be immune "adjuvants", continued investigation of their association with SAID is warranted because the similarities and differences between these groups will guide our understanding of environmental induction of autoimmunity.

Residents of Libby, MT have higher frequencies and titers of positive ANA tests, which correlated to the extent of exposure and the severity of disease [22]. AA characterized from the Libby cohort were initially described as recognizing more than one ENA [22]. However, the present characterization indicates that, in most cases, AA from the asbestos exposed cohort recognize a single antigen. The sensitivity and specificity of techniques for detecting specific AA are constantly being improved; therefore, the study reported in this chapter used some of the more advanced techniques and diagnostic platforms in order to better enable a more specific assessment of the serological profile.

The initial detection of AA has classically used indirect immunofluorescence for ANA on HEp-2 cell substrates. This screening test offers the appropriate level of sensitivity, however there are now more specific confirmatory tests for the detection and semi-quantification of ENA antibodies in human sera [37]. With the exception of antibodies to cytoplasmic antigens, such as Jo-1, ribo-P and Ro52, it is rare to have a positive anti-ENA antibody test in the absence of a positive ANA test. In order to correctly screen a patient for the presence of AA, it has been suggested that a two stage testing is performed that includes an initial ANA screening test followed by a confirmatory anti-ENA test [38]. Cytoplasmic staining, seen in 14% of the Libby samples, may become more clinically relevant as the specific target antigens are identified. The cytoplasmic pattern seen with the Libby samples was primarily filamentous, suggesting antibodies to cytoskeletal components, without evidence of antibodies to mitochondria, Golgi complex, endosomes, GW bodies or lysosomes [39]. All samples that were positive for cytoskeletal staining were also positive for ANA. Interestingly, autoreactivity to cytoskeletal proteins have been noted at high frequencies in RA patients. In a study comparing patients with RA, progressive SSc, or SLE with normal volunteers, the frequencies of fibrous or filamentous cytoplasmic staining were 76%, 30%, 6% and 4%, respectively [40].

The most common ALBIA ANA from the Libby cohort were reactive to chromatin, histones and Ro52. This AA profile is similar to those found in patients with SLE [41]. The homogeneous staining pattern, which was predominant in this population, is usually associated with antibodies to DNA, histone, or the macromolecular DNA/histone complex referred to as nucleosomes or chromatin. Previous data indicated that less than half of the ANA positive Libby subjects with homogeneous staining had positive tests to dsDNA, as measured by *Crithidia luciliae* testing [22]. The current study indicated that the antibodies targeted chromatin with some reactivity to histones. Antibodies to chromatin may occur earlier in a disease course, with antibodies to dsDNA and histone following due to epitope spreading. Interestingly, anti-histone AA have been reported in SSc patients exhibiting pulmonary fibrosis [42]. Anti-histone antibodies are also found in approximately 40% of patients with SLE, and are associated with symptomatic drug-induced lupus. Antibodies against certain components of histone, such as H2A-H2B dimer, are thought to be characteristic of drug-induced lupus while reactivity to the H1 and H2B subunits of histones is common in idiopathic SLE [43, 44]. Since the assay used to determine anti-histone reactivity was not specific for any one of the histones (except that H1 has been removed), the anti-histone antibodies observed could be against the H2A, H2B, H3 or H4 core subunits of the nucleosome. Therefore, further characterization may be needed to determine the specific core histones and their respective epitopes targeted by these antibodies. DIL generally resolves upon removal of the implicated drug, but since asbestos remains in the lung, the induced lupus would not likely resolve. Because patients with DIL often do not fulfill the criteria for idiopathic SLE, presenting with vague symptoms such as arthralgias, myalgia, malaise and fever, this could be an interesting explanation for the difficulty in identifying a discrete clinical autoimmune entity associated with asbestos exposure.

In addition to anti-chromatin antibodies, anti-Ro52 was the next most common autoantibody found in the Libby samples. These AAs have also been identified in patients with idiopathic SLE and other connective tissue diseases [45, 46]. A murine model of asbestos-induced autoimmunity was recently established to investigate the mechanisms by which asbestos triggers systemic autoimmunity [47]. Asbestos exposed mice developed positive antinuclear antibody tests and mild glomerulonephritis suggestive of a systemic lupus erythematosus (SLE)-like disease. Interestingly, the murine SLE-like disease was characterized by the production of AAs that recognize dsDNA and Ro52. These data support the premise that amphibole asbestos generates a serological SLE-like disease in both humans and in mice. Moreover, because humans and mice exposed to amphibole asbestos generate similar AA profiles, the alterations of the immune response by amphibole asbestos may be comparable. Therefore, the murine model of asbestos induced autoimmunity is both relevant and useful to study the immunological effects of amphibole asbestos. Further, the presence of antibodies to Ro52 raises the interesting question of its role in autoimmunity that was heightened when it was identified as an E3 ubiquitin ligase [48]. The possibility that autoantigens become antigenic due to proteolytic degradation has been postulated [49, 50]. It is possible that exposure to environmental toxins may cause protein misfolding leading to aberrant ubiquitination of targets by Ro52 (including self-ubiquitination) thus resulting in ineffective proteosomal degradation of target proteins, that may then lead to an autoimmune response. In addition, Ro52 has been shown to accumulate in apoptotic blebs during programmed cell death induced by a variety of oxidant challenges including asbestos [51, 52]. The data suggest that asbestos impairs proteolytic cleavage of Ro52 in murine macrophages, and the protein is then recognized by mouse autoantibodies as well as a commercial monoclonal antibodies raised against amino acids 141-280 of the 52 kD polypeptide by both immunocytochemistry and Western blotting of asbestos-treated cells undergoing apoptosis [51].

Because SAID patients often present with a specific pattern or selection of AA specificities, and also that some AA appear early in the course of the disease, it is possible and very intriguing that these AA might occur in distinct patterns following specific exposures. An association was shown between silica exposure and the production of anti-DNA and anti-Sm autoantibodies, both commonly found in lupus patients [53]. Remarkably, the autoantibody profiles in our asbestos-exposed cohort did not overlap reported profiles for silica-exposures except for topo-I. However, due to the wide range of antibodies, the presence of autoantibodies in controls, and variability between individuals, it would take larger number of samples from various exposures and compared to unexposed controls to see if a consistent pattern developed [54].

Silica exposure has been associated with the presence of RF and an increased risk of RA [55, 56]. In addition, there was some evidence of a higher rate of RA in Libby than might be expected [21]. Low titer IgM RF was present in 34% of the Libby subjects, compared to approximately 36% in Missoula samples [22]. Anti-CCP antibodies were seen in 6.6% of the Libby samples, where a frequency of 1-2% might be expected in a normal population. In order to determine the significance of this result, it would be important to follow up with additional samples compared to a gender and age matched set of samples from Missoula. The frequency of anti-CCP may be elevated in Libby particularly since this autoantibody appears to be predictive of incipient RA, which would be consistent with the epidemiological study. This is also interesting in view of the presence of AA to cytoskeletal components, which may also be a marker for RA [40]. However, a caveat is that the cases for RA in the study by Noonan, et al. [57], were self-reported so that although the surveys indicated that their RA was physician diagnosed, the reported cases may have included some non-RA patients, such as osteoarthritis. Finally, arthritis is an early symptom of SLE as well, often occurring prior to diagnosis suggesting that some of the RA cases could be evolving to that condition.

One of the anecdotal concerns of the Libby population has been the incidence of diseases not formally classified as rheumatoid, such as fibromyalgia and chronic fatigue syndrome (CFS). Although these diseases remain poorly defined serologically, there is some evidence of increased frequency of positive ANA tests in CFS patients [58, 59]. The diagnostic challenges associated with these diseases, especially in the presence of other chronic diseases, will make assessment of the true prevalence of these diseases in Libby a difficult task. Nevertheless, the presence of a high frequency of positive ANA that were not also positive by other tests for antibodies to ENA suggests that there may be unidentified antibodies in these subjects. Antibodies to nuclear envelope antigens were reported in CFS patients [59], giving a staining pattern that could be mistaken for a homogeneous pattern, which was the most common pattern seen in the Libby samples. However, other factors can cause positive ANA tests without reactivity to the ENAs tested in this study, including smoking or thyroid disease. There is no evidence of unusually high rates of thyroid disease or smoking in Libby, however, compared to other communities in Montana. Approximately 20-22% of adults in both Libby and Missoula smoke tobacco, according to the Montana Department of Public Health and Human Services, so smoking is unlikely to be the cause of ANA differences between these populations.

There is some evidence that AA appear prior to the onset of clinically overt disease [60]. A thorough analysis of an 80-patient cohort as well as a literature review in 1970, led by British researchers Turner-Warwick and Parkes, concluded that there was growing evidence not only that asbestos drives autoimmune responses, but also that there was an intriguing and potentially critical association of these asbestos-induced AA with the severity and progression of the pulmonary disease seen in the asbestos exposed subjects [8]. Interestingly, exposure to asbestos and silica lead to patterns of illness that are very similar to SAID including both pulmonary fibrosis and serum ANA [22, 61, 62]. Although the mechanisms leading to the progression of these conditions have not been fully explained, there is evidence that some of the lung pathologies seen with both asbestos and silica exposures are immunologically mediated [63-65]. Although many of the cells and mediators involved in the initiation of silicate-associated pulmonary fibrosis have been studied, the reasons for the chronic and progressive nature of silicosis and asbestosis remain unclear.

Interestingly, analysis of the data from the earlier study of AA in Libby subjects [22] showed a significant association of positive ANA tests with higher lung disease scores. In addition, when the CDC/ATSDR (Agency for Toxic Substances and Disease Registry) performed its screening in Libby during 2000-2001, of 7307 screening participants, 494 (6.7%) indicated that they had been diagnosed with either SLE, SSc, or RA [21]. Of those 494 participants from the Libby cohort with suspected SAID, 171 (35%) have had pleural and/or interstitial abnormalities indicated on chest radiographs that were confirmed by two B-readers. These data suggest that the proportion of radiographic abnormalities among those with suspected autoimmune disease (35%) was almost double the proportion of radiographic abnormalities among the entire Libby cohort (approximately 18%) [24]. These data are supported by a study by Tamura, *et al*, in which positive ANAs were more frequent in asbestos-exposed subjects who had pulmonary lesions [66]. A 3-year follow-up study of those patients demonstrated that positive ANAs were correlated with the progression of asbestosis [67]. Although it could be argued that AA are simply a result of the chronic lung inflammation in asbestos-exposed lungs, the alternate hypothesis is that there is an autoimmune component to these pulmonary pathologies.

This chapter reports that the only specificity that showed a significant association with scored pulmonary disease (ARD) was topo-I. Anti-topo-I was detected by two techniques: ALBIA (ENA8, INOVA Diagnostics) and ELISA (INOVA) (Table 1). The latter assay appeared more sensitive and revealed positive tests on eight subjects, compared to two by ALBIA. The results by ELISA were more consistent with ANA data of nucleolar staining. Therefore, all eight samples were used for subsequent analyses. An association between anti-topo-I and pulmonary disease has been reported [68], although that association is much stronger with subjects testing positive for anti-topo-I by immunodiffusion rather than by ELISA [69]. Two hypotheses have been proposed to explain this relationship. One is the possibility that the AA actually enter the cell where anti-DNA topoisomerase I is able to inhibit enzyme activity [70], resulting in cell death and therefore tissue damage. Second, anti-topo I antibodies from SSc patients have been shown to bind to fibroblasts and initiate proinflammatory/profibrotic cascades [71, 72]. These studies suggest that antibodies targeting various cell types can modulate cell function and therefore contribute to pathology.

The possible role of AA to fibroblasts, endothelial, and epithelial cells in vascular and fibrotic disorders is receiving considerable attention as the evidence of their pathogenicity expands. Antibodies to endothelial cells have been implicated in vasculitis [73], SSc [74], and SLE [75]. Anti-epithelial cell antibodies are being studied in cryptogenic fibrosing alveolitis [76] and non-allergic asthma [77]. Anti-fibroblast antibodies (AFA) have primarily been studied as a possible factor in the fibrosis of patients with SSc [78, 79]. However, despite the growing concern about an autoimmune process in these diseases, very few of the target antigens have been clearly identified, and the mechanism of lost tolerance to those antigens is unknown. Early techniques did not allow the sensitivity of detection of certain autoantibody specificities that is now available, and previous studies did not specifically link certain autoantibodies with these complex pulmonary/autoimmune combinations.

Table I. Data from 70 randomly selected Libby samples as described. Blank = no data

Patient	Age	Gender	Disease	Exposure	ANA score and pattern	SLE 9 Profile ALBIA	Topo-1 by ELISA	RF IgM
1	72	M	3	4	0	0		0
2	59	F	3	3	2 spkl	0		0
3	65	F	3	3	3 hom/spkl	SSB	Topo-1	0
4	48	M	3	1	0	0		0
5	54	M	2	4	1 spkl/cytsk	Ro52		0
7	47	F	0	3	3 nuc	Chromatin, Histone		0
8	48	F	1	3	0	RNP		0
9	65	M	2	4	3 hom	0		1
11	48	M	3	4	3 hom/cytsk	Topo-1	Topo-1	0
14	48	M	2	2	0	0		1
17	43	M	2	2	3 spkl	0		0
18	36	M	2	4	1 nuc	0	Topo-1	0
19	62	F	2	3	2 nuc/cytsk	0		0
36	57	M	3	3	2 nuc	0		1
38	61	M	3	2	3 hom	Chromatin		1
39	69	F	3	3	2 nuc/cytsk	Chromatin, Histone	Topo-1	1
40	78	M	3	4	2 nuc	0		1
41	43	M	3	4	2 cent	0		0
44	51	M	2	1	0	0		0
47	66	M	3	3	4 hom	0		0
49	49	F	1	3	0	0		0
50	63	F	2	3	3 hom	SSA-60		1
53	58	F	1	3	2 nuc/cytsk	0	Topo-1	1
58	60	M	3	1	0	RNP		1
60	53	M	1	4	4 hom/cytsp	Chromatin, Histone		1
65	73	F	3	3	2 hom	0		0
66	52	F	1	1	0	0		0
68	45	F	1	1	0	0		0
70	69	F	2	4	3 hom, cytsp	Chromatin		1
73	41	M	1	3	4 hom	0		0
74	44	M	0	3	1 nuc	Topo-1	Topo-1	0
77	55	F	2	3	3 hom/nuc	0	Topo-1	0
79	42	F	0	3	1 spkl	0		0
81	51	F	2	3	4 cent	0		1
83	32	F	1	1	0	0		0
86	59	M	2	3	1 spkl	0		0
89	56	M	2	3	2 hom/spkl	0		0
92	66	M	3	3	3 atyp	0		0
98	52	M		2	0	0		0
99	71	M	3	4	2 hom	0	Topo-1	0
100	66	M	2	3	1 hom/cytsk	0		0
102	64	M	2	3	1 spkl/cytsk	0		0
118	79	F	2	3	4 hom/cytsk	0		0
119	70	F	3	3	3 hom/nuc	0		1
120	79	M	3	2	2 hom	0		1
121	69	F	0	3	4 nuc	Chromatin, Histone		0
122	39	F	0	1	0	0		0
123	36	M	2	2	1 nuc	0		0
126	75	F	2	3	1 hom	0		1
127	60	F	0	3	2 spkl	0		0
129	50	M	0	4	3 spkl	0		0
135	62	M	3	3	3 nuc	0		0
136	44	F		1	4 spkl	0		1
142	62	M	2	0	0	0		1
164	39	F	1	3	3 spkl	0		1
167	33	M	3	4	0	0		1
176	99	F	2	3	0	Ro52		0
177	79	F	0	1	2spkl	0		1
180	62	F	3	3	2 spkl	0		0
185	49	F	0	4	1 spkl	0		0
190	44	F		3	0	0		1
196	66	M	1	4	0	0		0
198	35	M	1	3	0	0		0
207	69	M	3	3	0	0		0
224	49	F	0	1	2 spkl	0		0
225	41	M	0	1	2 hom	0		1
356					2 hom/nuc	Chromatin, Histone		1
360	53	M	2	4	2 hom/nuc	Ro52		0
366					1 hom/nuc	0		1
371	71	F	3	1	1 hom	0		0

New techniques allow exquisitely sensitive detection of large numbers of specificities, easily screened in large numbers of subjects. Modern radiographic techniques have also dramatically improved the ability to classify pulmonary outcomes of exposures compared to connective tissue diseases [80]. This chapter simply reports the presence of AFA in some asbestos-exposed subjects from Libby, illustrating the importance of follow up on these subjects to determine whether these antibodies might be markers for rapid progression or exacerbation of pleural or interstitial disease. An association of these antibodies with clinical progression might lead to excellent targets for therapeutic intervention.

Conclusion

The purpose of this study was to detect a serological signature in the asbestos exposed population of Libby, MT, and compare this profile with other known SAID autoantibody profiles, including those seen with silica exposure. While the variability in the samples makes comparisons difficult, autoantibody profiles of this asbestos-exposed population show similarities to those of patients with idiopathic SLE, drug-induced SLE, and scleroderma, due to the apparently high frequency of anti-topo-I. The presence of AFA may indicate a direct role for asbestos-induced AA in accelerating fibrotic manifestations of the exposure. This information may improve screening of asbestos-exposed populations and could serve to point toward diagnostic or prognostic markers relative to asbestos exposure. A marker that appears earlier after exposure and that is correlated with eventual autoimmune disease would be a great benefit. Future studies include the exploration of the specific autoantigen targets for the AFA in mouse and human models, and prospective study of this population to determine the relationship between ANA, AFA and clinical progression of both autoimmune and pulmonary pathologies. Finally, collaboration with medical doctors that treat and advise patients from Libby, MT would provide necessary clinical diagnostic data for future studies. Joining clinical observations and the serological characterization presented here has an excellent chance to help accurately characterize clinical autoimmune manifestations of asbestos exposure, and therefore to screen, diagnose and treat asbestos exposed individuals.

Acknowledgments

The authors gratefully acknowledge the Libby Center for Asbestos Related Diseases (Brad Black, M.D., Director) for assistance with sample acquisition, and Roger Diegel, M.D., Rheumatology, for his review of this Chapter.

References

[1] Bramwell, B. (1914). Diffuse scleroderma: its frequency; its occurrence in stone masons; its treatment by fibrolysis. *Edinburgh. Medical Journal, 12*, 387.

[2] Conrad, K., Mehlhorn, J., Luthke, K., Dorner, T., Frank, K. H. (1996). Systemic lupus erythematosus after heavy exposure to quartz dust in uranium mines: clinical and serological characteristics. *Lupus, 5*, 62-9.

[3] Sanchez-Roman, J., Wichmann, I., Salaberri, J., Varela, J. M., Nunez-Roldan, A. (1993). Multiple clinical and biological autoimmune manifestations in 50 workers after occupational exposure to silica. *Ann. Rheum. Dis, 52*, 534-8.

[4] Brown, J. M., Pfau, J. C., Pershouse, M. A., Holian, A. (2004). Silica, Apoptosis, and Autoimmunity. *Journal of Immunotoxicology, 1*, 177-187.

[5] Hess, E. V. (2002). Environmental chemicals and autoimmune disease: cause and effect. *Toxicology, 181-182*, 65-70.

[6] Parks, C. G., Cooper, G. S. (2006). Occupational exposures and risk of systemic lupus erythematosus: a review of the evidence and exposure assessment methods in population- and clinic-based studies. *Lupus, 15*, 728-36.

[7] Pernis, B., Paronetto, F. (1962). Adjuvant effects of silica (tridymite) on antibody production. *Proc. Soc. Exp. Biol. Med., 110*, 390-392.

[8] Turner-Warwick, M., Parkes, W. R. (1970). Circulating rheumatoid and antinuclear factors in asbestos workers. *Br. Med. J., 3*, 492-5.

[9] Conrad, K., Schlosser, W., Fritzler, M. J. (2007) The predictive relevance of autoantibodies. In *From Etiopathogenesis to the Prediction of Autoimmune Diseases: Relevance of Autoantibodies* (K. Conrad, E. K. L. Chan, M. J. Fritzler, U. Sack, Y. Schoenfeld and A. Wiik, eds), Pabst Scientific Publishers, Langerich, Germany 16-31.

[10] Mossman, B. T., Bignon, J., Corn, M., Seaton, A., Gee, J. B. (1990). Asbestos: scientific developments and implications for public policy. *Science, 247*, 294-301.

[11] Nicholson, W. J., Perkel, G., Selikoff, I. J. (1982). Occupational exposure to asbestos: population at risk and projected mortality--1980-2030. *Am. J. Ind. Med., 3*, 259-311.

[12] Joshi, T. K., Gupta, R. K. (2004). Asbestos in developing countries: magnitude of risk and its practical implications. *Int J Occup Med Environ Health, 17*, 179-85.

[13] Kazan-Allen, L. (2005). Asbestos and mesothelioma: worldwide trends. *Lung Cancer, 49 Suppl 1*, S3-8.

[14] Anderson, B. A., Dearwent, S. M., Durant, J. T., Dyken, J. J., Freed, J. A., Moore, S. M., Wheeler, J. S. (2005). Exposure pathway evaluations for sites that processed asbestos-contaminated vermiculite. *Int .J. Hyg. Environ. Health, 208*, 55-65.

[15] Bandli, B. R., Gunter, M. E. (2006). A review of scientific literature examining the mining history, geology, mineralogy, and amphibole asbestos health effects of the Rainy Creek igneous complex, Libby, Montana, USA. *Inhal. Toxicol., 18*, 949-62.

[16] Wright, R. S., Abraham, J. L., Harber, P., Burnett, B. R., Morris, P., West, P. (2002). Fatal asbestosis 50 years after brief high intensity exposure in a vermiculite expansion plant. *Am. J. Respir. Crit. Care Med., 165*, 1145-9.

[17] McDonald, J. C., Harris, J., Armstrong, B. (2004). Mortality in a cohort of vermiculite miners exposed to fibrous amphibole in Libby, Montana. *Occup. Environ. Med., 61*, 363-6.

[18] Whitehouse, A. C. (2004). Asbestos-related pleural disease due to tremolite associated with progressive loss of lung function: serial observations in 123 miners, family members, and residents of Libby, Montana. *Am. J. Ind. Med., 46*, 219-25.

[19] Meeker, G., Bern, A., Brownfield, I., Lowers, H., Sutley, S., Hoefen, T., Vance, J. (2003). The Composition and morphology of amphiboles from the Rainy Creek Complex, near Libby, Montana. *American Mineralogist, 88*, 1955-1969.

[20] Bernstein, D. M., Chevalier, J., Smith, P. (2005). Comparison of Calidria chrysotile asbestos to pure tremolite: final results of the inhalation biopersistence and histopathology examination following short-term exposure. *Inhal. Toxicol., 17*, 427-49.

[21] Noonan, C. W., Pfau, J. C., Larson, T. C., Spence, M. R. (2006). Nested case-control study of autoimmune disease in an asbestos-exposed population. *Environ. Health Perspect, 114*, 1243-7.

[22] Pfau, J. C., Sentissi, J. J., Weller, G., Putnam, E. A. (2005). Assessment of autoimmune responses associated with asbestos exposure in Libby, Montana, USA. *Environ. Health Perspect, 113*, 25-30.

[23] Horton, K., Kapil, V., Larson, T., Muravov, O., Melnikova, N., Anderson, B. (2006). A review of the federal government's health activities in response to asbestos-contaminated ore found in Libby, Montana. *Inhal. Toxicol, 18*, 925-40.

[24] Peipins, L. A., Lewin, M., Campolucci, S., Lybarger, J. A., Miller, A., Middleton, D., Weis, C., Spence, M., Black, B., Kapil, V. (2003). Radiographic abnormalities and exposure to asbestos-contaminated vermiculite in the community of Libby, Montana, USA. *Environ. Health Perspect, 111*, 1753-9.

[25] Sullivan, P. A. (2007). Vermiculite, respiratory disease, and asbestos exposure in Libby, Montana: update of a cohort mortality study. *Environ. Health Perspect., 115*, 579-85.

[26] Tan, E. M., Feltkamp, T. E., Smolen, J. S., Butcher, B., Dawkins, R., Fritzler, M. J., Gordon, T., Hardin, J. A., Kalden, J. R., Lahita, R. G., Maini, R. N., McDougal, J. S., Rothfield, N. F., Smeenk, R. J., Takasaki, Y., Wiik, A., Wilson, M. R., Koziol, J. A. (1997). Range of antinuclear antibodies in "healthy" individuals. *Arthritis Rheum., 40*, 1601-11.

[27] De Rycke, L., Peene, I., Hoffman, I. E., Kruithof, E., Union, A., Meheus, L., Lebeer, K., Wyns, B., Vincent, C., Mielants, H., Boullart, L., Serre, G., Veys, E. M., De Keyser, F. (2004). Rheumatoid factor and anticitrullinated protein antibodies in rheumatoid arthritis: diagnostic value, associations with radiological progression rate, and extra-articular manifestations. *Ann. Rheum. Dis., 63*, 1587-93.

[28] Vallyathan, V., Castranova, V., Pack, D., Leonard, S., Shumaker, J., Hubbs, A. F., Shoemaker, D. A., Ramsey, D. M., Pretty, J. R., McLaurin, J. L., et al. (1995). Freshly fractured quartz inhalation leads to enhanced lung injury and inflammation. Potential role of free radicals. *Am. J. Respir. Crit. Care Med., 152*, 1003-9.

[29] Webber, J. S., Getman, M., Ward, T. J. (2006). Evidence and reconstruction of airborne asbestos from unconventional environmental samples. *Inhal. Toxicol., 18*, 969-73.

[30] Ward, T. J., Spear, T., Hart, J., Noonan, C., Holian, A., Getman, M., Webber, J. S. (2006). Trees as reservoirs for amphibole fibers in Libby, Montana. *Sci. Total Environ., 367*, 460-5.

[31] Chong, S., Lee, K. S., Chung, M. J., Han, J., Kwon, O. J., Kim, T. S. (2006). Pneumoconiosis: comparison of imaging and pathologic findings. *Radiographics, 26*, 59-77.

[32] Honma, K., Abraham, J. L., Chiyotani, K., De Vuyst, P., Dumortier, P., Gibbs, A. R., Green, F. H., Hosoda, Y., Iwai, K., Williams, W. J., Kohyama, N., Ostiguy, G., Roggli, V. L., Shida, H., Taguchi, O., Vallyathan, V. (2004). Proposed criteria for mixed-dust pneumoconiosis: definition, descriptions, and guidelines for pathologic diagnosis and clinical correlation. *Hum. Pathol., 35*, 1515-23.

[33] Nishimura, Y., Miura, Y., Maeda, M., Hayashi, H., Dong, M., Katsuyama, H., Tomita, M., Hyodoh, F., Kusaka, M., Uesaka, A., Kuribayashi, K., Fukuoka, K., Nakano, T., Kashimoto, T., Osuki, T. (2006). Expression of the T cell receptor Vbeta repertoire in a human T cell resistant to asbestos-induced apoptosis and peripheral blood T cells from patients with silica and asbestos-related diseases. *Int. J. Immunopathol. Pharmacol., 19*, 795-805.

[34] Wu, P., Hyodoh, F., Hatayama, T., Sakaguchi, H., Hatada, S., Miura, Y., Takata-Tomokuni, A., Katsuyama, H., Otsuki, T. (2005). Induction of CD69 antigen expression in peripheral blood mononuclear cells on exposure to silica, but not by asbestos/chrysotile-A. *Immunol. Lett, 98*, 145-52.

[35] Blake, D. J., Bolin, C. M., Cox, D. P., Cardozo-Pelaez, F., Pfau, J. C. (2007). Internalization of Libby Amphibole Asbestos and Induction of Oxidative Stress in Murine Macrophages. *Toxicol Sci.*

[36] Mossman, B. T., Borm, P. J., Castranova, V., Costa, D. L., Donaldson, K., Kleeberger, S. R. (2007). Mechanisms of action of inhaled fibers, particles and nanoparticles in lung and cardiovascular diseases. *Part Fibre Toxicol, 4*, 4.

[37] Martins, T. B., Burlingame, R., von Muhlen, C. A., Jaskowski, T. D., Litwin, C. M., Hill, H. R. (2004). Evaluation of multiplexed fluorescent microsphere immunoassay for detection of autoantibodies to nuclear antigens. *Clin. Diagn. Lab. Immunol., 11*, 1054-9.

[38] Phan, T. G., Wong, R. C., Adelstein, S. (2002). Autoantibodies to extractable nuclear antigens: making detection and interpretation more meaningful. *Clin. Diagn. Lab. Immunol., 9*, 1-7.

[39] Stinton, L. M., Eystathioy, T., Selak, S., Chan, E. K., Fritzler, M. J. (2004). Autoantibodies to protein transport and messenger RNA processing pathways: endosomes, lysosomes, Golgi complex, proteasomes, assemblyosomes, exosomes, and GW bodies. *Clin. Immunol., 110*, 30-44.

[40] Shrivastav, M., Mittal, B., Aggarwal, A., Misra, R. (2002). Autoantibodies against cytoskeletal proteins in rheumatoid arthritis. *Clin Rheumatol, 21*, 505-10.

[41] D'Cruz, D. (2000). Autoimmune diseases associated with drugs, chemicals and environmental factors. *Toxicol Lett., 112-113*, 421-32.

[42] von Muhlen, C. A., Tan, E. M. (1995). Autoantibodies in the diagnosis of systemic rheumatic diseases. *Semin. Arthritis Rheum., 24*, 323-58.

[43] Gomez-Puerta, J. A., Burlingame, R. W., Cervera, R. (2006). Anti-chromatin (anti-nucleosome) antibodies. *Lupus, 15*, 408-11.

[44] Burlingame, R. W., Rubin, R. L. (1996). Autoantibody to the nucleosome subunit (H2A-H2B)-DNA is an early and ubiquitous feature of lupus-like conditions. *Mol. Biol. Rep., 23*, 159-66.

[45] Peene, I., Meheus, L., De Keyser, S., Humbel, R., Veys, E. M., De Keyser, F. (2002). Anti-Ro52 reactivity is an independent and additional serum marker in connective tissue disease. *Ann. Rheum. Dis., 61*, 929-33.

[46] Popovic, K., Brauner, S., Ek, M., Wahren-Herlenius, M., Nyberg, F. (2007). Fine specificity of the Ro/SSA autoantibody response in relation to serological and clinical findings in 96 patients with self-reported cutaneous symptoms induced by the sun. *Lupus, 16*, 10-7.

[47] Pfau, J. C., Sentissi, J. J., Blake, D. J., Li, S., Calderon-Garciduenas, L., Brown, J. M. (2007). Asbestos-Induced Autoimmunity in C57Bl/6 Mice. *Journal of Immunotoxicology, In Press.*

[48] Wada, K., Kamitani, T. (2006). Autoantigen Ro52 is an E3 ubiquitin ligase. *Biochem. Biophys. Res. Commun, 339*, 415-21.

[49] Chen, M., von Mikecz, A. (2005). Xenobiotic-induced recruitment of autoantigens to nuclear proteasomes suggests a role for altered antigen processing in scleroderma. *Ann. NY Acad. Sci., 1051*, 382-9.

[50] Rosen, A., Casciola-Rosen, L. (1999). Autoantigens as substrates for apoptotic proteases: implications for the pathogenesis of systemic autoimmune disease. *Cell Death Differ, 6*, 6-12.

[51] Blake, D. J., Wetzel, S. A., Pfau, J. C. (2008). Autoantibodies from mice exposed to Libby amphibole asbestos bind SSA/R052-enriched apoptotic blebs of murine macrophages. *Toxicology, In Press.*

[52] Saegusa, J., Kawano, S., Koshiba, M., Hayashi, N., Kosaka, H., Funasaka, Y., Kumagai, S. (2002). Oxidative stress mediates cell surface expression of SS-A/Ro antigen on keratinocytes. *Free Radic. Biol. Med., 32*, 1006-16.

[53] Parks, C. G., Cooper, G. S., Nylander-French, L. A., Sanderson, W. T., Dement, J. M., Cohen, P. L., Dooley, M. A., Treadwell, E. L., St Clair, E. W., Gilkeson, G. S., Hoppin, J. A., Savitz, D. A. (2002). Occupational exposure to crystalline silica and risk of systemic lupus erythematosus: a population-based, case-control study in the southeastern United States. *Arthritis Rheum., 46*, 1840-50.

[54] Cooper, G. S., Parks, C. G., Schur, P. S., Fraser, P. A. (2006). Occupational and environmental associations with antinuclear antibodies in a general population sample. *J Toxicol. Environ. Health A, 69*, 2063-9.

[55] Calvert, G. M., Rice, F. L., Boiano, J. M., Sheehy, J. W., Sanderson, W. T. (2003). Occupational silica exposure and risk of various diseases: an analysis using death certificates from 27 states of the United States. *Occup. Environ. Med., 60*, 122-9.

[56] Sluis-Cremer, G. K., Hessel, P. A., Hnizdo, E., Churchill, A. R. (1986). Relationship between silicosis and rheumatoid arthritis. *Thorax, 41*, 596-601.

[57] Heinlen, L. D., McClain, M. T., Merrill, J., Akbarali, Y. W., Edgerton, C. C., Harley, J. B., James, J. A. (2007). Clinical criteria for systemic lupus erythematosus precede diagnosis, and associated autoantibodies are present before clinical symptoms. *Arthritis Rheum., 56*, 2344-51.

[58] Nishikai, M. (2007). [Antinuclear antibodies in patients with chronic fatigue syndrome]. *Nippon Rinsho, 65*, 1067-70.

[59] Konstantinov, K., von Mikecz, A., Buchwald, D., Jones, J., Gerace, L., Tan, E. M. (1996). Autoantibodies to nuclear envelope antigens in chronic fatigue syndrome. *J. Clin. Invest, 98*, 1888-96.

[60] Arbuckle, M. R., McClain, M. T., Rubertone, M. V., Scofield, R. H., Dennis, G. J., James, J. A., Harley, J. B. (2003). Development of autoantibodies before the clinical onset of systemic lupus erythematosus. *N. Engl. J. Med., 349*, 1526-33.

[61] Cooper, G. S., Miller, F. W., Germolec, D. R. (2002). Occupational exposures and autoimmune diseases. *Int. Immunopharmacol., 2*, 303-13.

[62] Nigam, S. K., Suthar, A. M., Patel, M. M., Karnik, A. B., Dave, S. K., Kashyap, S. K., Venkaiah, K. (1993). Humoral immunological profile of workers exposed to asbestos in asbestos mines. *Indian J. Med. Res., 98*, 274-277.

[63] Hamilton, R. F., Iyer, L. L., Holian, A. (1996). Asbestos induces apoptosis in human alveolar macrophages. *Am. J. Physiol., 271*, L813-9.

[64] Holian, A., Uthman, M. O., Goltsova, T., Brown, S. D., Hamilton, R. F. (1997). Asbestos and silica-induced changes in human alveolar macrophage phenotype. *Environmental Health Perspectives, 105*, 1139-1142.

[65] Perkins, R. C., Scheule, R. K., Hamilton, R., Gomes, G., Freidman, G., Holian, A. (1993). Human alveolar macrophage cytokine release in response to in vitro and in vivo asbestos exposure. *Exp Lung Res, 19*, 55-65.

[66] Tamura, M., Liang, D., Tokuyama, T., Yoneda, T., Kasuga, H., Narita, N., Sada, K., Miyazaki, R., Okada, S. (1993). [Study on the relationship between appearance of autoantibodies and chest X-ray findings of asbestos plant employees]. *Sangyo Igaku, 35*, 406-12.

[67] Tamura, M., Tokuyama, T., Kasuga, H., Yoneda, T., Miyazaki, R., Narita, N. (1996). [Study on correlation between chest X-P course findings and change in antinuclear antibody in asbestos plant employees]. *Sangyo Eiseigaku Zasshi, 38*, 138-41.

[68] Jacobsen, S., Ullman, S., Shen, G. Q., Wiik, A., Halberg, P. (2001). Influence of clinical features, serum antinuclear antibodies, and lung function on survival of patients with systemic sclerosis. *J. Rheumatol., 28*, 2454-9.

[69] Basu, D., Reveille, J. D. (2005). Anti-scl-70. *Autoimmunity, 38*, 65-72.

[70] Samuels, D. S., Tojo, T., Homma, M., Shimizu, N. (1986). Inhibition of topoisomerase I by antibodies in sera from scleroderma patients. *FEBS Lett., 209*, 231-4.

[71] Henault, J., Tremblay, M., Clement, I., Raymond, Y., Senecal, J. L. (2004). Direct binding of anti-DNA topoisomerase I autoantibodies to the cell surface of fibroblasts in patients with systemic sclerosis. *Arthritis Rheum., 50*, 3265-74.

[72] Henault, J., Robitaille, G., Senecal, J. L., Raymond, Y. (2006). DNA topoisomerase I binding to fibroblasts induces monocyte adhesion and activation in the presence of anti-topoisomerase I autoantibodies from systemic sclerosis patients. *Arthritis Rheum., 54*, 963-73.

[73] Del Papa, N., Conforti, G., Gambini, D., La Rosa, L., Tincani, A., D'Cruz, D., Khamashta, M., Hughes, G. R., Balestrieri, G., Meroni, P. L. (1994). Characterization of the endothelial surface proteins recognized by anti-endothelial antibodies in primary and secondary autoimmune vasculitis. *Clin. Immunol. Immunopathol., 70*, 211-6.

[74] Ihn, H., Sato, S., Fujimoto, M., Igarashi, A., Yazawa, N., Kubo, M., Kikuchi, K., Takehara, K., Tamaki, K. (2000). Characterization of autoantibodies to endothelial cells in systemic sclerosis (SSc): association with pulmonary fibrosis. *Clin. Exp. Immunol., 119*, 203-9.

[75] Renaudineau, Y., Dugue, C., Dueymes, M., Youinou, P. (2002). Antiendothelial cell antibodies in systemic lupus erythematosus. *Autoimmun Rev., 1*, 365-72.

[76] Singh, S., du Bois, R. (2001). Autoantibodies in cryptogenic fibrosing alveolitis. *Respir. Res., 2*, 61-3.

[77] Nahm, D. H., Lee, Y. E., Yim, E. J., Park, H. S., Yim, H., Kang, Y., Kim, J. K. (2002). Identification of cytokeratin 18 as a bronchial epithelial autoantigen associated with nonallergic asthma. *Am. J. Respir. Crit. Care Med., 165*, 1536-9.

[78] Ronda, N., Gatti, R., Giacosa, R., Raschi, E., Testoni, C., Meroni, P. L., Buzio, C., Orlandini, G. (2002). Antifibroblast antibodies from systemic sclerosis patients are internalized by fibroblasts via a caveolin-linked pathway. *Arthritis Rheum., 46*, 1595-601.

[79] Chizzolini, C., Raschi, E., Rezzonico, R., Testoni, C., Mallone, R., Gabrielli, A., Facchini, A., Del Papa, N., Borghi, M. O., Dayer, J. M., Meroni, P. L. (2002). Autoantibodies to fibroblasts induce a proadhesive and proinflammatory fibroblast phenotype in patients with systemic sclerosis. *Arthritis Rheum., 46*, 1602-13.

[80] Muravov, O. I., Kaye, W. E., Lewin, M., Berkowitz, Z., Lybarger, J. A., Campolucci, S. S., Parker, J. E. (2005). The usefulness of computed tomography in detecting asbestos-related pleural abnormalities in people who had indeterminate chest radiographs: the Libby, MT, experience. *Int. J. Hyg. Environ. Health, 208*, 87-99.

Funding:
CDC 822092
NIH ES04804
NIH ES012596
NCRR P20 017670

In: Autoimmunity: Role, Regulation and Disorders
Editor: Fynn L. Vogel and L. F. Zimmermann
ISBN 978-1-60456-833-2

Chapter 12

Shared Variable Domain Elements among Anti-Collagen Antibodies Reactive with Goodpasture Epitopes

***Faustina N. Sackey*[1]*, Kendra L. Congdon*[1]*, Graham F. Brady*[1]*, Helmut Hopfer*[2]*, Ying Zhang*[1]*, Katherine M. Mackin*[1]*, Amy G. Clark*[1] *and Mary H. Foster*[*1]**

[1]Departments of Medicine and Research Service,
Duke University and Durham Veterans Affairs Medical Centers,
Durham, North Carolina
[2]Department of Pathology, University Hospital Hamburg-Eppendorf,
Hamburg, Germany

Abstract

Patients and rodents with Goodpasture's syndrome develop severe glomerulonephritis and lung hemorrhage due to binding of pathogenic autoantibodies to the non-collagenous NC1 domain of the alpha3 chain of type IV collagen. To gain insight into origins of anti-collagen autoimmunity and to identify potential targets for therapeutic intervention, we analyzed the variable domains of five anti-alpha3(IV)NC1 monoclonal autoantibodies (mAb) obtained by fusion of splenocytes from C57BL/6 and SJL mice immunized with alpha3(IV)NC1collagen. Sequencing reveals that all mAb are minimally mutated and share use of IGHV1 (previously J558) and IGKV3 (formerly Vkappa21) subgroup genes, despite their origins from three different mice and two different strains. Use of a conserved combination of unmutated IG genes suggests that a restricted germline-encoded optimal binding site conformation dominates the antibody response to alpha3(IV)NC1 antigen. Preferential expression of the IGKV3 subgroup was also previously reported among pathogenic autoantibodies reactive with type II collagen

[*] Address Correspondence to: Mary H. Foster, M.D, Nephrology Research, MSRBII. Duke University Medical Center. Box 103015. Durham, NC 27710. Phone 919-684-9788. Email: mhfoster@duke.edu. FAX 919-684-3011

in autoimmune arthritis, raising the possibility of structural similarities between seemingly disparate pathogenic collagen II and collagen IV epitopes. The C57BL/6- and SJL-derived anti-Goodpasture mAb differ in their use of D and J genes, using IGHD2-1 and IGHJ2 genes (IMGT® nomenclature, http://imgt.cines.fr) and IGHD1-1 and IGHJ4, respectively. However, both sets of mAb include four core amino acids with a conserved charge structure in the CDR3 of the heavy chain. The shared determinants present potential therapeutic targets on pathogenic anti-collagen B cells that escape central deletion *in vivo*.

Keywords: Goodpasture syndrome, anti-collagen autoimmunity, anti-GBM disease, autoantibody.

Introduction

Collagen is the main structural protein in vertebrates and a frequent target of autoimmune attack by anti-collagen antibodies and T cells. At least twenty collagen types with restricted tissue and organ distributions are formed by trimers of over 30 different collagen alpha chains. Several of these collagens bear epitopes targeted by pathogenic lymphocytes and antibodies [1]. Collagens types II and XI are attacked in experimental rheumatoid arthritis, types VII and XVII in autoimmune bullous skin diseases, and type V in pulmonary allograft rejection, whereas collagen chains alpha3(IV) and alpha5(IV) are the focus of injury in Goodpasture's syndrome and Alport's allograft immune nephritis, respectively [2-15]. The molecular basis of disease pathogenesis and of the propensity for failed tolerance is poorly understood. It is thus anticipated that identification of target epitopes and elucidation of antibody structure will provide key mechanistic insights and new therapeutic targets for these debilitating diseases.

Goodpasture's syndrome and its kidney-restricted counterpart, anti-glomerular basement membrane (GBM) disease, can be life threatening. Both entities are characterized by rapidly progressive glomerulonephritis and kidney failure due to anti-GBM autoantibodies [15]. Goodpasture's syndrome is further complicated by lung hemorrhage due to alveolar involvement. In patients, diagnosis depends on demonstration of circulating or organ-deposited anti-GBM antibodies that bind in a linear pattern along basement membrane. Major epitopes targeted by pathogenic antibodies have been localized to the non-collagenous globular (NC1) domain of the alpha3 chain of type IV collagen, hereafter alpha3(IV)NC1 or Goodpasture antigen [10, 11]. Experimental anti-GBM nephritis and Goodpasture's syndrome can be induced by passive transfer of anti-GBM antibodies (i.e., nephrotoxic nephritis) or by active immunization with alpha3(IV)NC1 (i.e., experimental autoimmune glomerulonephritis) [16, 17]. The clinical manifestations are explained by the highly restricted tissue distribution of the type IV alpha3-alpha4-alpha5 collagen protomer; this collagen isoform is found primarily in glomerular and alveolar basement membranes [18, 19]. The epitopes engaged by Goodpasture antibodies are conformational and sequestered within the native NC1 hexamer [19, 20], suggesting that unmasking is required for antibody deposition. Overlapping epitopes are targeted by a subset of pathogenic alloantibodies induced in Alport's patients receiving a renal allograft [13]. Individuals with Alport's hereditary nephritis have a mutation in the alpha3, alpha4, or alpha5 chain of type IV collagen. They thus fail to form the alpha3-alpha4-alpha5 protomer and lack the Goodpasture antigen, leading to alloimmunization upon transplantation with a normal kidney.

In contrast to the intense investigation that has elucidated the nature of the Goodpasture antigen, little is known about the structure or origin of Goodpasture autoantibodies or about regulation of the anti-collagen humoral immune response. To address these questions, we analyzed the variable domains of five anti-alpha3(IV)NC1 monoclonal autoantibodies (mAb) obtained by fusion of splenocytes from C57BL/6 and SJL mice immunized with alpha3(IV)NC1collagen. Herein we report the use of a conserved combination of immunoglobulin variable region genes by anti-alpha3(IV)NC1 mAb derived from mice of two different strains.

Materials and Methods

Monoclonal antibodies. SJL and C57BL/6 mice were immunized and boosted with recombinant human [21] or purified bovine (Wieslab, Lund, Sweden) alpha3(IV)NC1 antigen in adjuvant. After a final boost, spleen cells were harvested and fused with murine myeloma cells and selected in aminopterin using standard techniques [22]. Supernatants were screened for antigen binding by ELISA. Hybridomas producing anti-alpha3(IV) NC1 antibody were subcloned at least twice by limiting dilution.

Evaluation of Ig Binding Specificity and Competition ELISA. Hybridoma culture supernatants were tested for antibody production by ELISA as described [23]. To test antigen specificity, Immulon 2 HB 96-well microtiter plates (Thermo, Milford, MA) were coated overnight at 4°C with purified bovine alpha3(IV) NC1 antigen (Wieslab) at 200-400 ng/well in coating buffer (6M guanidine-HCl, 50 mM TRIS, pH 7.4) or in coating buffer alone to detect background binding. After blocking with 3% BSA in PBS for 30 minutes, supernatants were incubated at 50 ul per well at room temperature for 1 hour, then washed 3X with PBS. Alkaline phosphatase conjugated goat-anti-mouse-Ig diluted 1/2,000 in PBS was used as second step reagent. Assays were developed for 1 hour at room temperature, monitored at OD 405 nm, and values recorded as OD-antigen minus OD-diluent. Commercial (Sigma, St. Louis, MO and BD Biosciences, San Jose, CA) or laboratory-generated mouse IgM and IgG served as controls. IgM were purified from hybridoma or transfectant culture supernatants by ammonium sulfate precipitation followed by extensive dialysis against PBS. Purified Ig were stored before use at -20°C. Alkaline-phosphatase-labeled anti-mouse Ig second step antibodies were purchased from Roche Applied Sciences, Indianapolis, IN.

Subclones were tested for binding to the epitope bound by mouse anti-alpha3(IV)NC1 monoclonal IgG MAB3 (Wieslab) by competition ELISA. The dilution of MAB3 that gave submaximal binding to antigen was incubated with varying concentrations of purified mAb before plating on antigen-coated microplates. Bound Ig was detected with alkaline-phosphatase labeled goat anti-mouse-IgG.

Analysis of variable region genes expressed by anti-alpha3(IV)NC1 mAb: The rearranged variable region genes that encode anti-alpha3(IV)NC1 mAb were determined by RT-PCR of cDNA, essentially as previously described [23]. Briefly, cDNA was generated using a oligodT primer and total RNA extracted from hybridoma cells using TRIzol reagent (Invitrogen, Carlsbad, CA). Heavy chain variable region was amplified by PCR using a universal degenerate VH 5' primer and Cmu 3' primer. Light chain variable region was amplified using a set of 5' primers complementary to the first 18-25 nucleotides of Vk framework 1 (FR1) and a 3' primer complementary to Ck [23]. PCR product was ligated into TOPO PCR cloning vector (Invitrogen) and amplified as described [23]. Purified DNA from multiple colonies was sequenced at the Duke University DNA Core facility. Sequences were analyzed using BLAST software of National Center for Biotechnology Information (NCBI) (http//www.ncbi.nlm.nih.gov) and compared to sequences deposited in the public Ig gene database International ImMunoGeneTics Information System, IMGT, (http://imgt.cines.fr). Alignments were generated by the ClustalW software tool at the European Bioinformatics Institute (www.ebi.ac.uk/clustalw/index.html).

Primer sequences:
VH 5' primer: 5'-GGGAATTCGAGGTGCAGCTGCAGGAGTCTGG-3'
Cmu 3' primer: 5'-CTCTCGCAGGAGACGAGGGGGAA-3'
VkFR1 5' primer: 5'-GACATTGTGATGACACAGTCTCCATCCTAT-3'
Ckappa 3' primer: 5'-CTGCTCACTGGATGGTGGGA-3'

Results

Anti-Alpha3(IV)NC1 Monoclonal Antibodies

Fusion of splenocytes from six immunized mice and subsequent subcloning yielded five IgM mAb that bound strongly to alpha3(IV)NC1 collagen in ELISA. MAb 1C3, 1C4 and 1D4 were derived from the same B6 mouse, mAb 1G6 from a different B6 mouse, and mAb 159 from an SJL mouse. IgG anti-alpha3(IV)NC1 mAb were not recovered from any fusion despite high serum IgG titers and multiple fusions. None of three mAb tested inhibited antigen binding by murine mAb IgG MAB3 (not shown). MAB3 binds a non-pathogenic epitope of alpha3(IV)NC1 collagen [19].

Analysis of Heavy and Light Chain Variable Region Genes

The rearranged variable region genes that encode the heavy and light chains of the five anti-alpha3(IV)NC1 mAb were determined by sequence analysis of RT-PCR of cDNA using a universal degenerate VH 5' primer, Cmu 3' primer, a set of 5' primers complementary to the first 18-25 nucleotides of Vk framework 1 (FR1), and a Ck 3' primer, essentially as described [23]. The genes are listed in Figure 1 and key nucleotide and deduced amino acid sequences are shown in Figure 2.

MAb	IGHV subgroup	IGHD gene	IGHJ gene	IGKV subgroup	IGKJ gene
1G6	IGHV1	IGHD2-1#	IGHJ2	IGKV3	IGKJ2
1C3 cluster	IGHV1	IGHD2-1#	IGHJ2	IGKV3	IGKJ4
159	IGHV1	IGHD1-1	IGHJ4	IGKV3	IGKJ1

Figure 1. Genes used in the VH (V-D-J-REGION) and V-KAPPA (V-J-REGION) of the anti-alpha3(IV)NC1 monoclonal antibodies. The 1C3 cluster is comprised of three presumed clonally related mAb, 1C3, 1D4 and 1C4, that were isolated from the same mouse and that share near-identical heavy and light chains, including junctional sequences. Both the 1G6 and 1C3 cluster VH CDR3-IMGT can be accounted for by an IGHD2-1 gene translated in reading frame 3 combined with somatic additions.

It is likely that MAb 1C3, 1D4 and 1C4 were derived from the same B cell clone. These three mAb were generated from the same spleen and the nucleotide sequences of the VH domain (V-D-J-REGION), obtained for 1C3 and 1D4, are identical, including the V-D-J junction. The nucleotide sequences of the V-KAPPA domains (V-J-REGION) were also identical with the exception of three residues in the FR3-IMGT of 1C3, at positions 77 and 78 according to the IMGT unique numbering [24] (Figure 2b). These FR3-IMGT differences presumably arose by mutation during *in vivo* clonal expansion. Complete IGKJ sequence was obtained only for 1C4. For the purposes of further discussion, these three mAb are referred to as the 1C3 cluster; they are shown as a single sequence in Figure 2 with the exception of the light chain FR3-IMGT as noted above.

Variable gene classification was determined based on homology to sequences deposited in the National Center for Biotechnology Information (NCBI) (http//www.ncbi.nlm.nih.gov) and International ImMunoGeneTics Information System, IMGT, (http://imgt.cines.fr) databases [25]. IGHV sequences sharing at least 75% nucleotide identity are assigned to a subgroup.

Antibodies of the 1C3 cluster use an unmutated IGHV gene of the IGHV1 subgroup (previously J558). The 1C3 IGHV gene is 100% identical to an IGHV gene recovered from a C57BL/6 (Igh-b allotype) genomic DNA BAC clone incorporating a portion of mouse chromosome 12 (accession no. AC160990 and BN000872) [26] and to a B6-derived mRNA from LPS-stimulated spleen clone J558.B16 (accession no. AF296433) [27]. This unmutated IGHV gene is also used by anti-keratin autoantibody M51-0 from the autoimmune tight-skin (Tsk) mouse (accession no. U09597) [28]. The closest IGHD gene identified by the IMGT/V-QUEST tool [29] integrated with IMGT/JunctionAnalysis [30] is IGHD2-1 with 2 mutations, and with 4 nucleotides in the N-REGION. FR4 of the 1C3 antibody cluster is encoded by the IGHJ2 gene.

The light chain of antibodies of the 1C3 cluster uses a mutated gene of the IGKV3 subgroup, previously termed Vk21 family, and an IGKJ4 gene. The closest matched sequence in the databases is the germline gene IGKV3-10 (allele IGKV3-10*01), also retrieved from a BAC clone of B6 genomic DNA (accession no. AC153928).

```
                                                                          12                                          23          26
                                                                       L   V   K   P   G   A   S   V   K   M   S   C   K   A   S
1G6H                                                                   CTG GTG AAG CCT GGG GCT TCA GTG AAG ATG TCC TGT AAG GCT TCT
AF459881 (GL)                                                          --- --- --- --- --- --- --- --- --- --- --- --- --- --- ---
                                                                               R                           T       C
1C3*                                                                   --- --- -G- --- --- --- --- --- --- -C- --- --C --- --- ---
AC160990 (GL)                                                          --- --- -G- --- --- --- --- --- --- -C- --- --C --- --- ---
                                                                           A   R                           L       C
159                                                                    --- -C- AG- --- --- --- --- --- --- C-- --- --C --- --- ---
BN000872 (GL)                                                          --- -C- AG- --- --- --- --- --- --- C-- --- --C --- --- ---

                                                   39      41                                  50
                   G   Y   K   F   T   D   Y   Y   M   N   W   V   K   Q   S   H   G   K   S   L   E   W   I   G
1G6H               GGA TAC AAA TTC ACT GAC TAC TAT ATG AAC TGG GTG AAG CAG AGC CAT GGA AAG AGC CTT GAG TGG ATT GGA
AF459881 (GL)      --- --- -C- --- --- --- --- --- --- --- --- --- --- --- --- --- --- --- --- --- --- --- --- ---
                   G       T                       I                       R   P       Q   G                       A
1C3*               --C --- -CT --- --- --- --- --- --A --- --- --- --- --- --G -C- --- C-- G-A --- --- --- --- -C-
AC160990 (GL)      --C --- -CT --- --- --- --- --- --A --- --- --- --- --- --G -C- --- C-- G-A --- --- --- --- -C-
                   G       T       T   T   Y   G   I   S                   R   T       Q   G
159                --C --- -CC --- --A AC- --T GG- --A -G- --- --- --- --- --A AC- --- C-- G-- --- --- --- --- ---
BN000872 (GL)      --C --- -CC --- --A AG- --T GG- --A -G- --- --- --- --- --A AC- --- C-- G-- --- --- --- --- ---
                   ________________________________
                           CDR1-IMGT

                   55                                  66                      72  74
                   V   I   N   P   Y   N   G   G   T   N   Y   N   Q   K   F   K   G   K   A   T   L   T   V   D   K
1G6H               GTT ATT AAT CCT TAC AAC GGT GGT ACT AAC TAC AAC CAG AAG TTC AAG GGC AAG GCC ACA TTG ACT GTT GAC AAG
AF459881 (GL)      --- --- --- --- --- --- --- --- --- -G- --- --- --- --- --- --- --- --- --- --- --- --- --- --- ---
                   R       Y       G   S       N       Y       N   E                               L       A   E   K
1C3*               AGG --- T-- --- GGA -GT --- AA- --- T-- --- --T G-- --- --- --- --- --- --- --- C-- --- -CA --A --A
AC160990 (GL)      AGG --- T-- --- GGA -GT --- AA- --- T-- --- --T G-- --- --- --- --- --- --- --- C-- --- -CA --A --A
                   E       Y       R   S       N   A   Y       N   E                               L       A       K
159                -AG --- T-- --- AGA -GT --- AA- G-- T-- --- --T G-- --- --- --- --- --- --- --- C-- --- -CA --- --A
BN000872 (GL)      -AG --- T-- --- AGA -GT --- AA- A-- T-- --- --T G-- --- --- --- --- --- --- --- C-- --- -CA --- --A
                       ________________________________
                               CDR2-IMGT

                                           89                                                            104
                   S   S   S   T   A   Y   M   D   L   N   S   L   T   F   D   D   S   A   V   Y   Y   C   A   R
1G6H               TCC TCC AGC ACA GCC TAC ATG GAC CTC AAC AGC CTG ACA TTT GAT GAC TCT GCA GTC TAT TAC TGT GCA AGA
AF459881 (GL)      --- --- --- --- --- --- --- --G --- --- --- --- --- -C- --G --- --- --- --- --- --- --- --- ---
                               T               Q       S               S   E           A           F
1C3*               --- --- --- --T --- --- --- C-G --- -G- --- --- --- -C- --G --- --- --T --- --- -T- --- --- ---
AC160990 (GL)      --- --- --- --T --- --- --- C-G --- -G- --- --- --- -C- --G --- --- --T --- --- -T- --- --- ---
                                   A           E       R               S   E           A           F
159                --- --- --- --- --A --- --- --G --- CG- --- --- --- -C- --G --- --- --G --- --- -T- --- --- ---
BN000872 (GL)      --- --- --- --- --G --- --- --G --- CG- --- --- --- -C- --G --- --- --G --- --- -T- --- --- ---
                                                                                                         _______
IGHD2-1*01            C TAT GGT AAC TAC
N-regions          N1                      N2                                          118
                   P   P   Y   G   H   Y   G                       L   D   Y   W
1G6H               CCA CCC TAT GGC CAC TAC GGG                     CTT GAC TAC TGG      IGHJ2  CDR-IMGT lengths [8.8.12]
                   S       D   G   N   Y                           F   D   Y   W
1C3*               T--     G-- --T A-- ---                         T-- --- --- ---      IGHJ2  CDR-IMGT lengths [8.8.10]

IGHD1-1*01                         AC TAC GGT AGT AGC
N-regions                  N1                          N2
                           T   L   H   Y   G   S   S   P   L   A   M   D   Y   W
159                        A-- TTG CAC TAC GGT AGT AGC CCT CTT GCT ATG GAC TAC TGG      IGHJ4  CDR-IMGT lengths [8.8.15]
                   ____________________________________________________________
                                   CDR3-IMGT
```

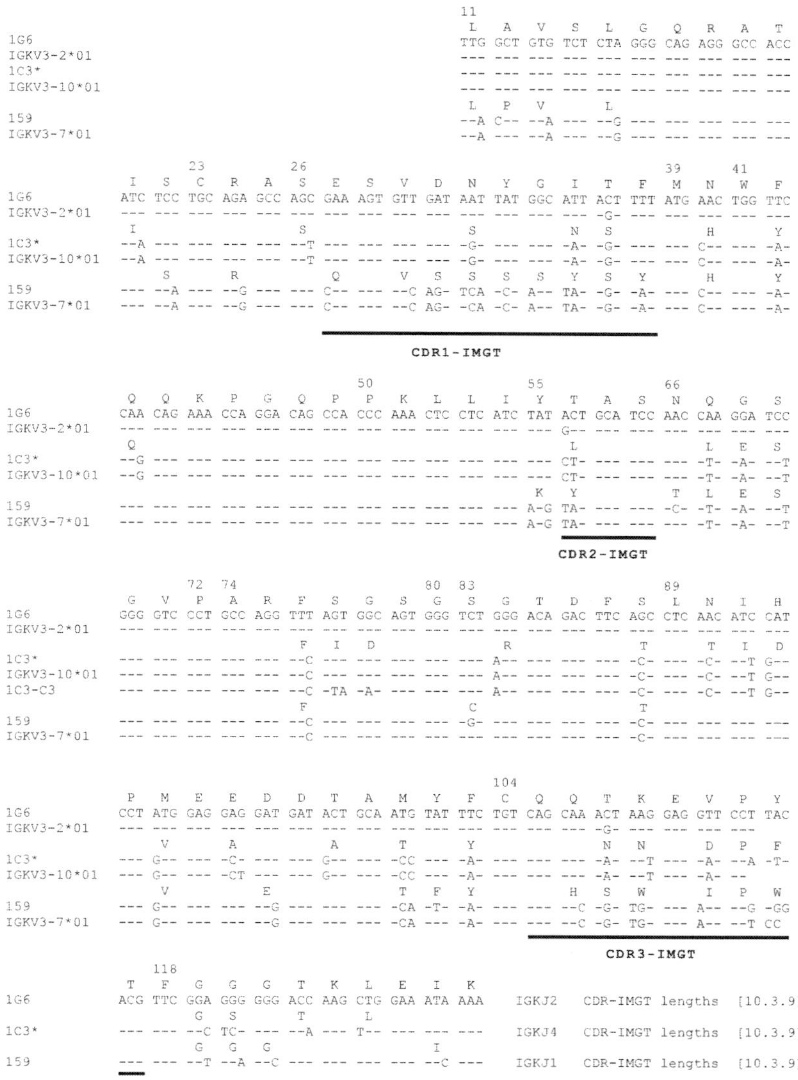

Figure 2. Sequences of rearranged heavy chain (a) and light chain (b) variable region genes of anti-alpha3(IV) NC1 collagen mAb derived from immunized mice. All sequences are compared with those of the prototype 1G6 anti-alpha3(IV) NC1 collagen IG. Dashes represent sequence identity with 1G6. 1C3* represents the three putative clonally related antibodies, 1C3, 1C4 and 1D4, with identical VH domain sequences. AF459881 and AC160990 are GenBank accession numbers for bacterial artificial chromosome (BAC) clones containing the corresponding B6 germline IGHV sequences. BN000872 is the EMBL accession number for the manually assembled 2.75 Mb C57BL/6 mouse *Igh* locus that incorporates all relevant BACs [26]. Germline IGKV sequences are from the IMGT/V-QUEST reference directory [29]. The IGHD2-1*01 and IGHD1-1*01 allele sequences encoding D-REGIONs are shown in (a). Empty spaces are introduced to maximize sequence homologies. Blanks at the 5' end of the IGH V-REGION denote sequence determined by degenerate PCR primers. CDR-IMGT are delineated according to the IMGT unique numbering for V-DOMAIN [24] and to IMGT/V-QUEST [29]. CDR-IMGT lengths are shown between brackets, separated by dots. The IGHJ and IGKJ genes are indicated; no mutations were found in these sequences. In (b), the FR3-IMGT is shown in which clone 1C3-C3 differs by three nucleotides from the other two presumed clonally related members of this cluster.

The IGKV consensus sequence for the 1C3 cluster has a single silent mutation t288>g according to the IMGT unique numbering [24] in the FR3-IMGT compared to the germline. The 1C3 mAb differs from the other two members of the cluster in having three additional closely grouped replacement mutations also in FR3-IMGT. The germline IGKV3-10 gene is reportedly used by an anti-DNA Ab (accession no. U30235).

Antibody 1G6 uses a mutated IGHV gene of the IGHV1 subgroup. The 1G6 IGHV gene has 98% identity (253/258 nucleotides) with IGHV1-19*01 using IMGT/V-QUEST [29]. This is a novel B6 germline gene based on comparison with a BAC clone incorporating C57BL/6 genomic DNA (accession no. AC073565), and was assigned the name J558.3A (accession no. AF459881) based on similarity between sequences recovered by single cell PCR from nine independent B cell isolates originating from five different B6 or B6.Sle1 mice and the sequence of the closest known germline gene J558.3 [31]. Assembly of the entire 2.5-Mb IGHV region sequence of the B6 strain was recently reported [26] and was included in our GenBank search. This and the IMGT/V-QUEST analysis indicate that 1G6 has 5 mutations from the germline sequence. These lead to 2 conservative framework changes (E90>D and E97>D, according to the IMGT unique numbering [24] and 3 non-conservative changes, one in CDR1-IMGT (T29>K) and two in FR3-IMGT (S66>N, S96>F), from hydroxyl to basic, amide and phenylalanine, respectively, according to the IMGT amino acid classes [32] and IMGT Aide-Mèmoire> Amino acids. The 1G6 IGHV CDR3-IMGT derives from a mutated IGHD-2-1*01 allele and 9 N-region nucleotide additions flanking the IGHD gene (Figure 2). One IGHD gene mutation is silent; the other replaces the germline-encoded asparagine with a histidine residue. 1G6 uses an unmutated IGHJ2 gene.

Antibody 1G6 uses a mutated IGKV3-2*01 allele and an IGKJ2 gene. The closest matched sequence in the IMGT/V-QUEST reference directory is X16954 from BALB/c. The same gene and allele in C57BL/6 has been located on a BAC clone (accession no. AC153612). There are three mutations (S35>T, A56>T and S107>T, localized in the CDR1-IMGT, CDR2-IMGT and CDR3-IMGT, respectively, with no change of the IMGT chemical classes for two of them [32]. Use of this IGKV germline sequence by anti-DNA autoantibodies isolated from BWF1 mice has been reported (accession no. Z22133).

The SJL-derived mAb 159 uses an IGHV gene of the IGHV1 subgroup that has 98% identity (261/264 nucleotides) with a C57BL/6 germline sequence (accession no. BN000872) [26]. Whether the 3 nucleotide differences represent the SJL germline allele or mutations is unknown. The C57BL/6 sequence is identical to that used by an antinuclear antibody from the B6.Sle1 strain (accession no. AY454455). The closest matched sequence in the IMGT/V-QUEST reference directory is C57BL/6-derived X02065 that shares 91% identity with Ab 159. The 159 IGHV CDR3-IMGT derives from an unmutated IGHD1-1*01 allele and 12 N-region nucleotide additions flanking the IGHD gene (Figure 2). 159 uses an unmutated IGHJ4 gene. SJL mAb 159 uses a IGKV3-7*01 allele and an IGKJ1 gene. The VK sequence shares 98% identity with IMGT/V-QUEST reference sequence K02158 from BALB/c and with the identical allele in C57BL/6 (259/262 nucleotides, accession no. AC153928). The SJL germline allele is not retrieved from the database search.

Strikingly, the VH CDR3-IMGT of all C57BL/6-derived antibodies is encoded by the IGHD2-1 gene translated in reading frame 3 and with a conservative replacement mutation that preserves the charge structure within the 4 a.a. IGHD2-1-gene-encoded core: YGHY,

DGNY, and YGNY in 1G6, the 1C3 cluster, and the germline sequence, respectively. Moreover, this core structure is preserved in the VH CDR3-IMGT of the SJL-derived mAb 159 as TLHY encoded by 7 N-region and 5 IGHD1-1-gene-encoded nucleotides.

Conclusion

We generated mAb against the Goodpasture antigen to gain insight into origins of anti-collagen autoimmunity and to identify potential targets for therapeutic intervention. Immunization with purified NC1 domains of alpha3(IV) collagen yielded five mAb that bound strongly to antigen in ELISA. Three mAb were derived from a single mouse and shared identical Ig heavy chains and near-identical Ig light chains, suggesting that they arose from a single clone in vivo. These Ig, in combination with mAb 1G6 and mAb 159, derived independently from different B6 and SJL immunized mice, share multiple gene features. All are encoded by IGHV1 and IGKV3 subgroup genes with minimal mutation. Moreover, all VH CDR3-IMGT have a 4 a.a. core with a preserved charge structure: YGHY, DGNY, and TLHY in mAb 1G6, 1C3, and 159, respectively.

This conserved use of a well-defined set of heavy and light chain IG genes among multiple mAb from different mice suggests that the mAb bind the same or similar epitopes on alpha3(IV)NC1 collagen. Shared use of minimally mutated IG genes is also interpreted to indicate that only certain IG gene combinations provide the strict structural requirements that ensure relatively high affinity antigen binding in the immediate antibody response. Such responses are described in the murine primary protective response to phosphocholine [33] and among human IgG against deadly *Haemophilus influenzae* type b [34]. For germline configurations that provide near-optimal antigen binding, subsequent random mutation would be inefficient at further increasing affinity. Use of shared sequences anticipates the presence of dominant idiotypic markers in the Goodpasture immune response [35]. Structural analysis of anti-alpha3(IV)NC1 mAb should provide insights to assist engineering of therapeutic blocking anti-idiotypic or antibody-like molecules.

The recovery of minimally mutated IgM also has implications regarding regulation of alpha3(IV)NC1-reactive B cells. This suggests that pathogenic autoreactivity was present in newly generated immature B cells in the bone marrow, such that mutation and affinity maturation within germinal centers was not essential. These cells thus were not deleted centrally, but exited the bone marrow either as functionally responsive or reversibly anergized B cells. This hypothesis and *in vivo* tolerogenesis of the Goodpasture antigen is currently being tested in our laboratory using autoantibody transgenic mice generated using a prototype mAb. Relevance to human anti-glomerular basement membrane disease is suggested by recent reports of recovery of low titers of natural anti-alpha3(IV)NC1 IG from normal human sera [36].

A striking bias toward use of several IGKV3 subgroup genes, often expressed unmutated, as well as biased use of the IGHV1 and IGKV3 subgroup gene combination was previously reported among IgG mAb reactive with collagen II epitopes [37-39]. Rodent immunization with heterologous collagen II induces self-reactive anti-collagen antibodies and a destructive arthritis. Transfer of immune serum IgG or combinations of anti-collagen II mAb induces destructive arthritis in naïve recipients. Preferential use of IGKV3 genes is particularly striking, given that this family is typically expressed in adult mouse spleen at low frequency [40]. The significance of biased IGHV1 subgroup use is less clear, because this large IGHV subgroup accounts for approximately 48% (52/110) of functional murine IGHV genes in the C57BL/6 strain [26]. Use of a similar IGHV and IGKV gene combination among anti-collagen antibodies reactive with different types of collagen raises the possibility of a structural relationship between pathogenic alpha3(IV)NC1 and collagen II epitopes. A molecular basis for this is not immediately obvious; the pathogenic Goodpasture alpha3(IV)NC1 epitopes reside within the globular non-collagenous portion of the type IV molecule, whereas most arthritogenic IgG bind to epitopes in the native collagen II triple helix formed by the repeated Gly-X-Y-Pro motif. Further dissection of the molecular and structural composition of pathogenic anti-collagen IG as described here will provide needed insight for development of new therapeutic targets for these debilitating autoimmune diseases.

Acknowledgments

This work was supported by a Department of Veterans Affairs Merit Review Grant, the Durham VAMC Research Service and Medical Research Institute, and National Institutes of Health Grant DK47424.

Nucleotide sequence data reported are available in the DDBJ/EMBL/GenBank databases under the accession number(s) – DQ889716, DQ889717, DQ889718, DQ889719, DQ889720, DQ889721, DQ889722, EF219161, EF219162.

This work was supported in part by the National Institutes of Health Grant DK47424, a VAMC Merit Award, the Durham VAMC Institute for Medical Research and the Research and Medical Media Services of the Durham VAMC. Dr. Raghu Kalluri (Harvard University) is gratefully acknowledged for provision of recombinant human alpha3(IV)NC1. We thank the Duke University Comprehensive Cancer Center Hybridoma and Cell Culture and DNA sequencing facilities and Dr. Carol Wikstrand for their expertise. The experiments comply with the current laws of the country in which experiments were performed.

References

[1] Myllyharju, J. and Kivirikko, K. I., Collagens and collagen-related diseases. *Ann. Med.* 2001. 33: 7-21.

[2] Luross, J. A. and Williams, N. A., The genetic and immunopathological processes underlying collagen-induced arthritis. *Immunology* 2001. 103: 407-416.

[3] Haque, M. A., Mizobuchi, T., Yasufuku, K., Fujisawa, T., Brutkiewicz, R. R., Zheng, Y., Woods, K., Smith, G. N., Cummings, O. W., Heidler, K. M., Blum, J. S. and Wilkes, D. S., Evidence for immune responses to a self-antigen in lung transplantation:

role of type V collagen-specific T cells in the pathogenesis of lung allograft rejection. *J. Immunol.* 2002. 169: 1542-1549.

[4] Burlingham, W. J., Love, R. B., Jankowska-Gan, E., Haynes, L. D., Xu, Q., Bobadilla, J. L., Meyer, K. C., Hayney, M. S., Braun, R. K., Greenspan, D. S., Gopalakrishnan, B., Cai, J., Brand, D. D., Yoshida, S., Cummings, O. W. and Wilkes, D. S., IL-17-dependent cellular immunity to collagen type V predisposes to obliterative bronchiolitis in human lung transplants. *J. Clin. Invest* 2007. 117: 3498-3506.

[5] Moll, R. and Moll, I., Epidermal adhesion molecules and basement membrane components as target structures of autoimmunity. *Virchows Arch.* 1998: 487-504.

[6] Xu, L., Robinson, N., Miller, S. D. and Chan, L. S., Characterization of BALB/c mice B lymphocyte autoimmune responses to skin basement membrane component type XVII collagen, the target antigen of autoimmune skin disease bullous pemphigoid. *Immunol. Lett* 2001. 77: 105-111.

[7] Gammon, W. R. and Briggaman, R. A., Epidermolysis bullosa acquisita and bullous systemic lupus erythematosus. Diseases of autoimmunity to type VII collagen. *Dermatologic Clinics* 1993. 11: 535-547.

[8] Brainwood, D., Kashtan, C., Gubler, M. C. and Turner, A. N., Targets of alloantibodies in Alport anti-glomerular basement membrane disease after renal transplantation. *Kidney Int.* 1998. 53: 762-766.

[9] Ghohestani, R., Hudson, B., Claudy, A. and Uitto, J., The alpha 5 chain of type IV collagen is the target of IgG autoantibodies in a novel autoimmune disease with subepidermal blisters and renal insufficiency. *J. Biol. Chem.* 2000. 275: 16002-16006.

[10] Wieslander, J., Barr, J. F., Butkowski, R. J., Edwards, S. J., Bygren, P., Heinegard, D. and Hudson, B. G., Goodpasture antigen of the glomerular basement membrane: localization to noncollagenous regions of type IV collagen. *Proc. Natl. Acad. Sci. USA* 1984. 81: 3838-3842.

[11] Saus, J., Wieslander, J., Langeveld, J., Quinones, S. and Hudson, B., Identification of the Goodpasture antigen as the alpha 3(IV) chain of collagen IV. *J. Biol. Chem.* 1988. 263: 13374-13380.

[12] Schulte, S., Unger, C., Mo, J. A., Wendler, O., Bauer, E., Frischholz, S., von der Mark, K., Kalden, J. R., Holmdahl, R. and Burkhardt, H., Arthritis-related B cell epitopes in collagen II are conformation-dependent and sterically privileged in accessible sites of cartilage collagen fibrils. *J. Biol. Chem.* 1998. 273: 1551-1561.

[13] Wang, X. P., Fogo, A. B., Colon, S., Giannico, G., Abul-Ezz, S. R., Miner, J. H. and Borza, D. B., Distinct epitopes for anti-glomerular basement membrane alport alloantibodies and goodpasture autoantibodies within the noncollagenous domain of alpha3(IV) collagen: a janus-faced antigen. *J. Am. Soc. Nephrol.* 2005. 16: 3563-3571.

[14] Borza, D. B., Chedid, M. F., Colon, S., Lager, D. J., Leung, N. and Fervenza, F. C., Recurrent Goodpasture's disease secondary to a monoclonal IgA1-kappa antibody autoreactive with the alpha1/alpha2 chains of type IV collagen. *Am. J. Kidney Dis.* 2005. 45: 397-406.

[15] Hudson, B. G., Tryggvason, K., Sundaramoorthy, M. and Neilson, E. G., Alport's syndrome, Goodpasture's syndrome, and type IV collagen. *N. Engl. J. Med.* 2003. 348: 2543-2556.

[16] Lerner, R. A., Glassock, R. J. and Dixon, F. J., The role of anti-glomerular basement membrane antibody in the pathogenesis of human glomerulonephritis. *J. Exp. Med.* 1967. 126: 989-1004.

[17] Sado, Y., Boutaud, A., Kagawa, M., Naito, I., Ninomiya, Y. and Hudson, B., Induction of anti-GBM nephritis in rats by recombinant alpha 3(IV)NC1 and alpha 4(IV)NC1 of type IV collagen. *Kidney Int* 1998. 53: 664-671.

[18] Kalluri, R., Cantley, L., Kerjaschki, D. and Neilson, E., Reactive oxygen species expose cryptic epitopes associated with autoimmune goodpasture syndrome. *J. Biol. Chem.* 2000. 275: 20027-20032.

[19] Borza, D. B., Netzer, K. O., Leinonen, A., Todd, P., Cervera, J., Saus, J. and Hudson, B. G., The goodpasture autoantigen. Identification of multiple cryptic epitopes on the NC1 domain of the alpha3(IV) collagen chain. *J. Biol. Chem.* 2000. 275: 6030-6037.

[20] Borza, D. B., Bondar, O., Colon, S., Todd, P., Sado, Y., Neilson, E. G. and Hudson, B. G., Goodpasture autoantibodies unmask cryptic epitopes by selectively dissociating autoantigen complexes lacking structural reinforcement: novel mechanisms for immune privilege and autoimmune pathogenesis. *J. Biol. Chem.* 2005. 280: 27147-27154.

[21] Kalluri, R., Danoff, T. M., Okada, H. and Neilson, E. G., Susceptibility to anti-glomerular basement membrane disease and Goodpasture Syndrome is linked to MHC class II genes and the emergence of T cell-mediated immunity in mice. *J. Clin. Invest* 1997. 100: 2263-2275.

[22] Harlow, E. and Lane, D., *Antibodies: A Laboratory Manual*. Cold Spring Harbor Laboratory, New York: 1988.

[23] Fitzsimons, M. M., Chen, H. and Foster, M. H., Diverse endogenous light chains contribute to basement membrane reactivity in nonautoimmune mice transgenic for an anti-laminin Ig heavy chain. *Immunogenetics* 2000. 51: 20-29.

[24] Lefranc, M. P., Pommie, C., Ruiz, M., Giudicelli, V., Foulquier, E., Truong, L., Thouvenin-Contet, V. and Lefranc, G., IMGT unique numbering for immunoglobulin and T cell receptor variable domains and Ig superfamily V-like domains. *Dev. Comp Immunol* 2003. 27: 55-77.

[25] Lefranc, M. P., Giudicelli, V., Kaas, Q., Duprat, E., Jabado-Michaloud, J., Scaviner, D., Ginestoux, C., Clement, O., Chaume, D. and Lefranc, G., IMGT, the international ImMunoGeneTics information system. *Nucleic Acids Res.* 2005. 33: D593-597.

[26] Johnston, C. M., Wood, A. L., Bolland, D. J. and Corcoran, A. E., Complete sequence assembly and characterization of the C57BL/6 mouse Ig heavy chain V region. *J. Immunol.* 2006. 176: 4221-4234.

[27] Haines, B. B., Angeles, C. V., Parmelee, A. P., McLean, P. A. and Brodeur, P. H., Germline diversity of the expressed BALB/c VhJ558 gene family. *Mol. Immunol.* 2001. 38: 9-18.

[28] Kasturi, K. N., Yio, X. Y. and Bona, C. A., Molecular characterization of J558 genes encoding tight-skin mouse autoantibodies: identical heavy-chain variable genes code for antibodies with different specificities. *Proc. Natl. Acad. Sci. USA* 1994. 91: 8067-8071.

[29] Giudicelli, V., Chaume, D. and Lefranc, M. P., IMGT/V-QUEST, an integrated software program for immunoglobulin and T cell receptor V-J and V-D-J rearrangement analysis. *Nucleic Acids Res.* 2004. 32: W435-440.

[30] Yousfi Monod, M., Giudicelli, V., Chaume, D. and Lefranc, M. P., IMGT/JunctionAnalysis: the first tool for the analysis of the immunoglobulin and T cell receptor complex V-J and V-D-J JUNCTIONs. *Bioinformatics* 2004. 20 Suppl 1: I379-I385.

[31] Chang, S. and Mohan, C., Identification of novel VH1/J558 immunoglobulin germline genes of C57BL/6 (Igh b) allotype. *Mol. Immunol.* 2005. 42: 1293-1301.

[32] Pommie, C., Levadoux, S., Sabatier, R., Lefranc, G. and Lefranc, M. P., IMGT standardized criteria for statistical analysis of immunoglobulin V-REGION amino acid properties. *J. Mol. Recognit* 2004. 17: 17-32.

[33] Claflin, J. and Berry, J., Genetics of the phosphocholine-specific antibody response to Streptococcus pneumoniae. Germ-line but not mutated T15 antibodies are dominantly selected. *J. Immunol.* 1988. 141: 4012-4019.

[34] Hougs, L., Juul, L., Svejgaard, A. and Barington, T., Structural requirements of the major protective antibody to Haemophilus influenzae type b. *Infect. Immun.* 1999. 67: 2503-2514.

[35] Meyers, K. E., Kinniry, P. A., Kalluri, R., Neilson, E. G. and Madaio, M. P., Human Goodpasture anti-alpha3(IV)NC1 autoantibodies share structural determinants. *Kidney Int.* 1998. 53: 402-407.

[36] Cui, Z., Wang, H. and Zhao, M., Natural autoantibodies against glomerular basement membrane exist in normal human sera. *Kidney Int.* 2006. 69: 894-899.

[37] Mo, J. A., Bona, C. A. and Holmdahl, R., Variable region gene selection of immunoglobulin G-expressing B cells with specificity for a defined epitope on type II collagen. *Eur. J Immunol.* 1993. 23: 2503-2510.

[38] Mo, J. A. and Holmdahl, R., The B cell response to autologous type II collagen: biased V gene repertoire with V gene sharing and epitope shift. *J Immunol* 1996. 157: 2440-2448.

[39] Ye, X. J., Marion, T. N., Terato, K., Aelion, J. A., Cremer, M. A., Tillman, D. M., Krug, M. S., Jackson, B. and Yoo, T. J., Variable-region gene family usage for type II collagen autoantibodies in arthritis-susceptible DBA/1 mice. *Clin. Immunol. Immunopathol.* 1996. 78: 263-275.

[40] Kaushik, A., Schulze, D. H., Bona, C. and Kelsoe, G., Murine V kappa gene expression does not follow the VH paradigm. *J. Exp. Med.* 1989. 169: 1859-1864.

Index

A

AA, 32, 68, 250, 255, 259, 260, 261, 262, 264
abdominal, 68, 197
aberrant, 153, 155, 161, 162, 166, 180, 238, 260
abnormalities, 33, 154, 162, 163, 167, 210, 236, 237, 239, 244, 245, 251, 255, 262, 266, 270
abortion, 238, 244, 245
absorbents, 257
AC, 109, 166, 197
access, 128, 173
accessibility, 170
accidental, 78
accounting, 14
ACE, 37
acetic acid, 132
acetylcholine, 108, 153, 164, 172, 181
Achilles heel, 81
acid, 72, 107, 113, 125, 131, 134, 135, 138, 142, 144, 172, 176, 180, 193
acoustic, 241
acquired immunity, 229
ACR, 62
ACTH, 111
actin, 89, 92, 102, 170, 183
activated receptors, 49
activation, 12, 15, 18, 20, 28, 29, 31, 33, 47, 50, 55, 60, 67, 69, 71, 73, 74, 75, 84, 111, 113, 127, 131, 132, 133, 135, 152, 163, 164, 166, 169, 171, 173, 174, 175, 178, 180, 183, 186, 189, 190, 192, 195, 196, 198, 204, 207, 217, 219, 221, 223, 224, 225, 226, 227, 229, 230, 231, 232, 258, 269
activation state, 207
activators, 71, 134, 183
active site, 141
acute, 61, 86, 88, 98, 100, 101, 106, 107, 110, 114, 116, 118, 119, 120, 123, 130, 134, 137, 138, 140, 143, 184, 189, 193, 196
acute infection, 98, 107
acylated, 124
ADAM33, 2, 11, 29, 54
Adams, 88, 105, 122, 149
adaptive immune system, 205, 209, 210, 223, 224
adenosine deaminase, 34
adenovirus, 86, 170, 179
adhesion, 25, 26, 32, 51, 52, 54, 55, 60, 67, 111, 140, 143, 155, 166, 179, 197, 269, 281
adipocyte, 21
adipose, 21
adiposity, 50
administration, 105, 109, 114, 155, 183, 239
ADP, 190, 196
adsorption, 90
adult, 147, 163, 196, 280
adventitia, 63
aetiology, 36, 49, 68
AF, 167, 244
age, 2, 21, 50, 60, 61, 62, 115, 116, 130, 144, 153, 154, 156, 157, 218, 219, 236, 237, 239, 241, 243, 251, 254, 261
agent, 77, 78, 80, 84, 85, 89, 90, 93, 96, 97, 100, 101, 138, 155
agents 49, 78, 79, 80, 84, 85, 86, 88, 89, 90, 92, 95, 97, 101, 102, 103, 104, 105, 108, 111, 115, 132, 141, 148, 155, 174
aggregates, 92, 98, 99, 204
aggregation, 69, 98
aid, 123
AIDS, 77, 84, 85, 86, 87, 88, 89, 91, 92, 93, 98, 99, 105, 106, 107, 108, 109, 110, 111, 112, 113, 114
air, 249

airways, 54, 163
alanine, 21, 50, 112, 123, 128, 139, 144
Alberta, 247
albumin, 198
alkaline, 273
allele, 6, 8, 9, 12, 13, 14, 15, 16, 17, 19, 21, 22, 24, 25, 26, 30, 31, 32, 34, 51, 275, 277, 278
alleles, 2, 4, 5, 7, 8, 9, 10, 12, 15, 19, 21, 43, 57, 154, 216, 218
allergic, 106, 109, 114, 115, 116, 142, 145, 149, 150, 262
allergic asthma, 262
allergy, 230
alloantibodies, 272, 281
allogeneic, 107, 206, 224, 238
allograft, 15, 45, 177, 272, 273, 281
allosteric, 203
alpha, 1, 11, 35, 36, 44, 47, 56, 57, 73, 124, 125, 133, 135, 147, 177, 180, 181, 272, 281, 282
alternative, 5, 8, 29, 34, 106, 152, 162, 163, 165, 191, 215
alters, 31, 35, 123, 178, 228, 237
aluminium, 204
alveolar macrophage, 269
alveolitis, 262, 270
amelioration, 109
amide, 278
amino, 25, 26, 30, 35, 49, 106, 112, 115, 116, 128, 144, 172, 193, 199, 201, 260, 272, 274, 278, 283
amino acid, 25, 26, 30, 35, 49, 106, 112, 115, 116, 128, 144, 172, 193, 199, 201, 260, 272, 274, 278, 283
amino acids, 106, 115, 116, 128, 144, 172, 201, 260, 272
ammonium, 273
amorphous, 248
Amsterdam, 149
amylase, 161, 166
anaemia, 85
analog, 112, 147
anatomy, 138
ANCA, 26
anemia, 240
angiotensin, 142
animal models, 78, 79, 81, 83, 97, 101, 102, 104, 154, 155
animals, 18, 47, 92, 96, 97, 101, 102, 120, 152, 156, 157, 176, 192, 207
ankylosing spondylitis, 172, 181
ANOVA, 157, 159, 253
antenatal exposure, 241
anti-apoptotic, 151, 155, 162
antibiotics, 86, 252
Antibodies, 77, 107, 113, 252, 253, 256, 259, 261, 262, 271, 274, 275, 282
antibody, 74, 77, 78, 80, 81, 82, 83, 84, 87, 88, 89, 90, 91, 92, 93, 94, 95, 96, 97, 98, 99, 100, 102, 103, 104, 105, 111, 112, 113, 121, 122, 153, 159, 172, 173, 181, 190, 191, 192, 193, 198, 199, 204, 205, 209, 210, 216, 217, 225, 238, 244, 245, 247, 248, 252, 259, 260, 265, 269, 271, 272, 273, 275, 278, 279, 281, 282, 283
anti-cancer, 228
anticardiolipin, 238
antidiabetic, 21, 36
antigen presenting cells, 155, 172, 173, 176
antigen-presenting cell, 31, 55, 87, 130, 169, 182, 203, 230
Antigens, 1, 51, 93
antigen-specific cells, 174
anti-HIV, 88, 91, 106
anti-idiotypic, 80, 81, 84, 87, 89, 90, 91, 105, 111, 112, 279
anti-inflammatory, 21, 151, 155
antinuclear antibodies, 249, 266, 268, 269
antioxidant, 20, 59, 61, 155
anti-platelet, 108
antisense, 80, 81, 112, 113
antisera, 210
anti-TNFα, 219
anti-tumor, 225, 227
antiviral, 18, 47, 74, 75, 110, 177, 186
aortic aneurysm, 197
APC, 172, 185, 203, 204, 206, 209, 210, 216, 221, 223
APL, 180
apoptosis, 15, 18, 19, 25, 31, 35, 46, 49, 51, 55, 56, 151, 152, 153, 154, 155, 157, 158, 159, 161, 162, 165, 166, 167, 171, 195, 196, 203, 231, 259, 260, 267, 269
apoptotic, 153, 154, 157, 158, 160, 163, 164, 191, 209, 260, 268
application, 4, 38, 90, 104, 167
aqueous solution, 121, 123, 141
ARC, 225
Argentina, 45
arginine, 26, 35, 67, 128, 138, 216, 231
argument, 7
arrest, 182
ART, 236, 238, 239

artery, 61, 68, 197
arthritis, 60, 71, 72, 73, 74, 75, 93, 97, 168, 184, 187, 215, 261, 272, 279, 280, 283
artificial, 121, 123, 127, 216, 277
asbestos 247, 248, 249, 250, 251, 255, 258, 259, 260, 261, 262, 264, 265, 266, 267, 268, 269, 270
asbestosis, 249, 258, 262, 265
Asian, 18, 47, 48
asparagines, 193
aspirin, 239, 245
assaults, 190
assessment, 9, 246, 249, 259, 261, 265
associations, 7, 8, 9, 51, 52, 60, 61, 237, 249, 266, 268
assumptions, 5, 78
asthma, 3, 29, 54, 270
astrocytes, 56, 135, 182
astroglial, 142
asymptomatic, 69, 166, 245
atherogenesis, 185
atherosclerosis, 59, 60, 61, 62, 66, 67, 68, 69
atrophy, 46, 155, 163, 171
attachment, 26, 170, 192
attacks, 130, 138
attention, 61, 160, 190, 262
atypical, 144
audiology, 241
Australia, 109
autoantigens, 114, 151, 155, 157, 163, 253, 255, 260, 268
201, 202, 206, 217, 223, 224, 225, 230, 231, 243, 247, 248, 251, 262, 264, 265, 266, 268, 269, 280, 281
autoimmune diseases, ix, xi, xii, 7, 13, 15, 19, 20, 29, 30, 35, 37, 56, 61, 62, 77, 78, 79, 81, 82, 83, 84, 85, 87, 89, 92, 93, 94, 95, 96, 97, 98, 99, 100, 101, 102, 103, 104, 105, 106, 109, 130, 172, 177, 178, 201, 202, 206, 223, 224, 225, 230, 247, 248, 259, 280
autoimmune disorders, vii, x, 3, 31, 151, 152, 155, 248
autoimmune manifestations, 215, 264, 265
autoimmune responses, 178, 247, 250, 261, 266, 281
autonomous, 211
autophagy, 52
autoreactive T cells, 96, 171, 174, 178
availability, 6, 15, 67, 127, 136, 240
axonal, 149

B

B lymphocytes, 153, 154, 155, 170
BAC, 275, 277, 278
Bacillus, 129
bacteria, 79, 111, 128, 129, 130, 132, 136, 138, 149, 171, 177, 209
bacterial, 72, 73, 75, 90, 96, 105, 111, 121, 122, 130, 131, 132, 141, 161, 175, 187, 206, 229, 277
bacterial infection, 130, 161, 187
bacterium, 128
barrier, 3, 130, 132, 196, 198
basal lamina, 164
basement membrane, 161, 272, 279, 281, 282, 283
Bax, 46, 166
Bayesian, 8
B-cell, 51, 73, 74, 75, 81, 135, 161, 181, 228
B-cell lymphoma, 181
bcl-2, 166
behavior, 163
beneficial effect, x, 61, 152, 155, 162, 239
benefits, 37
beta, 2, 14, 18, 19, 20, 21, 26, 35, 47, 49, 105, 106, 107, 123, 124, 134, 135, 142, 146, 176, 177, 180, 183, 184, 186, 187
bias, 7, 9, 46, 178, 184, 279
bifurcation, 62
bilateral, 251
binding, 12, 14, 15, 19, 21, 25, 28, 29, 32, 33, 35, 44, 52, 55, 56, 68, 80, 90, 104, 111, 112, 113, 147, 153, 170, 174, 177, 179, 189, 190, 191, 193, 194, 198, 201, 202, 203, 216, 219, 221, 230, 231, 237, 256, 257, 269, 271, 273, 274, 279
binding globulin, 68, 237
bioassay, 218
bioavailability, 61, 69
biochemical, 140, 244
biologic, 181
biological, 5, 17, 29, 174, 216, 243, 259, 265
biologically, 141, 248, 257
biology, 44, 78, 184, 229
biomarkers, 62, 66, 67, 165
biomedical, 7, 189
biopsies, 154, 165
biopsy, 110
birth, 130, 236, 239
birth rate, 236, 239
black, 218
bladder, 33
bleeding, 107

blocks, 3, 6, 13, 36, 42, 43, 193, 194
blood, 2, 73, 88, 92, 116, 130, 134, 135, 136, 144, 147, 148, 150, 191, 251
blood clot, 88, 92
blood glucose, 2
blood transfusion, 88
blood vessels, 116
blood-brain barrier, 130, 134, 147, 148, 150
B-lymphocytes, 183
body fat, 53
body fluid, 205
body mass index, 49
body weight, 156
boiling, 216
bonds, 219
bone, 21, 50, 60, 68, 105, 212, 215, 217, 233, 279
bone marrow, 105, 212, 233, 279
Boston, 110
botulinum, 167
bovine, 147, 273
bowel, 197
brain, 116, 136, 138, 141, 142, 143, 145, 146, 148, 190, 211, 241
brain injury, 142
Brazil, 236
Brazilian, 140
breakdown, 12, 98, 130, 148, 215
breast, 33
British, 24, 261
bronchial hyperresponsiveness, 29, 54
bronchiolitis, 281
Brooklyn, 189
buffer, 252, 273
building blocks, 204
bullous pemphigoid, 281
burn, 190, 193, 195

C

C reactive protein, 63
Ca^{2+}, 35
calcification, 61, 69
calcium, 31, 32, 164, 174, 183
California, 115
cAMP, 25
Canada, 225
cancer, 3, 44, 53, 55, 181, 184, 185, 204, 228, 229, 258
cancer cells, 204
cancers, 33, 248
candidates, 1, 5, 18, 19, 32, 34, 162
capacity, 59, 61, 73, 164, 185, 203, 206, 210, 212, 213, 221
CAR, 170, 179
carbohydrate, 32, 51, 125
CARD15, 8, 42
cardiac function, 196
cardiac myocytes, 180
cardiomyopathy, 173, 182
cardiovascular, 59, 60, 61, 62, 67, 68, 69, 195, 267
cardiovascular disease, 59, 60, 61, 68, 267
cardiovascular morbidity, 60
cardiovascular risk, 59, 62, 69
carotid arteries, 62
carrier, 135, 217
cartilage, 215, 216, 281
case study, 111
caspase, 18, 134, 142, 161, 165, 166, 177
caspases, 171
castration, 121, 123, 127, 141, 143
CAT, 83, 84, 87, 97
catalase, 20
catalytic, 29
cations, 250
Caucasian, 12, 37, 47, 251
Caucasians, 17, 18, 19, 24, 50
causal relationship, 238
causation, 37, 84
CBP, 186
CCR, 74, 75
CD19, 207, 221, 222
CD1d, 177, 186, 209, 212, 218, 219, 221, 222, 224, 225, 226, 230, 231, 232
CD4, 14, 15, 16, 18, 30, 31, 35, 36, 37, 44, 45, 46, 55, 57, 87, 88, 91, 97, 106, 107, 108, 111, 112, 113, 114, 153, 154, 168, 173, 174, 175, 176, 177, 178, 180, 182, 185, 186, 187, 203, 204, 205, 207, 210, 212, 215, 217, 218, 219, 223, 224, 225, 226, 230, 231, 232, 233, 234
CD40, 176, 178, 183, 204, 206, 221, 222
CD45, 203, 227
CD5, 238, 245
CD8+, 18, 174, 175, 187, 204, 205, 207, 210, 217, 218, 221, 224, 228, 229, 234
CD95, 31
CDC, 262, 270
cDNA, 274
CDR, 277
cell adhesion, 32
cell culture, 182

cell cycle, 53, 171, 180
cell death, 12, 15, 135, 143, 145, 152, 153, 160, 190, 193, 198, 260, 262
cell differentiation, 163, 204, 218
cell division, 160
cell growth, 182, 210
cell invasion, 132
cell killing, 177, 213, 231
cell line, 15, 32, 100, 138, 140, 155, 164, 216, 221, 222
cell lines, 15, 32, 100, 138, 140, 216, 221, 222
cell signaling, 28, 53
cell surface, 26, 29, 88, 189, 193, 194, 201, 202, 211, 212, 213, 256, 268, 269
cellular immunity, 96, 281
central nervous system, 35, 115, 116, 130, 148
ceramics, 257
cerebral cortex, 137
cerebrospinal fluid, 140, 144, 145, 146, 148
CFA, 139, 209
Chagas disease, 86
chemical, 122, 141, 150, 215, 278
chemicals, 265, 267
chemoattractants, 192, 197
chemokine, 74, 75, 145, 162, 174, 183
chemokine receptor, 74, 145, 174, 183
chemokines, 75, 99, 155, 171, 183
chemotaxis, 193, 199
chest radiograph, 262, 270
child development, 246
childbearing, 236, 237, 243
childhood, 2, 37, 114
children, 2, 108, 114, 241, 246
Chinese, 18
chlorpromazine, 251
cholesterol, 63, 66, 67, 69
chromatin, 14, 248, 252, 253, 254, 259, 260, 267
chromosome, 2, 11, 13, 14, 15, 16, 17, 18, 22, 25, 26, 27, 29, 30, 32, 33, 34, 35, 38, 39, 45, 47, 51, 53, 54, 56, 236, 275, 277
chromosomes, 6, 10
chronic, 2, 28, 59, 60, 71, 72, 74, 86, 95, 98, 100, 106, 109, 110, 113, 118, 119, 120, 130, 131, 132, 138, 145, 147, 161, 165, 167, 183, 215, 240, 241, 245, 261, 262, 268, 269
chronic disease, 2, 261
chronic fatigue syndrome, 261, 268, 269
chronic obstructive pulmonary disease, 161, 167
circulation, 26
civil war, 77, 88, 91, 95, 103
classes, 193, 278
classical, 32, 60, 61, 62, 106, 132, 153, 177, 191, 202, 213, 218, 223, 224, 225
classification, 69, 275
classified, 253, 255, 258, 261
cleavage, 13, 30, 173, 260
clinical, 2, 18, 21, 37, 60, 61, 62, 66, 67, 69, 77, 96, 108, 109, 110, 113, 115, 127, 130, 131, 132, 134, 135, 136, 140, 144, 145, 148, 151, 153, 163, 170, 179, 184, 242, 244, 247, 249, 250, 251, 252, 260, 264, 265, 267, 268, 269, 272
clinical symptoms, 96, 153, 268
clinical syndrome, 170
clinical trials, 69
clone, 192, 275, 277, 278, 279
clones, 141, 150, 171, 172, 181, 193, 216, 224, 277
cloning, 213, 274
clustering, 2
clusters, 2, 31
CMV, 85, 89, 91, 92, 107
CNS, 115, 116, 119, 120, 121, 127, 130, 131, 132, 134, 135, 136, 140, 141, 143, 145, 146, 148, 149, 184
CO2, 157, 252
coagulation, 105, 237
coagulation factors, 237
codes, 32
coding, 5, 7, 11, 22, 40
codon, 17, 18, 21, 25, 26, 30, 35, 50, 193
cofactors, 88, 91, 97
cognitive deficit, 241
cognitive deficits, 241
cohort, 17, 250, 253, 259, 260, 261, 262, 265, 266
collaboration, 3, 204, 212, 215, 217, 264
Collaboration, 204
collagen, 97, 187, 215, 271, 272, 273, 274, 277, 279, 280, 281, 282, 283
Colorado, 250
coma, 119
commercial, 249, 260
communities, 251, 261
community, 36, 247, 249, 250, 266
competition, 273
compilation, 254
complement, 5, 78, 80, 93, 96, 103, 183, 189, 190, 191, 192, 194, 197, 198, 215, 236
complement pathway, 198, 215
complement system, 189, 197
complementarity, 77, 80, 81, 82, 84, 87, 89, 90, 91, 93, 98, 103, 104, 106, 110, 111, 112

complementary, 77, 78, 80, 81, 82, 83, 84, 87, 88, 89, 90, 91, 92, 93, 94, 95, 96, 97, 98, 99, 100, 102, 103, 104, 109, 110, 111, 113, 163, 171, 274
complex interactions, 60
complexity, 55, 175, 195, 249
complications, 33, 38, 62, 84, 103, 151, 190, 235, 240, 245, 250
components, 44, 72, 78, 96, 100, 101, 132, 134, 164, 204, 209, 213, 217, 247, 253, 258, 259, 261, 281
composition, 21, 131, 136, 280
compounds, 130, 132, 135, 136, 155, 219, 221
computed tomography, 270
concentration, 13, 31, 130, 135, 136, 156, 225
conception, 239, 242
concordance, 2
confidence interval, 241
confidentiality, 250
conformational, 170, 226, 272
confusion, 77, 82, 83
connective tissue, 152, 249, 250, 260, 264, 268
connective tissue diseases, 250, 260, 264
consensus, 10, 39, 278
consent, 62
consumption, 155, 157, 225, 258
contamination, 249, 250
contingency, 253
continuous data, 63
control, 3, 9, 12, 14, 16, 22, 23, 25, 27, 29, 30, 32, 34, 37, 42, 45, 46, 49, 61, 62, 71, 72, 108, 131, 136, 149, 151, 158, 159, 160, 163, 169, 173, 193, 194, 203, 218, 224, 225, 226, 236, 240, 247, 250, 252, 266, 268
control group, 62, 236
controlled, 45, 85, 109, 133, 187, 204, 209, 210, 211, 224, 236, 240, 242
controlled studies, 85
controlled trials, 240
convergence, 107
conversion, 216, 231
COPD, 161
Copenhagen, 70
corpus callosum, 137
correlation, 61, 66, 67, 85, 101, 134, 143, 161, 165, 167, 172, 216, 255, 267, 269
correlations, 37, 61, 85, 134
cortex, 137
cost saving, 9
costimulatory signal, 30, 31, 54
costs, 248
couples, 236
coupling, 180, 215
coverage, 7, 10
coxsackievirus, 106, 108, 170, 172, 173, 174, 175, 176, 179, 181, 182, 184, 185, 186
C-reactive protein, 61, 69
critically ill, 113
criticism, 240
crosslinking, 225
cross-linking, 174, 178
cross-sectional study, 134
7
Cross-talk, 227, 229
CRP, 61, 63, 190
crust, 248
crystal structure, 51
crystalline, 248, 257, 258, 268
CSF, 130, 134, 135, 136, 145, 147, 150
C-terminus, 127
culture, 212, 217, 218, 273
cycles, 161
cyclin D1, 173, 182
cystatins, 161
cystine, 135, 140
cytokine, 14, 15, 16, 22, 29, 32, 33, 73, 155, 162, 164, 166, 174, 176, 177, 184, 185, 197, 202, 204, 223, 233, 269
cytokine receptor, 204
cytokine response, 174
cytokines, 19, 20, 21, 28, 29, 35, 36, 71, 72, 135, 140, 141, 155, 171, 172, 174, 175, 176, 177, 178, 184, 185, 186, 191, 204, 205, 209, 210, 211, 215, 218, 225, 234
cytomegalovirus, 18, 85, 86, 88, 89, 91, 92, 93, 103, 105, 172
cytometry, 211, 213
cytoplasm, 29, 170, 171
cytoplasmic tail, 202
cytoskeleton, 193
cytosolic, 30, 176
cytotoxic, 1, 3, 18, 52, 114, 153, 168, 177, 180, 204, 210, 213, 224, 226
cytotoxicity, 31, 165, 171, 177, 204, 210, 211, 213, 236

D

DAD, 90
danger, 206, 210
database, 6, 251, 274, 278
DD, 108, 111, 245

death, 20, 49, 61, 98, 160, 163, 167, 191, 193, 204, 218, 268
deaths, 60, 190
decay, 179, 183
defects, 5, 28, 88, 161, 172, 219, 229
defense, 174, 184, 186, 190, 203, 215
defense mechanisms, 190
deficiency, 15, 45, 55, 57, 105, 106, 107, 108, 114, 240, 246
deficit, 241, 251
deficits, 246, 251
definition, 4, 115, 122, 150, 267
degenerate, 274, 277
degradation, 20, 133, 164, 173, 260
degrading, 144
degree, 2, 6, 10, 85, 95, 128, 154, 202
delivery, 150, 227, 241, 242
delta, 169, 184, 185, 186, 187
demand, 21
demographic data, 238
demyelinating disease, 85, 103, 112, 138
demyelination, 115, 142, 143, 147, 148
demyelinization, 85
dendritic cell, 25, 32, 51, 57, 73, 74, 75, 87, 109, 134, 144, 155, 168, 172, 174, 175, 176, 177, 178, 180, 184, 186, 187, 201, 204, 217, 227, 230, 232, 233, 234
density, 6, 10, 25, 39, 40, 43, 59, 62, 170, 180, 252
dephosphorylation, 27, 28, 29, 53
deposition, 72, 106, 192, 215, 247, 272
deposits, 236
depression, 236
derivatives, 139, 141
destruction, x, 2, 18, 20, 21, 52, 60, 98, 99, 151, 152, 163, 211, 215, 217
detection, 8, 63, 67, 152, 157, 163, 259, 262, 264, 267
developing countries, 249, 265
developing nations, 248
dexamethasone, 33
diabetes mellitus, 37, 38, 43, 49, 182
diabetic, 13, 17, 21, 22, 33, 38, 44, 50, 51, 52, 55, 61, 163, 167, 168, 231, 232, 233
diabetic nephropathy, 51
diabetic patients, 13, 44, 50
diagnostic, 98, 161, 215, 248, 259, 261, 264, 266
dialysis, 273
diastolic blood pressure, 63
diet, 155
dietary, 152, 156, 160, 162
differentiation, 21, 30, 31, 33, 46, 54, 55, 56, 75, 152, 161, 162, 176, 185, 204, 218, 222, 237
diffusion, 90, 103
digestion, 78, 127, 136
dilated cardiomyopathy, 106, 107
diluent, 273
dimer, 259
dimeric, 51
dimerization, 26
dimorphism, 35
dinucleotides, 14, 72
dipeptides, 111, 139, 145
disability, 60, 61
discomfort, 152
discordance, 153, 158
discrete variable, 63
discrimination, 72, 73, 203, 227
disease activity, 106, 134, 140, 142, 143, 144, 147
disease gene, 4, 37, 40
disease model, 85, 102
disease progression, 156
diseases, 4, 5, 21, 32, 37, 52, 61, 77, 78, 84, 85, 93, 96, 97, 98, 101, 102, 104, 161, 164, 178, 181, 190, 223, 247, 249, 250, 261, 267
disequilibrium, 3, 9, 13, 19, 36, 40, 42, 43, 113
disintegrin, 2, 11, 29, 54
disorder, 28, 236, 249
dissociation, 239
distribution, 137, 254, 272
disulfide, 30
diversity, 86, 164, 282
DNA, 3, 6, 7, 8, 19, 21, 38, 42, 44, 45, 72, 73, 75, 80, 81, 85, 104, 113, 157, 172, 175, 185, 206, 256, 259, 260, 262, 267, 269, 274, 275, 278, 280
DNA polymerase, 3, 172
DNA repair, 19
DNA sequencing, 280
doctors, 264
domain structure, 32
dominance, 187
donor, 25, 102, 236
Doppler, 62, 64, 65, 66, 67
down-regulation, 88, 177, 211
drug-induced, 251, 259, 264
drug-induced lupus, 251, 259
drug-related, 42
drugs, 21, 36, 62, 132, 193, 251, 267
dry, 151, 152, 153, 251
dry eyes, 151, 152, 153
dsRNA, 71, 72, 73, 74, 176

duration, 3, 60, 62, 180, 191
dust, 265, 267
dysfunctional, 153
dyslipidemia, 68
dysregulated, 62, 162
dysregulation, 153, 154, 160, 161, 231
dystrophin, 173, 182

E

EAE, 88, 92, 95, 96, 97, 98, 102, 115, 116, 117, 118, 119, 120, 121, 122, 123, 124, 125, 129, 131, 132, 136, 137, 138, 139, 140, 141, 143, 144, 145, 146, 147, 148, 149, 150, 201, 223
earth, 248
ECM, 134, 162, 163
efficacy, 239
EGCG, 151, 152, 155, 156, 157, 160, 161, 162
EGF, 33, 196
Einstein, 96, 110, 116, 119, 141, 147
elderly, 166
electrical, 258
electron, 26
electron microscopy, 26
ELISA, 63, 90, 193, 222, 252, 254, 255, 256, 257, 262, 273, 274, 279
embryo, 236, 238, 244
embryonic, 211
embryos, 229
emergency response, 249
emitters, 202
employees, 269
employment, 3, 11
encephalomyelitis, 46, 106, 107, 109, 112, 114, 115, 116, 140, 141, 142, 143, 144, 145, 146, 149, 150, 184
encoding, 3, 15, 18, 25, 26, 27, 32, 33, 34, 201, 205, 210, 211, 277, 282
endogenous, 135, 141, 181, 195, 210, 218, 224, 282
endometriosis, 236, 243
Endothelial, 52, 67, 68, 69
endothelial cell, 26, 60, 67, 170, 179, 262, 270
endothelial dysfunction, 60
endothelium, 26, 52, 67, 135, 140, 155
energy, 202
engagement, 14, 226, 232
engineering, 279
enteric, 170
enterovirus, 170, 172, 180, 181
envelope, 109, 114, 183, 261, 269
environment, 9, 19, 156, 163, 207, 209, 211, 224, 237, 238, 242, 258
environmental, 2, 61, 85, 152, 155, 206, 224, 247, 248, 249, 259, 260, 266, 267, 268
environmental factors, 2, 85, 155, 267
Environmental Protection Agency, 249, 250
enzymatic, 62, 67
enzyme, 17, 29, 54, 67, 90, 130, 140, 262
enzymes, 20, 131, 149, 215
EPA, 249
ependymal, 56
ependymal cell, 56
epidemiological, 37, 67, 81, 84, 106, 155, 240, 247, 248, 261
epidemiology, 37, 42, 107, 115, 250
epidermal, 33, 155, 161, 165, 168
epidermal growth factor receptor, 33
epidermis, 174, 183
epistasis, 19
epithelia, 153, 161
epithelial cell, 153, 155, 157, 160, 161, 162, 167, 170, 185, 196, 226, 262
epithelial regeneration, 162, 166
epithelium, 151, 152, 153, 158, 160, 166, 171
epitope, 25, 81, 105, 140, 143, 145, 147, 150, 173, 181, 192, 209, 216, 259, 273, 274, 283
epitopes, 51, 90, 93, 120, 140, 143, 144, 148, 172, 173, 182, 191, 192, 215, 217, 260, 272, 279, 281, 282
Epstein Barr, 86, 172
Epstein-Barr virus, 85, 86, 104, 105, 106, 174, 183
equilibrium, 9
ErbB2, 55
ErbB3, 55
erectile dysfunction, 33, 55
Erk, 28, 53
ERK1, 196
erythrocyte sedimentation rate, 61, 63
erythropoietin, 85
ES, 68, 226, 233
ESR, 61, 63, 66
ester, 69
esterase, 197, 198
estimating, 8
estradiol, 237
estrogen, 19, 184, 236
ethnicity, 251
etiology, 2, 4, 11, 19, 34, 36, 37, 100, 101, 104, 147, 161, 237
eukaryotic, 71, 170, 193

eukaryotic cell, 193
Europe, 37
European, 17, 21, 25, 39, 43, 251, 274
evidence, 2, 3, 4, 5, 13, 14, 17, 21, 26, 27, 32, 33, 39, 47, 48, 53, 60, 61, 77, 80, 81, 82, 83, 84, 86, 87, 89, 90, 91, 98, 99, 110, 123, 127, 129, 132, 137, 142, 145, 146, 148, 155, 161, 166, 172, 174, 178, 181, 182, 185, 191, 193, 210, 217, 245, 251, 259, 261, 262, 265
evolution, 90, 141, 186, 202, 225
excitement, 36
exclusion, 244, 251
exercise, 21
exocrine, 153, 154, 162, 167, 168
exogenous, 2, 140, 218, 224
exons, 27, 31
experimental allergic encephalomyelitis, 84, 88, 93, 95, 107, 110, 111, 114, 187
experimental autoimmune encephalomyelitis, 15, 105, 106, 108, 109, 184, 201
experimental design, 11
expertise, 280
exposure, 77, 88, 101, 136, 156, 172, 173, 190, 247, 248, 249, 250, 251, 253, 255, 256, 258, 259, 260, 261, 264, 265, 266, 267, 268, 269
Exposure, 251, 255, 265
extracellular, 30, 133, 136, 143, 161, 162, 166, 170, 175, 203
extracellular matrix, 133, 161, 162, 166
extravasation, 26
extrinsic, 191

F

failure, 103, 162, 164, 237, 242, 243, 244
false, 8, 9, 38, 42
false positive, 38
familial, 2
family, 3, 5, 9, 11, 12, 13, 19, 21, 22, 25, 29, 30, 32, 33, 36, 43, 53, 133, 135, 161, 164, 169, 177, 197, 230, 258, 265, 275, 280, 282, 283
family members, 33, 265
Fas, 15, 26, 46, 153, 166, 211, 218
FasL, 26, 153, 218
FBG, 215, 216, 217
feces, 116
federal government, 266
feedback, 19, 130
females, 237
fertility, 239
fertilization, 29, 237, 243, 244
fetal, 238, 240, 244, 245, 246, 252
fetal brain, 246
fetal growth, 244
fetus, 235
fever, 86, 89, 260
fibers, 194, 248, 249, 250, 258, 266, 267
fibrate, 68
fibrils, 281
fibrin, 215, 216
fibrinogen, 215, 216, 217, 231
fibroblast, 18, 161, 252, 256, 257, 262, 270
fibroblast proliferation, 161
fibroblasts, 54, 140, 248, 256, 262, 269, 270
fibromyalgia, 261
fibrosis, 153, 161, 167, 249, 250, 251, 259, 261, 262, 270
filament, 199
Finland, 51, 182, 243
Finns, 51
fire, 258
fish, 202
flank, 4
flooring, 258
flow, 156, 211, 213
flow rate, 156
Flt3, 233
fluid, 132, 139, 153
fluorescence, 252
follicular, 51, 243
follicular fluid, 243
Ford, 144, 145, 147
forest fires, 251
Fox, 152, 153, 155, 160, 164
Foxp3, 186, 226, 231
fractionation, 212
fragmentation, 157
France, 201, 225
free radicals, 266
frontal lobes, 137
FSH, 237
fuel, 99
functional changes, 26, 167
fungi, 171
fusion, 182, 271, 273, 274

G

gadolinium, 134
Gamma, 187

ganglia, 137
ganglion, 145
gangliosides, 90
gas, 131
gas chromatograph, 131
gastric, 164
gastritis, 28
gastrointestinal, 196
G-CSF, 176
GenBank, 277, 278, 280
gender, 261
gene, 1, 3, 4, 5, 7, 8, 10, 11, 12, 13, 14, 15, 16, 17, 18, 19, 21, 22, 25, 26, 27, 29, 30, 32, 33, 34, 35, 36, 38, 39, 42, 44, 45, 46, 47, 48, 49, 50, 51, 52, 53, 54, 55, 56, 57, 81, 128, 133, 166, 176, 183, 184, 185, 193, 195, 196, 197, 201, 202, 223, 229, 242, 274, 275, 278, 279, 282, 283
gene combinations, 279
gene expression, 14, 15, 21, 176, 183, 185, 196, 229, 283
gene mapping, 242
generation, 43, 62, 110, 169, 173, 178, 180, 226, 227, 233
genes, 1, 2, 3, 4, 5, 10, 11, 12, 13, 14, 15, 17, 19, 21, 29, 33, 34, 36, 37, 40, 42, 43, 45, 49, 53, 56, 178, 187, 205, 210, 223, 233, 271, 273, 274, 277, 279, 282, 283
genetic, 1, 2, 3, 4, 5, 7, 9, 10, 11, 14, 17, 18, 21, 36, 37, 39, 40, 42, 43, 49, 54, 56, 61, 106, 155, 163, 165, 236, 280
genetic abnormalities, 163
genetic code, 106
genetic factors, 236
genetic marker, 9, 37
genetic traits, 39
genetics, 1, 3, 7, 11, 36, 38, 39, 85
genome, 1, 3, 4, 5, 6, 7, 8, 10, 11, 38, 39, 40, 41, 42, 43, 46, 51, 55, 56, 169, 170
genome sequences, 10
genomes, 7, 171
genomic, 4, 5, 6, 16, 26, 27, 33, 41, 44, 46, 165, 194, 210, 275, 278
genomic instability, 210
genomic regions, 4, 6, 16, 41
genotype, 6, 8, 10, 26, 40, 42, 144
geology, 265
Georgia, 151
germ line, 201, 202
Germany, 156, 265, 271
gestation, 239, 240, 241
gestational diabetes, 241
Gibbs, 41, 267
gland, 151, 153, 154, 155, 157, 160, 162, 163, 164, 165, 166, 167, 168, 172
glass, 257
glial cells, 185
gliosis, 135
glomerulonephritis, 140, 260, 271, 272, 282
glucagon, 104, 111
glucose, 21, 50, 156, 157
glutamate, 128, 135, 140, 142, 149
glutamic acid, 135, 150, 172, 181, 182
glutamine, 35, 128
glycine, 26, 123, 128, 148
glycolipid antigens, 177
glycolipids, 80, 186, 206, 209, 210, 215, 218, 219, 220, 221, 222, 223, 224, 225, 232
glycoprotein, 26, 89, 92, 109, 112, 113, 114, 117, 132, 148, 170, 183, 197, 216
glycoproteins, 80, 113, 114, 116, 142, 175
glycosyl, 183, 231
glycosylation, 15, 45
GM-CSF, 217, 219, 233
goals, 11
Golgi complex, 259, 267
GPI, 85, 170
grafting, 187
gram negative, 177
gram-negative bacteria, 130, 175
gram-positive bacteria, 124, 129, 175
granulocyte, 196
granulomas, 187
granulosa cells, 243
granzyme, 153
Graves disease, 85
green tea, 152, 155, 163, 165
groups, 3, 6, 62, 63, 84, 108, 113, 132, 136, 144, 156, 157, 177, 218, 223, 241, 253, 255, 259
growth, 14, 29, 133, 169, 173, 179, 187, 228
growth factor, 29, 133
guidelines, 267
Guinea, 116, 117, 118, 119, 120, 124, 126, 139
gut, 128, 129, 130, 131, 132, 136, 138, 149, 173, 192, 198

H

H. pylori, 113
H1, 260
H_2, 254

Haj, 53
half-life, 15
handling, 251
haplotype, 2, 8, 12, 40, 42, 43, 45, 52, 210
haplotypes, 6, 7, 8, 42, 224
HapMap, 3, 6, 10, 11, 38, 52
harm, 202
harmful, 72, 204, 206, 223, 225, 249
Harvard, 280
hazards, 258
HCV, 92
HDL, 63, 66, 67, 69
head, 218
health, 152, 198, 203, 247, 248, 249, 250, 258, 265, 266
Health and Human Services, 261
health effects, 248, 265
health problems, 250
healthcare, 248
hearing, 246
heart, 86, 92, 95, 103, 106, 179, 180, 182, 185, 190, 191
Heart, 70, 107, 113, 169, 195, 196
heart disease, 86, 103, 106, 179, 182, 185, 190
heart failure, 106, 180
heat, 19, 49, 190, 210, 258
heat shock protein, 190
heating, 258
Helicobacter pylori, 106, 113
helix, 280
helper cells, 87, 218, 225
hemorrhage, 271, 272
hepatic necrosis, 28
hepatitis, 72, 88, 89, 91, 103, 107, 172, 209
Hepatitis B, 129
hepatitis C, 107, 172
Hepatitis C virus, 181
hepatocytes, 33
HER3, 55
hereditary nephritis, 273
heritability, 4
herpes, 79, 85, 86, 107, 108, 172, 181
herpes simplex, 85, 86, 107, 172, 181
herpes virus, 79, 85, 86
herpesviruses, 183
heterogeneity, 3, 19, 238
heterogeneous, 34, 60, 114, 149, 237
heterozygotes, 9
high risk, 61, 68, 108
high-risk, 2, 18
histidine, 278
histological, 115, 132, 136
histology, 115, 136, 194
histone, 14, 44, 248, 252, 254, 259
histopathology, 165, 266
HIV, 85, 86, 87, 88, 91, 92, 93, 97, 103, 105, 106, 107, 108, 109, 110, 111, 112, 113, 114, 171, 173, 174, 182, 183
HIV infection, 87, 105, 110, 112
HIV-1, 86, 107, 109, 112, 113, 182, 183
HLA, 1, 2, 3, 11, 16, 18, 37, 38, 48, 107, 143, 155, 172, 181, 216, 229, 231
HNF, 49
Holland, 53, 149
homeostasis, 15, 21, 35, 37, 44, 45, 67, 154, 161, 162, 164
homogeneous, 251, 253, 255, 259, 261
homolog, 32
homology, 89, 104, 107, 142, 143, 172, 180, 182, 193, 275
homosexuals, 105
Honda, 54, 55
hormonal control, 131, 138, 149
hormone, 68, 140, 171, 237, 239, 240, 243, 244
horse, 196
host, 72, 74, 78, 79, 80, 81, 84, 91, 93, 94, 95, 101, 102, 106, 122, 144, 170, 173, 174, 177, 179, 180, 184, 190, 229, 230
host tissue, 84
HRP, 159, 252
human genome, 3, 6, 40, 43, 52
human immunodeficiency virus, 105, 107, 108
human leukocyte antigen, 181
human subjects, 26, 144
humans, 14, 15, 18, 34, 43, 45, 114, 128, 138, 145, 154, 160, 175, 176, 177, 190, 216, 234, 247, 248, 249, 250, 260
hybridoma, 216, 217, 218, 219, 220, 273, 274
hydrogen peroxide, 159
hydrolysis, 191
hydroxyl, 278
hypercholesterolemia, 61
hypergammaglobulinemia, 88, 91
hyperglycemia, 218
hyperplasia, 73, 160, 161, 215
hyperproliferation, 161
hypersensitivity, 121, 178
hypertension, 3, 33, 61, 240, 244
Hypertension, 63
hypothalamus, 142

hypothesis, 31, 36, 67, 135, 136, 156, 163, 182, 191, 192, 203, 209, 238, 262, 279
hypothyroidism, 235, 237, 239, 240, 241, 243, 245
hypoxia, 190, 193, 195, 198
hypoxic, 190, 192, 193, 195
hypoxic cells, 191, 192

I

ICAM, 22, 24, 25, 26, 31, 50, 51, 52, 134, 140, 144
ICD, 12
ice, 212
icosahedral, 169
ICSI, 236, 242
id, 94
identification, 1, 3, 4, 11, 36, 39, 40, 43, 45, 61, 68, 189, 192, 228, 272
identity, 5, 10, 275, 277, 278
idiopathic, 2, 92, 98, 108, 111, 113, 114, 161, 167, 236, 260, 264
idiopathic thrombocytopenic purpura, 108, 113, 114
IFA, 209
IFN, 28, 47, 50, 71, 73, 74, 75, 170, 175, 176, 179, 180, 185, 186, 211, 229, 230
IFNγ, 173, 204, 205, 212, 213, 218, 221, 224, 233
IgE, 171
IgG, 109, 154, 167, 171, 252, 255, 273, 274, 279, 281
images, 64, 65, 66
imbalances, 190
immune activation, 73, 184
immune cells, 28, 30, 132, 135, 136, 205, 207, 210, 212, 216, 224, 228
immune disorders, 151
immune function, 32, 95
immune regulation, 34, 37, 82, 94, 176, 184, 186, 204, 226
immune response, 18, 19, 28, 72, 74, 77, 78, 80, 81, 83, 84, 87, 88, 94, 95, 98, 102, 112, 121, 135, 141, 154, 165, 169, 171, 172, 173, 177, 178, 184, 186, 187, 190, 194, 195, 198, 202, 203, 204, 205, 206, 209, 210, 215, 219, 225, 226, 227, 228, 230, 231, 260, 273, 279, 280
immune system, 35, 72, 73, 77, 78, 81, 82, 83, 84, 87, 88, 89, 91, 93, 94, 103, 112, 128, 129, 131, 136, 153, 154, 169, 180, 189, 190, 193, 194, 201, 202, 204, 205, 206, 209, 210, 213, 227, 229, 230, 238, 239
immunity, 18, 60, 71, 75, 88, 94, 112, 172, 173, 175, 176, 177, 183, 184, 185, 187, 194, 201, 206, 207, 209, 219, 223, 225, 227, 228, 229, 231, 243, 282
immunization, 107, 112, 143, 207, 210, 215, 219, 230, 245, 272, 279
immunocytochemistry, 148, 260
immunodeficiency, 35, 57, 107
immunodeficient, 166, 228
immunoediting, 229
immunofluorescence, 252, 259
immunogen, 121, 122, 123, 125, 127, 128, 129, 130, 138
immunogenicity, 180
immunoglobulin, 26, 30, 108, 135, 170, 174, 192, 239, 245, 273, 282, 283
immunoglobulin G, 245, 283
immunoglobulins, 179, 192, 198, 205, 239, 247
immunohistochemical, 165
immunohistochemistry, 157
immunological, 78, 83, 88, 93, 95, 98, 104, 109, 115, 120, 130, 132, 143, 203, 226, 227, 236, 248, 260, 269
immunology, 115, 227
immunomodulatory, 19
immunopathogenesis, 107
immunopathology, 144
immunoregulation, 178, 185
immunostimulant, 121, 122, 123
immunostimulatory, 72
immunosuppression, 178
immunosuppressive, 85, 174, 178
immunosurveillance, 230
Immunotherapy, 185, 233
impurities, 121
in situ, 73, 157, 166, 191
in vitro, 14, 21, 29, 44, 57, 62, 105, 112, 157, 179, 193, 207, 213, 215, 233, 236, 243, 244, 245, 269
in vitro fertilization, 244, 245
in vivo, 15, 19, 74, 84, 135, 179, 183, 192, 198, 208, 213, 227, 228, 229, 232, 233, 269, 272, 275, 279
inactivation, 170
inactive, 117, 123, 135, 216
incidence, 2, 21, 22, 37, 61, 85, 93, 119, 190, 220, 228, 245, 261
India, 113
Indian, 114, 269
indication, 103
indicators, 142
indices, 157, 158, 160
inducer, 122, 178

inducible protein, 176
induction, 13, 15, 18, 20, 28, 31, 83, 88, 89, 93, 96, 97, 100, 101, 104, 107, 109, 111, 120, 121, 122, 123, 124, 129, 130, 138, 140, 143, 144, 145, 146, 149, 150, 152, 153, 165, 173, 174, 178, 183, 184, 185, 186, 187, 197, 205, 207, 209, 212, 215, 216, 217, 221, 223, 236, 258, 259
industry, 248
inert, 72
infancy, 2, 37
infection, 62, 71, 72, 73, 74, 80, 85, 86, 89, 90, 91, 92, 94, 98, 100, 101, 104, 105, 106, 108, 112, 128, 138, 169, 170, 171, 173, 174, 176, 177, 178, 179, 181, 182, 187, 198, 204
infections, viii, ix, x, 18, 47, 71, 72, 77, 81, 82, 83, 84, 85, 86, 88, 89, 91, 101, 103, 104, 111, 130, 138, 140, 169, 170, 171, 172, 173, 174, 176, 178, 185, 209
infectious, 78, 79, 80, 84, 85, 88, 89, 92, 97, 101, 102, 103, 104, 107, 108, 110, 111, 114, 121, 150, 174, 180, 187, 194
infertile, 236, 237, 243, 244
infertility, 235, 236, 237, 238, 239, 242, 243, 244
inflammation, 27, 28, 59, 60, 61, 68, 71, 72, 73, 74, 132, 134, 137, 154, 161, 169, 171, 183, 185, 187, 189, 193, 195, 196, 197, 198, 230, 233, 262, 266
inflammatory, 3, 8, 19, 20, 26, 28, 29, 35, 52, 53, 59, 60, 61, 62, 72, 73, 74, 93, 106, 109, 110, 115, 130, 132, 134, 135, 140, 142, 145, 146, 153, 155, 161, 162, 163, 174, 176, 177, 178, 182, 185, 187, 189, 190, 191, 192, 193, 197, 204, 215, 218, 255
inflammatory arthritis, 59
inflammatory bowel disease, 3, 8, 26, 52
inflammatory cells, 74, 191, 192
inflammatory disease, 26, 35, 53, 60, 62, 215, 255
inflammatory mediators, 61
inflammatory response, 20, 28, 29, 60, 72, 130, 140, 145, 155, 178, 185, 189, 190, 191, 197
influenza, 72, 79, 85, 88, 186, 187
Information System, 274, 275
inguinal, 210
inhalation, 157, 266
inheritance, 2
inherited, 9, 49
inhibition, 27, 28, 88, 114, 130, 149, 154, 172, 183, 196, 198, 230
inhibitor, 135, 146, 167, 191, 197, 198
inhibitors, 19, 55, 133, 141, 144, 193, 198
inhibitory, 178, 183, 186, 201, 202, 210, 211, 213, 224, 225
initiation, 60, 73, 90, 115, 122, 131, 136, 152, 158, 160, 165, 170, 191, 193, 204, 215, 262
injection, 71, 73, 117, 118, 120, 122, 142, 143, 146, 205, 221, 236
iinjury, 106, 137, 143, 147, 161, 164, 167, 173, 189, 190, 191, 192, 193, 194, 195, 196, 197, 198, 199, 266, 272
innate immunity, 32, 47, 55, 74, 106, 173, 180, 185, 194, 195, 227
inoculation, 187
iNOS, 185
inositol, 227
insemination, 236
insight, 39, 84, 154, 250, 271, 279, 280
insulation, 249, 257
insulin, 1, 2, 3, 5, 8, 18, 21, 27, 29, 33, 37, 38, 42, 43, 49, 50, 53, 55, 104, 150, 151, 202
insulin sensitivity, 21, 49, 50
insulin signaling, 27, 53
insulin-like growth factor, 55
insulin-producing cells, 18
integrin, 26, 174, 203
integrity, 78, 148, 161, 165, 198
intelligence quotient, , 235
intensity, 69, 175, 252, 253, 265
intensive care unit, 241
interaction, 26, 98, 112, 123, 127, 154, 155, 162, 172, 192, 202, 211, 216, 224, 226, 231
Interaction, 105, 179, 183
interactions, 19, 26, 29, 39, 103, 108, 113, 123, 171, 174, 178, 180, 186, 198, 201, 202, 203, 204, 205, 215, 223, 224, 225, 226, 227, 235, 237, 257
intercellular adhesion molecule, 22, 25, 30, 50, 51, 52, 135
interferon, 1, 11, 16, 17, 18, 46, 73, 75, 135, 140, 153, 163, 172, 176, 177, 185, 186, 187, 211, 229
interferon (IFN), 18
interferon gamma, 140
interferons, 176, 177, 211
interleukin, 1, 11, 15, 35, 36, 44, 45, 56, 57, 109, 133, 135, 172, 175, 180
Interleukin-1, 134, 135, 141, 142, 149
interleukin-2, 2, 15, 44, 45, 56, 172
interleukin-6, 135
internal ribosome entry site (IRES), 170
internalization, 173, 174, 226
international, 3, 38, 69, 282
interpretation, 61, 102, 236, 267
interstitial, 250, 251, 262, 264
interval, 19, 45

intervention, 157, 239, 264, 271, 279
intestine, 196, 197
intima, 60, 61, 62, 63
intracellular signaling, 162, 202
intracranial, 107
intracytoplasmic sperm injection, 242
intravenous, 199, 239, 245
intrinsic, 79, 152, 229, 233
intron, 12, 25, 27, 29, 32, 33, 34
inversions, 251
Investigations, 48, 52, 53, 54
iodine, 240, 241
ion channels, 183
ions, 259
IP-10, 176
IR, 27, 111, 195
Ireland, 40, 230
irritability, 119
IRs, 224
ischemia, 189, 190, 192, 195, 196, 197, 198, 199
ischemic, 67, 68, 70, 148, 189, 190, 193, 194, 195, 196, 198
ischemic heart disease, 67, 70
ischemic preconditioning, 196
ischemic stroke, 68
isoforms, 33, 35
isolation, 102, 147
isoleucine, 35
isoniazid, 251
Israel, 107
Italy, 59, 106, 235
IVF, 236, 237

J

JAMA, 244
Japanese, 18, 19, 23, 26, 35, 48, 177
JNK, 172, 180
joint damage, 60
joints, 60, 73, 74
Jordan, 232
Jun, 47, 107, 109, 112, 114, 168
Jung, 166
juvenile idiopathic arthritis, 48

K

kainic acid, 137
kappa, 47, 281, 283
kappa B, 47
keratin, 275
keratinocytes, 155, 161, 165, 268
Ki-67, 158, 159
kidney failure, 272
killer cells, 186, 202, 229, 230
killing, 177, 210
kinase, 27, 28, 30, 33, 55, 73, 170, 172, 174, 179, 185, 195
kinase activity, 27, 33
kinases, 18, 28, 33, 53, 170, 175, 177, 183, 190, 203
King, 56, 167
knockout, 15, 197
Korean, 18

L

labeling, 154, 165
labor, 1
labor-intensive, 1
lactation, 243
Lactobacillus, 129
laminin, 166, 282
large-scale, 2, 3, 9, 11, 36, 42, 46
laser, 162, 254
latency, 180, 249
lattice, 56
laws, 280
LDL, 59, 62, 63, 64, 65, 66, 67
lead, 7, 9, 26, 28, 31, 33, 87, 135, 155, 161, 162, 189, 190, 239, 241, 260, 261, 264, 278
lectin, 32, 33, 55, 189, 190, 191, 192, 194, 198
lesions, 119, 132, 134, 135, 137, 142, 148, 149, 155, 161, 165, 229, 262
leucine, 175
leukemia, 32
leukocyte, 26, 67, 140, 170, 197
leukocytes, 72, 73, 135, 140, 144, 170, 184, 211
leukocytic cells, 116
LFA, 26, 30, 31, 52, 55
liberal, 8
lifetime, 2
ligand, 25, 31, 33, 35, 44, 74, 75, 89, 174, 175, 183, 185, 193, 202, 203, 204, 209, 213, 227, 233
ligands, 55, 74, 175, 181, 203, 206, 211, 224, 226
likelihood, 8
limitation, 8, 9, 67, 129, 241
limitations, 68, 79
Lincoln, 56, 243, 251
linear, 62, 143, 272

linkage, 1, 2, 3, 4, 5, 11, 13, 19, 36, 39, 43, 51, 53
linkage mapping, 4
links, 174
lipases, 190
lipid, 30, 31, 49, 55, 196, 218, 226, 232
lipid metabolism, 49
lipid peroxidation, 196
lipid rafts, 31
lipids, 137, 190, 204, 212, 230
lipopolysaccharides, 130, 132, 150
lipoprotein, 68, 119, 121, 132, 175
lipoproteins, 59, 62, 206
literature, 176, 248, 261, 265
liver, 187
LM, 107, 108, 111, 164, 226, 227
localization, 145, 148, 199, 281
location, 5, 17, 25, 27, 115, 128, 136
locus, 2, 3, 4, 5, 11, 13, 15, 19, 21, 22, 27, 29, 33, 35, 38, 42, 43, 44, 45, 46, 48, 53, 56, 231, 277
LOD, 11
London, 46, 147, 225
long period, 258
longitudinal studies, 135
longitudinal study, 134, 135
losses, 10
low molecular weight, 146
low-density, 68, 69, 227
low-density lipoprotein, 68, 69
low-dose aspirin, 245
LPS, 111, 150, 175, 223, 275
lumen, 62
lung, 54, 161, 196, 197, 198, 248, 249, 250, 251, 252, 253, 255, 256, 260, 262, 265, 266, 267, 269, 271, 272, 280, 281
lung cancer, 249, 250
lung disease, 161, 248, 251, 253, 255, 256, 262
lung function, 54, 265, 269
lupus, 110, 113, 152, 165, 260, 265, 267
luteinizing hormone, 140
lymph, 46, 92, 210, 212, 216, 218, 233
lymph node, 46, 92, 212, 216, 218, 233
lymphocyte, 1, 26, 30, 35, 45, 54, 83, 98, 99, 100, 109, 110, 111, 151, 152, 154, 158, 230, 238, 281
lymphocytes, 14, 26, 52, 83, 87, 92, 95, 98, 99, 100, 102, 103, 107, 121, 145, 153, 155, 160, 169, 171, 187, 201, 202, 228, 230, 231, 245, 272
lymphoid, 3, 38, 48, 52, 56, 171, 173, 175, 177, 215
lymphoid organs, 171, 173, 215
lymphoid tissue, 175
lymphoma, 207, 209, 211, 215, 225, 228, 230
lymphomas, 201
lysine, 138
lysis, 18
lysosomes, 259, 267
lysozyme, 78

M

mAb, 207, 211, 212, 213, 219, 222, 271, 273, 274, 275, 277, 278, 279
machinery, 202, 211
macrophage, 50, 59, 60, 74, 75, 182
macrophage inflammatory protein, 74, 75
macrophages, 18, 28, 60, 87, 106, 153, 183, 203, 204, 206, 209, 210, 211, 215, 216, 218, 223, 225, 227, 228, 229, 231, 260, 268
Madison, 54
magnetic resonance imaging, 115, 132, 143, 148
maintenance, 57, 152, 178, 180, 215, 224
Maintenance, 151
major histocompatibility complex, 33, 171, 182, 229, 234
Major Histocompatibility Complex (MHC), 2
malaise, 260
malignancy, 62
malignant, 229, 249, 250
Mammalian, 45, 56
mammalian cells, 72
mammals, 17, 116, 133
management, 60, 67, 242
manufacturer, 63, 157, 159, 252
MAPK, 165, 172
mapping, 4, 6, 10, 38, 43, 44, 45, 50, 51
marketing, 249
marrow, 21, 233, 279
mass spectrometry, 131
mast cells, 191, 197, 215
maternal, 238, 240, 244, 245, 246
maternal age, 238, 244
matrix, 29, 133, 141, 143, 144, 145, 147, 155, 164, 166, 167, 168
matrix metalloproteinase, 133, 141, 143, 145, 147, 155, 164, 166, 167, 168
maturation, 14, 171, 174, 187, 218, 222, 224, 230, 279
Mb, 34, 277, 278
MBP, 90, 96, 109, 118, 119, 121, 125, 126, 127, 132, 136, 138, 139, 140, 142, 143, 146, 150
MDA, 71
meanings, 78

measles, 85, 89, 93, 103, 107
measurement, 62, 236
measures, 8, 9, 21, 61
media, 60, 61, 63, 252
median, 63, 239
mediators, 44, 262
medication, 63
medications, 251
medicine, 2, 37, 195
medulla oblongata, 137
MEK, 196
melanoma, 46, 176, 209, 211, 213, 228, 229, 230
membranes, 141, 272
memory, 35, 172, 180, 209, 216
men, 60, 61, 69, 112, 113, 114, 116, 236
Mendel, 105, 116, 119, 120, 143, 144, 145
Mendelian disorders, 7
menorrhagia, 237, 243
menstrual, 235, 237
menstruation, 243
mesenchymal stromal cells, 180
mesothelioma, 250, 265
messenger RNA, 147, 170, 267
meta-analysis, 22, 44
metabolic, 49, 50, 61, 133
metabolism, 33, 61, 62, 129, 132, 150
metalloproteinase, 141, 145, 146, 166, 167
metastasis, 229, 230
methanol, 159
methionine, 18
methylation, 14, 44, 53, 75
metric, 10
MHC, 15, 32, 81, 83, 87, 88, 91, 105, 107, 108, 111, 113, 171, 172, 173, 174, 177, 180, 201, 202, 203, 204, 205, 210, 211, 214, 216, 218, 219, 223, 224, 225, 226, 230, 231, 233, 282
microarray, 36
microbes, 82, 90, 110, 172, 175, 178, 184
microbial, 78, 79, 81, 82, 83, 90, 91, 92, 93, 94, 121, 169, 172, 173, 174, 175, 176, 177, 178, 227
microbial agents, 173, 177
microchimerism, 238
microglia, 135, 182
microorganisms, 120, 131, 136, 182, 190, 209, 215
microscope, 252
migration, 67, 99, 161, 171
mimicking, 87, 88, 90, 91, 102
mimicry, 77, 78, 79, 81, 83, 84, 89, 90, 104, 105, 106, 107, 109, 111, 113, 149, 150, 172, 178, 180, 181, 182
mineralogy, 265
minerals, 248
mines, 265, 269
mining, 247, 249, 257, 265
MIP, 74, 75
miscarriage, 235, 238, 239, 240, 244, 245
misleading, 93, 135
mitochondrial, 190, 195
mitogen, 183, 196
mitogen-activated protein kinase, 183, 196
mitogenic, 121
MMP, 133, 134, 135, 137, 149, 161, 163, 166, 183
MMP-2, 134
MMP-3, 133, 134
MMP-9, 133, 134, 135, 137, 149, 163, 166, 183
MMPs, 133, 134, 162
MND, 254
modalities, 248
models, 37, 43, 61, 82, 97, 101, 140, 154, 163, 166, 174, 189, 191, 193, 211, 213, 238, 264
modulation, 50, 152, 239
MOG, 119, 120, 132, 143, 144
moieties, 202
molar ratio, 120
molecular mechanisms, 4, 20, 248
molecular mimicry, 18, 77, 78, 79, 80, 81, 82, 83, 84, 87, 101, 102, 103, 111, 112, 128, 129, 182
molecular structure, 204
molecular weight, 202
molecules, 12, 26, 29, 32, 52, 60, 81, 99, 104, 107, 113, 115, 127, 129, 130, 132, 143, 149, 153, 154, 155, 168, 169, 170, 172, 173, 174, 175, 177, 178, 190, 201, 202, 203, 204, 206, 209, 210, 211, 212, 213, 215, 216, 218, 221, 223, 224, 225, 279, 281
monkeys, 106, 119, 138, 141, 143, 146
monoclonal, 26, 51, 52, 79, 105, 112, 181, 189, 197, 205, 260, 271, 273, 275, 281
monoclonal antibodies, 26, 51, 52, 79, 181, 205, 260, 275
monoclonal antibody, 197
monocytes, 14, 26, 28, 30, 60, 61, 74, 75, 135, 140, 183
monogenic, 4
monomeric, 143
mononuclear cell, 28, 134, 144, 147, 148
monozygotic twins, 2
Montana, 247, 249, 250, 251, 261, 265, 266
morbidity, 4, 60, 190, 193, 235
morphological, 191
morphology, 154, 258, 266

mortality, 4, 60, 61, 68, 119, 190, 250, 265, 266
mortality rate, 190
Moscow, 1
mothers, 241
mouse, 7, 15, 28, 35, 41, 45, 50, 53, 56, 117, 120, 121, 142, 144, 151, 154, 155, 156, 158, 159, 160, 161, 162, 163, 165, 167, 168, 184, 185, 192, 197, 205, 209, 215, 216, 217, 230, 231, 260, 264, 273, 274, 275, 277, 279, 280, 282
mouse model, 155, 160, 162, 165, 167, 168
mouth, 151, 152, 153
movement, 170
MRI, 115, 132, 134, 142, 144, 148, 149
mRNA, 17, 25, 29, 31, 32, 51, 72, 73, 105, 133, 134, 135, 142, 144, 148, 149, 150, 170, 174, 175, 275
MS, ix, 35, 36, 85, 90, 112, 115, 116, 119, 121, 127, 129, 130, 131, 132, 133, 134, 135, 136, 137, 138, 140, 141, 142, 143, 144, 145, 146, 147, 148, 149, 150, 195, 228, 230, 244
mucosal barrier, 173, 196
mucus, 161
multicellular organisms, 190
multi-ethnic, 69
multiple sclerosis, 35, 56, 57, 77, 85, 88, 89, 105, 106, 108, 109, 116, 138, 146, 147, 149, 172, 176, 177, 187
mumps, 18
murine model, 165, 196, 248, 260
muscarinic receptor, 154, 155
muscle, 29, 89, 191, 192, 194
musculoskeletal, 60, 75
mutagenesis, 112
mutation, 7, 8, 273, 275, 278, 279
mutations, 69, 275, 277, 278
myalgia, 260
myasthenia gravis, 97, 99, 172, 181
mycobacteria, 85, 89, 91, 93, 209, 210
Mycobacterium, 86, 108, 122, 125
myelin, 89, 90, 92, 93, 95, 96, 102, 105, 107, 108, 109, 111, 114, 115, 116, 118, 119, 121, 122, 123, 124, 125, 127, 128, 131, 132, 136, 137, 138, 140, 141, 142, 143, 144, 145, 146, 147, 148, 149, 150, 172, 180, 181, 228
myelin antigens, 131, 136, 144, 147, 148
myelin basic protein, 89, 90, 92, 93, 95, 96, 102, 105, 107, 108, 109, 111, 114, 116, 118, 122, 123, 124, 125, 128, 132, 137, 138, 141, 145, 146, 147, 148, 149, 150, 172, 180, 181, 228
myelin oligodendrocyte glycoprotein, 140, 143, 145
myelination, 141
myeloid, 175, 233
myeloma, 273
myocardial infarction, 190, 196, 197
myocardial ischemia, 195
myocarditis, 28, 77, 84, 85, 86, 89, 92, 93, 96, 98, 102, 106, 107, 108, 109, 110, 111, 113, 114, 172, 179, 184, 185, 186
myocardium, 110, 196
myocyte, 28, 173, 196
myopathies, 85
myosin, 85, 89, 92, 97, 102, 108, 114, 172, 181, 189, 192, 194

N

NAc, 124
N-acety, 125, 138, 144
nanoparticles, 267
Nash, 41, 69
National Academy of Sciences, 42, 44, 47, 51
National Institutes of Health, 6, 280
natural, 30, 78, 112, 153, 155, 169, 174, 176, 177, 186, 187, 189, 190, 191, 192, 193, 194, 198, 201, 204, 206, 207, 209, 223, 229, 230, 231, 232, 243, 279
natural killer, 30, 153, 169, 177, 186, 187, 204, 229, 230, 232
natural killer cell, 153, 169, 186
natural selection, 78
necrosis, 14, 133, 135, 147, 198, 233
negative selection, 4, 193, 201, 202, 218
neonatal, 15, 46, 113, 240, 244, 245
neoplasia, 164
neoplasms, 166
neoplastic, 121
nephritis, 28, 272, 282
nephropathy, 99, 108
nephrotoxic, 272
nerves, 145
nervous system, 33, 116, 138, 147
network, 19, 82, 107, 112, 113, 114, 205, 224
neural development, 235
neural tissue, 148
neuritis, 143
neurogenesis, 29
neurological disease, 139, 146
neurons, 35, 56
neuropathy, 110
neutralization, 88, 94
neutrophil, 26, 197, 198

neutrophils, 191, 196, 204, 215
New England, 57
New Jersey, 45
New South Wales, 109
New York, 38, 44, 45, 47, 48, 56, 110, 141, 189, 195, 282
NFkB, 47, 175, 176, 177, 178
NF-kB, 19, 190. 196,
NF-κB, 18
NHL, 241
nickel, 178, 187
Nielsen, 226
NIH, 270
nitric oxide (NO), 18, 59, 61, 65, 66, 69, 145, 175
nitric oxide synthase, 145
Nitrite, 63
NK, 30, 31, 32, 55, 177, 186, 187, 201, 202, 204, 205, 207, 210, 211, 212, 213, 214, 224, 225, 226, 227, 228, 229, 232, 236
NK cells, 31, 177, 204, 207, 211, 212, 213, 214, 224, 227, 229
NK-cell, 225, 236
NMDA, 145
NMR, 123, 125, 141, 142, 146
NO, 28, 60, 61, 62, 63, 64, 65, 66, 67, 69, 135
NO synthase, 67, 135
non-binding, 202
non-nuclear, 256
non-obese diabetic, x, 14, 50, 140, 151, 163, 167, 231, 233
non-polymorphic, 218
nontoxic, 105
normal, 77, 84, 92, 93, 95, 98, 103, 109, 112, 117, 125, 129, 130, 135, 136, 142, 146, 153, 155, 160, 161, 162, 163, 165, 171, 173, 177, 183, 203, 204, 211, 213, 215, 218, 219, 240, 241, 253, 259, 261, 273, 279, 283
North America, 49, 54
North Carolina, 271
Norway, 125
NSC, 211, 212, 213, 221, 226
N-terminal, 18, 51
nuclear, 12, 21, 29, 34, 53, 85, 89, 109, 110, 123, 157, 159, 175, 247, 252, 261, 267, 268, 269
nuclear family, 12
nuclear magnetic resonance, 89, 123
nucleic acid, 72, 73, 74, 75, 113
nucleosome, 260, 267
nucleotide sequence, 193, 275
nucleotides, 169, 274, 275, 277, 278, 279
nucleus, 29, 53, 56
nutrients, 209
nutrition, 204

O

Obese, 154, 232
obesity, 28, 53
obligations, 216
observations, 87, 136, 149, 152, 153, 154, 160, 162, 192, 209, 264, 265
obstruction, 236, 242
occlusion, 197
occupational, 248, 265
Odds Ratio, 3
oil, 121, 122, 123, 142
oligodendrocytes, 136, 137, 143, 146, 147, 148, 150
oligomenorrhea, 237
oligomer, 105
oligomerization, 177
Oncogene, 32, 46, 184
oocytes, 236, 237
opposition, 177
optic neuritis, 116, 146
optical, 256
optical density, 256
OR, 12, 16, 17, 18, 19, 21, 25, 27, 29, 32, 34, 241
oral, 114, 152, 164, 165
orchitis, 121, 142
ordinal data, 253, 255
organ, 13, 17, 30, 79, 83, 84, 109, 112, 153, 180, 197, 198, 238, 272
organism, 95, 115, 128, 217
ornithine, 67
osteoarthritis, 71, 72, 261
osteoblasts, 21
ovarian, 15, 46, 236, 237, 243, 245
ovarian failure, 236
overload, , 59, 61
ovulation, 236
oxidants, 196
oxidative, 20, 59, 61, 62, 69, 259
oxidative stress, 20, 59, 61, 62, 69, 259
oxide, 67, 163, 175, 185, 257
oxides, 248, 257
oxygen, 190, 282

P

P13K, 196
p38, 172, 180, 183, 185, 196
packaging, 34, 180
PAI-1, 134, 146
pairing, 78
pancreas, 2, 19, 26, 52
pancreatic, 19, 26, 35, 49, 50, 52, 211, 217, 218, 231, 232, 233
pancreatic acinar cell, 211
pancreatic islet, 50, 217
pandemic, 88
paper, 202, 223, 241
paradigm shift, 101
paradoxical, 67
paraffin-embedded, 157
paralysis, 116
parasite, 106, 228
parasites, 171, 209
parenchyma, 130, 140
parents, 21, 43
parotid gland, 160, 161, 163
PARP, 190, 191
particles, 91, 204, 267
passive, 272
paternal, 238
pathogenesis, 1, 2, 4, 5, 11, 13, 14, 17, 20, 25, 34, 52, 54, 57, 67, 68, 91, 98, 105, 106, 107, 111, 112, 113, 140, 143, 147, 154, 163, 167, 185, 190, 191, 195, 196, 237, 268, 272, 281, 282
pathogenic, 5, 18, 29, 47, 71, 86, 128, 172, 173, 178, 182, 190, 192, 193, 199, 218, 225, 232, 237, 245, 250, 271, 272, 274, 279, 280
pathogenic agents, 86
pathogens, 100, 128, 175, 189, 190, 203, 229
pathologic diagnosis, 267
pathology, 17, 37, 60, 131, 136, 152, 156, 161, 162, 164, 249, 262
pathophysiological mechanisms, 37
pathophysiology, 5, 152, 154
pathways, 18, 33, 36, 45, 133, 160, 165, 172, 174, 175, 177, 178, 182, 186, 190, 191, 227, 255
pattern recognition, 55
PCR, 274, 277, 278
penetrance, 2, 5
penis, 55
peptidase, 137, 142
peptide, 81, 89, 92, 95, 97, 107, 108, 109, 111, 113, 114, 116, 118, 119, 120, 121, 122, 123, 124, 125, 126, 127, 128, 138, 141, 143, 144, 145, 146, 149, 150, 161, 173, 181, 193, 194, 201, 202, 203, 204, 208, 211, 212, 213, 215, 216, 223, 224, 225, 226, 231, 248
peptides, 29, 80, 95, 96, 106, 109, 111, 112, 115, 117, 120, 121, 122, 123, 128, 136, 144, 146, 147, 149, 150, 164, 172, 173, 181, 182, 194, 199, 201, 202, 203, 209, 210, 211, 215, 216, 218, 223, 225, 226, 230, 232
percentile, 241
perception, 195
perforin, 153, 177, 218
perinatal, 241
Peripheral, 110, 131, 133, 142, 171
peripheral blood, 14, 26, 30, 62, 75, 144, 149, 267
peripheral blood mononuclear cell, 26, 267
peripheral nerve, 146
peritoneum, 212
perivascular cuffing, 77, 84, 97, 98, 100, 136
permeability, 150, 195, 197, 198
permit, 9, 179
Peroxisome, 49
peroxynitrite, 61
personal, 134, 249, 250
personal communication, 134, 250
pertussis, 89, 96, 97, 105, 108, 118, 122, 125, 126, 139, 183
pesticides, 250
pH, 169, 273
phage, 193
phagocytic, 203, 218
phagocytosis, 204
pharmaceutical industry, 130, 132
pharmacogenetics, 2, 37
pharmacological, 61
phenotype, 2, 9, 21, 42, 178, 221, 232, 269, 270
phenotypes, 4, 7, 40
phenotypic, 59, 60
phenylalanine, 128, 278
Philadelphia, 179, 195
phone, 77
phosphatases, 203
phosphate, 252
phosphodiesterase, 25
phospholipids, 105
phosphoprotein, 107
phosphorylates, 30, 175
phosphorylation, 19, 27, 31, 33, 170, 172, 203, 226
physical activity, 50
physical interaction, 171

physical properties, 169
Physicians, 105, 106, 113, 250
physiological, 5, 29, 57, 133, 202
physiology, 195
pig, 110, 116, 118, 119, 120, 121, 125, 138, 148, 149, 179
pigs, 88, 92, 110, 117, 119, 120, 122, 124, 125, 138, 142, 147, 150
pituitary, 237
PKC, 19, 183
placebo, 239, 242
placental, 238, 240, 241
planning, 101
plants, 190, 195
plaque, 61
plaques, 250, 251
plasma, 105, 108, 134, 135, 140, 142, 146, 175, 204
plasma cells, 204
plasma membrane, 140, 175
plasminogen, 134, 141, 146
platelet, 30, 55, 67, 89, 92, 112, 113, 114
platforms, 6, 7, 8, 36, 259
play, 16, 18, 25, 29, 34, 62, 93, 96, 99, 174, 203, 205, 215, 223, 224
pleasure, 225
pleural, 250, 251, 262, 264, 265, 270
PMA, 218
pneumoconiosis, 267
pneumonia, 86
polarization, 185
polarized, 170
poliovirus, 179, 180
poly(ADP-ribose) polymerase, 191
polycystic ovary syndrome, 243
polygenes, 50
polymerase, 171, 179, 190, 196
polymorphism, 7, 10, 17, 18, 19, 22, 23, 24, 25, 26, 30, 32, 35, 43, 46, 48, 49, 50, 51, 184, 224
polymorphisms, 12, 14, 25, 27, 48, 49, 51, 53, 56
polymorphonuclear, 140, 211
polypeptide, 202, 260
polypeptides, 135
polyphenols, 151, 152, 163, 165
Polyphenols, 151, 155
polysaccharides, 132
poor, 5, 122, 161, 217
population, 2, 3, 4, 5, 6, 9, 11, 12, 13, 14, 19, 25, 36, 42, 43, 48, 49, 59, 60, 61, 67, 68, 71, 72, 85, 140, 163, 169, 177, 178, 212, 237, 240, 242, 243, 247, 248, 250, 251, 253, 259, 261, 264, 265, 266, 268
pore, 195
pores, 170
positive correlation, 66
postpartum, 240, 244
postpartum period, 244
post-translational, 223
post-translational modifications, 223
potassium, 18
power, 5, 8, 9, 10, 11, 249
PPD, 105
precipitation, 273
preconditioning, 195
precursor cells, 204
prediction, 2, 37, 61, 87, 96, 99, 102
predictors, 112
prednisone, 245
pre-existing, 94, 95, 192
preference, 128
pregnancy, 235, 236, 238, 239, 240, 241, 242, 243, 244, 245, 246
pregnant women, 238, 239, 240, 241, 244, 245
premature delivery, 240
premature ovarian failure, 237
prenatal care, 241
preparation, 121, 157, 219, 221
pressure, 8, 210, 213, 229
prevention, 50, 61, 78, 93, 94, 95, 96, 105, 114, 150, 196, 231
preventive, 61, 219, 248
prices, 6
primary progressive multiple sclerosis, 57
priming, 152, 198, 204, 218
probability, 8, 42, 121, 172, 174, 253
probands, 21
procedures, 64, 67, 90, 120, 159, 236
processing pathways, 267
producers, 177, 231
production, 15, 18, 28, 31, 59, 61, 67, 69, 71, 72, 73, 74, 88, 105, 111, 120, 122, 130, 134, 135, 140, 143, 148, 149, 153, 155, 173, 174, 175, 176, 178, 183, 184, 185, 190, 204, 209, 219, 221, 223, 224, 225, 228, 229, 237, 249, 260, 265, 273
progenitor cells, 161
progenitors, 233
progeny, 171, 177, 241, 245
progesterone, 237
prognosis, 142
prognostic marker, 67, 248, 264
program, 283
progressive, 53, 115, 132, 161, 240, 259, 262, 265

proinflammatory, 20, 21, 28, 71, 155, 192, 262, 270
pro-inflammatory, 174, 175, 176, 184
prokaryotic, 72
prolactin, 29, 237, 243
proliferation, 13, 14, 15, 16, 30, 31, 33, 54, 56, 67, 94, 135, 142, 152, 160, 161, 162, 165, 174, 208, 224, 230
promote, 18, 60, 135, 170, 175, 176, 177, 178, 198
promoter, 47, 48, 186
property, 73, 130
prostaglandin, 114
prostate, 33
proteases, 136, 170, 173, 190, 268
protection, 96, 192, 193, 207, 210, 219, 223, 225, 228, 258
protein family, 19
protein kinase C (PKC), 30, 31, 180
protein misfolding, 260
protein sequence, 193
protein structure, 223
protein synthesis, 161, 170, 179
protein tyrosine phosphatases, 53
proteinase, 110, 141, 198
protein-protein interactions, 173
Proteins, 32, 118, 126, 129, 161
proteolipid protein, 116, 140, 141, 142, 147, 149
proteolysis, 131, 148, 182
protocol, 159, 252
protocols, 156, 250
prototype, 277, 279
proximal, 62
proxy, 6
Pseudomonas aeruginosa, 104
psoriasis, 29, 54, 59, 161
Psoriasis, 168
psoriatic arthritis, , 59, 60, 63, 64, 65, 66, 68, 69, 75
psychological development, 246
PTPs, 27
puberty, 130
public, 226, 249, 265, 274
purpura, 77, 84, 86, 92, 93, 111
P-value, 13, 34

Q

QTL, 46
quality control, 9
quality of life, 152
quartile, 63
quartz, 265, 266
Quebec, 42
questionnaire, 251
quinidine, 251
Quinones, 281

R

radiological, 266
RAGE, 113
random, 9, 43, 90, 193, 224, 279
range, 6, 32, 36, 63, 78, 88, 153, 160, 202, 230, 255, 260
RANTES, 176
rapidly progressive glomerulonephritis, 272
rat, 18, 55, 69, 116, 117, 118, 120, 125, 138, 140, 141, 142, 145, 147, 150, 161, 163, 167, 184, 195, 196, 197, 198, 217
rats, 18, 33, 105, 106, 109, 112, 114, 118, 119, 120, 123, 125, 138, 139, 144, 148, 195, 197, 198, 282
reactive oxygen species (ROS), 62, 190
reactivity, 96, 109, 143, 148, 172, 177, 182, 190, 201, 202, 203, 204, 207, 217, 218, 221, 224, 253, 254, 259, 261, 268, 282
reading, 170, 275, 278
reagent, 273, 274
reagents, 252
reality, 103
reasoning, 193
receptors, 28, 29, 31, 35, 55, 71, 73, 74, 80, 81, 130, 135, 170, 174, 175, 177, 178, 182, 184, 185, 186, 190, 195, 197, 201, 202, 203, 204, 205, 206, 209, 210, 213, 223, 224, 225, 226, 227, 229, 237, 243
recognition, 18, 30, 32, 55, 74, 75, 113, 114, 149, 174, 178, 181, 184, 186, 190, 192, 194, 198, 203, 212, 213, 226, 227, 229, 230, 231, 232, 238
recombination, 7, 35
reconcile, 96
reconstruction, 266
recovery, 198, 279
recruiting, 177
red blood cells, 205
redistribution, 179
redox, 62, 69
reduction, 8, 15, 130, 153, 157, 161, 163, 240
refractory, 108
regeneration, 163, 167
regional, 46
Registry, 250, 251, 262
regression, 228
regular, 125, 235

regulation, 12, 14, 16, 19, 27, 29, 35, 44, 53, 55, 69, 82, 104, 174, 184, 186, 201, 202, 211, 214, 224, 231, 233, 273, 279
regulations, 204
regulators, 211, 218
Reimann, 230
reinforcement, 282
rejection, 230, 238, 272, 281
relapses, 115, 129, 132, 133, 145
relationship, 17, 42, 111, 140, 142, 153, 164, 191, 241, 244, 262, 264, 269, 280
relatives, 2
relevance, 26, 32, 44, 265
remission, 74
remodeling, 14, 61, 161, 166, 167
renal, 211, 273, 281
reoxygenation, 195
repair, 161, 167
reperfusion, 189, 190, 192, 193, 194, 195, 196, 197, 198, 199
replication, 11, 39, 72, 171, 173, 174, 179, 180, 185
reproduction, 242, 243, 244
reproductive age, 156, 235, 237
research, 2, 3, 37, 100, 103, 104, 135, 184, 189, 241
research design, 37
researchers, 135, 250, 261
reservoirs, 266
residues, 32, 112, 113, 121, 128, 216, 275
resistance, 15, 27, 106, 140, 197, 229, 230
resolution, 10, 40, 179, 187
resources, 1, 36
respiratory, 240, 241, 266
respiratory distress syndrome, 240, 241
restitution, 196
restoration, 94, 240
retinoic acid, 176
retroviruses, 108
RF, xii, 248, 249, 252, 255, 261
rheumatic, 59, 61, 62, 67, 68, 69, 77, 84, 86, 89, 93, 101, 102, 106, 110, 111, 113, 114, 151, 172, 250, 267
rheumatic diseases, 59, 61, 68, 69, 267
rheumatic fever, 77, 84, 86, 89, 93, 106, 110, 113, 114
rheumatic heart disease, 86, 101, 102, 106, 110, 111, 172
rheumatoid arthritis, 3, 46, 48, 49, 56, 59, 60, 63, 64, 65, 66, 68, 69, 75, 85, 93, 99, 151, 176, 201, 223, 248, 249, 266, 267, 268, 272
rheumatoid factor, 60, 99, 105, 248, 249
ribose, 190, 196
ribosomal, 72
ribosomal RNA, 72
risk, 2, 4, 5, 10, 12, 17, 18, 20, 21, 22, 25, 26, 32, 47, 48, 51, 56, 57, 59, 60, 61, 62, 66, 67, 68, 70, 85, 88, 102, 105, 127, 152, 163, 204, 235, 236, 237, 238, 239, 240, 241, 244, 250, 261, 265, 268
risk factors, 5, 59, 60, 61, 62, 66, 67, 68, 105
risks, 61, 78, 102, 103, 248
RNA, 12, 15, 18, 19, 34, 47, 56, 71, 72, 73, 74, 75, 134, 169, 170, 175, 176, 179, 180, 186, 206, 274
RNA processing, 19
RNAs, 34, 171
rodents, 160, 271
Rome, 59
room temperature, 159, 273
ROS, 62, 191
rotavirus, 18
RP, 110, 167
rubella, 18, 72, 86, 108, 182
Russia, 1

S

sacrifice, 7
safety, 103, 162, 224
saline, 92, 117, 139, 141, 143, 194, 252
saliva, 152, 153, 161, 163
Salivary gland, 164, 165
salivary glands, 153, 157, 160, 164, 166, 167
Salmonella, 129, 209
salt, 204
sample, 3, 4, 8, 10, 11, 25, 40, 157, 236, 238, 248, 250, 251, 258, 264, 268
satisfaction, 101
savings, 9
science, 184
scientific, 265
scleroderma, 248, 264, 268, 269
sclerosis, 85, 115
scores, 194, 253, 256, 262
search, 8, 27, 38, 40, 48, 50, 90, 138, 194, 278
searching, 3, 5, 7, 104, 128
secrete, 60, 144, 153
secretion, 44, 134, 153, 154, 155, 204
sediment, 258
seizures, 119
selecting, 6, 11
Self, 78, 87, 110, 171, 192, 215, 223, 228
self-antigens, 82, 83, 84, 190, 199

self-recognition, 180
self-report, 261, 268
semen, 88
senescence, 243
sensitivity, 9, 21, 55, 153, 173, 255, 259, 262
sensitization, 119, 147, 230
sensorineural hearing loss, 241
sequencing, 10, 41, 45
series, 121, 203, 225
serine, 15, 30, 31, 128, 134, 147
serotonin, 111, 121, 130, 132, 147
serum, 13, 28, 60, 62, 63, 64, 65, 66, 69, 105, 109, 132, 134, 135, 140, 144, 145, 151, 152, 156, 157, 163, 167, 189, 192, 215, 216, 237, 238, 240, 241, 247, 248, 250, 251, 252, 253, 254, 255, 256, 257, 261, 268, 269, 274, 279
serum albumin, 215, 216
severity, 56, 155, 190, 237, 240, 248, 255, 259, 261
sex, 60, 62, 68, 237, 251
shaping, 209
shares, 34, 59, 60, 278
sharing, 106, 275, 283
Sheep, 119
shock, 19, 49, 195, 197
short-term, 266
siblings, 21, 22
signal transduction, 19, 26, 29, 30, 49, 53, 175, 180, 183, 203
signaling, , 5, 14, 16, 19, 21, 27, 28, 29, 31, 32, 33, 35, 45, 53, 55, 56, 67, 69, 71, 75, 162, 164, 169, 174, 175, 176, 177, 178, 180, 182, 183, 185, 187, 190, 203, 210, 227
signaling pathway, 5, 19, 28, 53, 71, 162, 183, 187, 227
signalling, 167, 184, 185, 230
signals, 14, 152, 162, 173, 176, 179, 210
signs, 116, 118, 119, 134, 136
silica, 248, 257, 258, 260, 261, 264, 265, 267, 268, 269
silicates, 258, 259
silicon, 248, 257
silicosis, 258, 262, 268
similarity, 108, 111, 172, 278
single nucleotide polymorphism, 6, 40, 42, 44, 48, 49
sites, 28, 98, 111, 120, 138, 147, 173, 177, 249, 258, 265, 281
Sjogren, 85, 99, 151, 152, 155, 156, 163, 165, 166, 172, 181
skeletal muscle, 191, 193, 197, 198, 199, 217
skin, 59, 60, 68, 155, 160, 165, 168, 173, 183, 272, 275, 281, 282
skin diseases, 272
SLE, 3, 19, 31, 104, 248, 250, 252, 259, 260, 261, 262, 264
sleep, 121, 145
small intestine, 195, 196, 197, 198
smoke, 63, 251, 261
smooth muscle, 67
snake venom, 29
SNP, 6, 7, 10, 11, 13, 16, 17, 19, 25, 29, 30, 31, 32, 34, 35, 36, 42, 43
SNPs, 3, 6, 7, 8, 10, 11, 12, 13, 14, 16, 17, 27, 29, 32, 33, 34, 35, 36, 40, 42, 43, 44, 46
software, 252, 253, 274, 283
soil, 249, 258
spasticity, 119
Spearman rank correlation coefficient, 64
species, 26, 72, 88, 90, 116, 118, 119, 120, 121, 122, 125, 128, 138, 175, 177, 195, 198, 202, 216, 223, 282
specificity, 9, 54, 81, 106, 109, 112, 122, 134, 136, 145, 146, 185, 186, 205, 228, 255, 259, 262, 268, 273, 283
spectroscopy, 89, 141
spectrum, 11, 39, 138, 190, 250
speculation, 239
sperm, 88, 91, 105, 107, 109, 111, 236
spermatid, 56
spermatozoa, 114
SPF, 205, 206, 207, 208, 209, 224
spinal cord, 122, 137, 142, 147
spirometry, 251
spleen, 16, 210, 211, 212, 213, 215, 216, 219, 222, 273, 275, 280
splenectomy, 107
sponges, 218
spontaneous abortion, 239, 244, 245
SSB, 153
St. Louis, 156, 195, 273
stability, 170
stabilization, 170
stages, 8, 141, 149, 157, 215
standard deviation, 222
standards, 3, 248
statistical analysis, 158, 251, 283
statistics, 195
steady state, 15
Stem cell, 197
stenosis, 69

sterile, 190, 195
steroids, 147
stimulant, 125
stimulus, 223
strain, 15, 92, 119, 163, 183, 224, 278, 280
strains, 15, 45, 56, 123, 149, 154, 179, 184, 205, 209, 213, 215, 216, 219, 233, 271, 273
strategic, 5
strategies, 3, 8, 37, 41, 211, 229
stratification, 5, 9, 42
strength, 13, 34, 79
streptavidin, 159
streptococci, 79, 86, 89, 92, 93, 101, 102, 107
stress, 20, 61, 69, 189, 268
stroke, 190, 195
stroma, 164, 203, 213
stromal cells, 203
structural changes, 203, 210
structural formation, 170
structural gene, 15
structural protein, 272
subdomains, 30
subgroups, 9
subjective, 153
substances, 121, 151
substitution, 7, 18, 21, 25, 30, 49, 50, 144
substrates, 27, 28, 29, 259, 268
suffering, 238, 241
sugar, 32, 150, 202, 218
sulfate, 15, 45, 273
Sun, 198
Superfund, 249
supernatant, 221, 222, 223
superoxide, 20, 61
supply, 190, 249
suppression, 14, 16, 19, 22, 33, 78, 87, 88, 94, 95, 96, 97, 111, 114, 138, 147, 163, 178
suppressor, 32, 33, 44, 106, 108, 127, 186
Surgery, 196, 199
surgical, 195, 236
surveillance, 223, 224
survival, 14, 16, 36, 45, 57, 149, 162, 176, 186, 193, 196, 269
surviving, 215, 222
susceptibility, 1, 2, 3, 4, 5, 11, 13, 14, 15, 19, 21, 22, 27, 29, 30, 32, 33, 34, 35, 37, 38, 39, 40, 43, 45, 46, 47, 48, 49, 50, 52, 54, 56, 198, 223, 242
susceptibility genes, 3, 19, 38, 50, 223, 242
Sweden, 63, 71, 273
Switzerland, 63
symptom, 261
symptoms, 72, 74, 77, 93, 97, 98, 116, 120, 136, 155, 161, 165, 250, 260, 268
synapse, 203, 227
syndrome, 35, 45, 85, 86, 99, 105, 107, 108, 113, 151, 152, 163, 164, 165, 166, 167, 168, 172, 181, 237, 271, 272, 281, 282
synergistic effect, 109
synovial fluid, 71, 72
synthesis, 69, 114, 141, 148, 149, 168, 170, 183, 212, 219
synthetic, 29, 107, 109, 117, 120, 122, 140, 141, 144, 145, 146, 147, 150, 193
synthetic oligopeptides, 147
systematic, 9
systemic lupus erythematosus, (SLE) 49, 55, 85, 99, 104, 107, 113, 247, 248, 249, 260, 265, 268, 269, 270, 281
systemic sclerosis, 35, 56, 248, 269, 270
systems, 77, 78, 127, 128, 138, 150, 210, 211
systolic blood pressure, 63

T

T lymphocytes, 18, 30, 35, 36, 54, 60, 91, 114, 153, 171, 175, 201, 202, 204, 210
T regulatory cells, x, 169, 176, 178, 185, 187
tandem repeats, 8
targets, 28, 36, 87, 89, 91, 92, 104, 114, 167, 171, 189, 192, 230, 250, 254, 260, 264, 271, 279
T-cell receptor, 14, 31, 78, 146, 186, 201, 211, 226
T-cells, 14, 46, 52, 57, 82, 93, 94, 96, 186, 238
TCR, 30, 31, 187, 201, 202, 203, 205, 207, 208, 209, 210, 211, 216, 218, 223, 224, 225, 226, 228, 231, 232
Tea, 151, 155
technological, 1, 36
technology, 10, 161
temperature, 273
temporal, 137
tensile strength, 258
testis, 34
testosterone, 237
TGF, 105, 180, 184
TGFβ, 176, 225
Th cells, 204, 215, 224
T-helper cell, 87
theoretical, 9, 82, 147

theory, 77, 78, 79, 80, 81, 82, 83, 84, 86, 87, 90, 93, 94, 95, 96, 97, 98, 99, 100, 101, 102, 103, 104, 107, 110, 111, 114, 150
therapeutic, 28, 36, 45, 115, 138, 193, 194, 196, 248, 264, 271, 272, 279, 280
therapeutic approaches, 36
therapeutic interventions, 196
therapeutic targets, 272, 280
therapy, 44, 68, 138, 147, 167, 177, 184, 197, 219, 245
thiazolidinediones, 21
thioredoxin, 69
Thomson, 37, 38, 48
thoracotomy, 157
threat, 78
threatened abortion, 239, 245
threatening, 272
threonine, 35
thresholds, 8, 227
thrombocytopenia, 77, 84, 85, 86, 89, 92, 93, 98, 107, 111, 112, 113
thrombocytopenic purpura, 105, 106, 114
thrombotic, 105
thymocytes, 203, 218, 226
thymus, 14, 16, 146, 171, 176, 180, 201, 202, 203, 209, 212, 217, 223, 230
thyroglobulin, 85, 238, 245
thyroid, 3, 19, 85, 235, 236, 237, 238, 239, 240, 242, 243, 244, 245, 246, 261
thyroid gland, 235
thyroiditis, 97, 223, 240, 241, 243, 245
tight junction, 132, 170, 179
time, 7, 50, 67, 74, 83, 89, 94, 122, 130, 131, 136, 160, 164, 171, 209, 213, 216, 223, 240, 242, 247
timing, 94
TIMP, 133, 134, 144, 149
TIR, 175
tissue, 28, 60, 61, 83, 90, 98, 99, 119, 120, 131, 133, 139, 141, 142, 143, 146, 152, 153, 154, 161, 162, 163, 166, 167, 171, 173, 189, 192, 193, 194, 198, 202, 262, 272
tissue homeostasis, 162
TLR, 174, 175, 176, 178, 184, 185, 190, 204, 209
TLR2, 175, 176
TLR3, 71, 73, 175, 176
TLR4, 175, 176
TLR9, 175
TNF, 18, 28, 29, 133, 134, 144, 165, 174, 179, 183, 196, 197, 211, 231
TNF-α, 231
tobacco, 261
tolerance, 14, 15, 35, 36, 77, 82, 83, 93, 94, 95, 97, 107, 108, 114, 171, 172, 174, 177, 178, 180, 184, 186, 187, 203, 209, 215, 217, 226, 230, 231, 238, 262, 272
Toll-like, 113, 184, 185, 186, 195, 206, 209, 227
tomato, 195
Tongue, 129
toxic, 258
toxin, 96, 105, 167, 183
TPA, 25, 51
TPO, 245
tracking, 257
traits, 4, 7, 49
transcript, 33, 54
transcription, 14, 15, 19, 21, 29, 49, 53, 74, 104, 133, 166, 176, 184, 186
transcription factor, 19, 21, 49, 74, 176, 186
transcriptional, 14, 19, 21, 29, 33
transducer, 62
transduction, 30, 183
transfer, 14, 21, 22, 69, 96, 102, 106, 207, 210, 219, 233, 244, 251, 272
transformation, 177
transforming growth factor, 135
transgenic, 205, 207, 209, 211, 216, 218, 219, 228, 232, 279, 282
transgenic mice, 207, 211, 216, 219, 228, 279
transition, 195
translation, 170
translocation, 175
transmembrane, 26, 30, 179, 202
transmission, 9, 42, 43, 51, 111, 202
transplantation, 84, 177, 190, 197, 273, 280, 281
transport, 34, 132, 267
transportation, 249
trauma, 190
Tregs, 16, 36, 185
trend, 32, 238
trial, 138, 240, 242
triggers, 47, 71, 86, 100, 132, 152, 154, 224, 227, 240, 260
triglycerides, 66
trophoblast, 243
tropism, 182
Trp, 117, 125, 147
trypsin, 140, 147, 216
tryptophan, 92, 116, 117, 119, 122, 123, 124, 125, 126, 128, 130, 132, 138, 148, 149, 150
TSH, 237, 238, 240, 241, 242, 243

tuberculosis, 97, 108, 122, 187
tubular, 211
tumor, 14, 53, 135, 140, 143, 203, 204, 206, 207, 209, 210, 211, 212, 213, 219, 223, 224, 225, 228, 229, 230, 231
tumor cells, 203, 204, 206, 207, 209, 210, 211, 212, 213, 224, 225, 229, 230
tumor growth, 228, 229
tumor necrosis factor, 53, 135, 140, 143
tumors, 33, 201, 229
tumour, 230
turnover, 29, 136
type 1 diabetes, 1, 2, 14, 17, 20, 23, 24, 27, 37, 38, 39, 42, 44, 45, 46, 47, 48, 49, 50, 51, 52, 53, 55, 56, 104, 172, 178, 181, 187, 223
type 2 diabetes, 3, 43, 49, 53, 68
type I IFNs, 75
tyrosine, 1, 3, 11, 15, 26, 27, 28, 30, 31, 33, 38, 48, 52, 53, 172, 183, 185, 203, 226
Tyrosine, 26

U

U.S. Geological Survey, 258
ubiquitin, 1, 11, 18, 48, 173, 260, 268
Ubiquitin, 18, 182
ubiquitous, 79, 190, 257, 267
ultrasonography, 62
ultrasound, 62, 69
United Kingdom, 50
United States, 6, 190, 242, 249, 268
unmasking, 272
UPR, 225
uranium, 265
urea, 67
urinary, 130, 132, 156, 157
urine, 116, 130, 132, 145, 156

V

vaccination, 209
vaccine, 44, 84, 102, 103, 139, 141, 210
vaccines, 78, 84, 88, 96, 102, 103, 104, 114, 140, 28
validity, 47, 48, 128
valine, 18, 35
values, 8, 9, 64, 133, 135, 158, 237, 239, 241, 245, 252, 273
variability, 125, 136, 202, 261, 264
variable, 8, 21, 115, 116, 131, 136, 175, 187, 202, 223, 224, 271, 273, 274, 277, 282
variables, 63, 134
variance, 14, 131, 136
variation, 6, 10, 11, 17, 26, 42, 46, 149, 238
vascular, 60, 61, 67, 69, 98, 140, 145, 155, 190, 191, 195, 262
vascular cell adhesion molecule, 145
vascular disease, 195
vascular surgery, 190
vascular wall, 98
vasculature, 98, 99, 100
vasculitis, 85, 262, 269
vasoactive intestinal peptide, 19
vector, 274
vermiculite, 247, 249, 250, 258, 265, 266
Vermont, 169
vertebrates, 31, 272
vertigo, 116
vessels, 52
VIP, 19
viral, 18, 32, 71, 72, 73, 74, 75, 80, 86, 90, 91, 108, 110, 127, 130, 132, 138, 143, 148, 149, 150, 155, 161, 170, 173, 176, 180, 181, 185, 204, 206
viral infection, 18, 71, 72, 73, 74, 86, 108, 148, 155, 161, 204
virus, 18, 47, 74, 80, 85, 86, 87, 89, 91, 92, 93, 97, 102, 103, 104, 107, 109, 111, 112, 113, 114, 138, 142, 143, 145, 169, 170, 172, 173, 174, 176, 177, 178, 179, 180, 181, 184, 186, 209
virus infection, 86, 89, 107, 109, 114, 169, 173, 177, 178, 186
virus replication, 177
viruses, 18, 47, 71, 75, 79, 80, 86, 88, 89, 90, 91, 92, 93, 107, 111, 128, 169, 170, 171, 176, 179, 185, 186, 229
visible, 253
vision, 116
vomiting, 116
vulnerability, 148

W

war, 77, 91, 103, 228
waste, 127
water, 142, 152, 156, 157, 160
weakness, 116
Weinberg, 9
well-being, 250
wells, 253

white matter, 134, 142, 147
wild type, 193, 212
winning, 95, 228
winter, 251
women, 60, 61, 67, 69, 116, 235, 236, 237, 238, 239, 240, 241, 242, 243, 244, 245
wood burning, 251
workers, 248, 265, 269
wound healing, 161
wound repair, 163

X

Xenobiotic, 268
xerostomia, 152
X-ray, 269

Y

YAC, 213
yield, 81, 101
Young Finns Study, 68

Z

Zimbabwe, 110
Zn, 20